SAGE was founded in 1965 by Sara Miller McCune to support the dissemination of usable knowledge by publishing innovative and high-quality research and teaching content. Today, we publish over 900 journals, including those of more than 400 learned societies, more than 800 new books per year, and a growing range of library products including archives, data, case studies, reports, and video. SAGE remains majority-owned by our founder, and after Sara's lifetime will become owned by a charitable trust that secures our continued independence.

Los Angeles | London | New Delhi | Singapore | Washington DC | Melbourne

Advance Praise

This collection of essays fills the need for a comprehensive book on disability studies in South Asia. Covering a range of topics from the history of disability activism to philosophical and cultural issues in relationship to the disabled body and mind, the book has a strong through-line of calling for greater attention to disability and promoting a biopolitical approach to a previously disregarded group of people who make up a fifth of the population.

—Lennard J. Davis, Distinguished Professor of Liberal Arts and Sciences, University of Illinois at Chicago

I have known Anita Ghai for over two decades now. She is one of the most fiery and outspoken advocates we have in the Indian disability movement. She has dedicated her life to creating a body of knowledge that speaks of her commitment to the cause of disability in general, and women and girls with disabilities in particular. This is an exemplary contribution in a scenario where scholarship on disability issues is just not there. Her latest work, *Disability in South Asia: Knowledge and Experience*, is another such effort in this direction. I am confident that this publication will generate a discussion and trigger actions that will pave the way for better and dignified lives for people with disabilities not just in India but the whole of the South Asian region.

—Javed Abidi, Chairperson, Disabled People's International (India) (DPII) and National Centre for Promotion of Employment for Disabled People (NCPEDP) Asia Pacific

Anita Ghai has orchestrated a collection that will enrich disability studies scholarship everywhere, bringing forward a wonderful variety of work from, and about, South Asia. This collection represents new engagements with various impairment experiences while theorizing powerful colonial systems of knowing. A must-read *Disability in South Asia* revolutionizes the connections between disability studies in the Global South and in the Global North by enacting a vital promise to nurture scholars and activists in a re-examination of the meaning of disability. Readers of *Disability in South Asia* are invited to carry forward this promise by joining the developing need to question the peripheral existence of those living with disability and engaged in disability studies.

—Tanya Titchkosky, Professor of Disability Studies, Department of Social Justice Education, OISE, University of Toronto, Canada; author of *Disability, Self, and Society*; *Reading and Writing Disability Differently* and *The Question of Access: Disability, Space, Meaning*

Disability in South Asia is an essential text that captures a crucial moment in time of the development of critical disability studies—a time when the dominance of Western European and North American disability theory is contested and replaced instead with new forms of critical thinking and activism.

—Professor Dan Goodley, iHuman, University of Sheffield

This book has brought together writers on disability whose activism and theorizing are integral to each other as they capture the multiplicity of arenas in which activists and scholars are engaging. A collection of powerful statements on disability with great insights, it sets before us a line of serious enquiry. It is a book sorely needed and inspiring and will be a rare resource for every disability studies classroom and on the reading list of disability organizations and activists.

—Asha Hans, Co-Chair, Pakistan India People's Forum for Peace and Democracy

Disability in South Asia

Disability in South Asia
Knowledge and Experience

Edited by
Anita Ghai

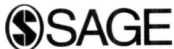

Los Angeles | London | New Delhi
Singapore | Washington DC | Melbourne

Copyright © Anita Ghai, 2018

All rights reserved. No part of this book may be reproduced or utilised in any form or by any means, electronic or mechanical, including photocopying, recording, or by any information storage or retrieval system, without permission in writing from the publisher.

First published in 2018 by

SAGE Publications India Pvt Ltd
B1/I-1 Mohan Cooperative Industrial Area
Mathura Road, New Delhi 110 044, India
www.sagepub.in

SAGE Publications Inc
2455 Teller Road
Thousand Oaks, California 91320, USA

SAGE Publications Ltd
1 Oliver's Yard, 55 City Road
London EC1Y 1SP, United Kingdom

SAGE Publications Asia-Pacific Pte Ltd
3 Church Street
#10-04 Samsung Hub
Singapore 049483

Published by Vivek Mehra for SAGE Publications India Pvt Ltd, typeset in 10.5/13 pts Bembo by Zaza Eunice, Hosur, Tamil Nadu, India and printed at Chaman Enterprises, New Delhi.

Library of Congress Cataloging-in-Publication Data

Name: Ghai, Anita, editor.
Title: Disability in South Asia: knowledge and experience/edited by Anita
  Ghai.
Description: New Delhi, India;Thousand Oaks, California: SAGE Publications
  India, 2018. | Includes bibliographical references and index.
Identifiers: LCCN 2018038628| ISBN 9789352807079 (pbk. : alk. paper) | ISBN
  9789352807086 (epub 2.0) | ISBN 9789352807093 (ebook)
Subjects: LCSH: People with disabilities—South Asia. | Sociology of
  disability—South Asia. | Disabilities—South Asia.
Classification: LCC HV1559.S63 D57 2018 | DDC 305.9/080954—dc23 LC record available at
https://lccn.loc.gov/2018038628

ISBN: 978-93-528-0707-9 (HB)

SAGE Team: Abhijit Baroi, Guneet Kaur Gulati and Ritu Chopra

To

Dr B. R. Ambedkar's vision of social justice and equity

so that

concerted efforts are made to include people with disabilities

in the ambit of this vision

Thank you for choosing a SAGE product!
If you have any comment, observation or feedback,
I would like to personally hear from you.

Please write to me at **contactceo@sagepub.in**

Vivek Mehra, Managing Director and CEO, SAGE India.

Bulk Sales

SAGE India offers special discounts
for purchase of books in bulk.
We also make available special imprints
and excerpts from our books on demand.

For orders and enquiries, write to us at

Marketing Department
SAGE Publications India Pvt Ltd
B1/I-1, Mchan Cooperative Industrial Area
Mathura Road, Post Bag 7
New Delhi 110044, India

E-mail us at **marketing@sagepub.in**

Subscribe to our mailing list
Write to **marketing@sagepub.in**

This book is also available as an e-book.

Contents

Foreword by Shyam Menon — xi
Acknowledgements — xiii
Introduction: Epistemological and Academic Concerns of Disability in the Global South by Anita Ghai — xvii

Part 1: Historical and Theoretical Perspectives on Disability Studies

Chapter 1	Disability Rights Law and Origin of Disability Rights Movement in India: Contesting Views by *Jagdish Chander*	3
Chapter 2	Emergence of Disability Rights Movement in India: From Charity to Self-advocacy by *Meenu Bhambhani*	21
Chapter 3	Refocusing and the Paradigm Shift: From Disability to Studies in Ableism by *Fiona Kumari Campbell*	38
Chapter 4	Disability within Rawlsian Framework of Justice: Challenging the Injustice Rationale by *Deepa Palaniappan and Valerian Rodrigues*	58
Chapter 5	Disability Studies as Resistance: The Politics of Estrangement by *Tanmoy Bhattacharya*	75

Part 2: Disability, Body, Care and Sexuality

Chapter 6	Experiencing the Body: Femininity, Sexuality and Disabled Women in India by *Nandini Ghosh*	101
Chapter 7	Emergence of Epistemological Questions of Crip Queer across Shifting	

Chapter 8	Geo/Bio-political Terrain by *Janet Price and Niluka Gunawardena*	118
	Ethics and Practice of Care: A Focus on Disability by *Upali Chakravarti*	146

Part 3: Knowing the Self and Writing Life

Chapter 9	Privilege or Marginalization: Narrative of a Disability Rights Activist by *Nidhi Goyal*	163
Chapter 10	Journey So Far: My Life with an Impairment by *Sameer Chaturvedi*	183
Chapter 11	Narratives of Growing with A-typicality by *Asha Singh*	196
Chapter 12	Life-writing and Disabled Self in the Works of Oliver W. Sacks by *Sandeep R. Singh*	214
Chapter 13	Blind Culture and Cosmologies: Notes from Ved Mehta's Continent of India by *Hemachandran Karah*	227

Part 4: Disability in Literature and Culture

Chapter 14	Disability across Cultures by *Shubhangi Vaidya*	245
Chapter 15	Corporeality and Cultural Difference by *Shilpaa Anand*	262
Chapter 16	Interrogating Normalcy, Decolonizing Disability: Corporeal Difference in the Post-colonial Indian English Novel by *Someshwar Sati*	278
Chapter 17	Jataka Katha Goes On: Materiality as Metaphor by *Santosh Kumar*	295

Part 5: Disability, Family Epistemologies and Resistance to Shame within the Indian Context

Chapter 18	Disability, Family Epistemologies and Resistance to Shame within the Indian Context by *Shridevi Rao*	313

Chapter 19	Inclusive Education in India: Concept, Practice and the Way Forward by *Ankur Madan*	330
Chapter 20	The Emancipatory Potential of a Structural Understanding of Disability: A Response to Linda Ware by *Suchaita Tenneti*	349
Chapter 21	Disability at Work? Media Representations, CSR and Diversity by *Arun Kumar and Nivedita Kothiyal*	359

Part 6: Legal Discourses of Disability in India

| Chapter 22 | A Disability Studies Reading of the Law for Persons with Disabilities in India by *Amita Dhanda* | 383 |
| Chapter 23 | Reimagining Kinship in Disability-specific Domesticity: Legal Understanding of Care and Companionship by *Rukmini Sen* | 401 |

Part 7: Constructing Disability as Diversity

| Chapter 24 | Disability as Diversity: An Alternative Perspective by *Shanti Auluck* | 413 |
| Chapter 25 | Unification of Disability in Diversity: A Different Voice by *Anita Ghai* | 422 |

About the Editor and Contributors   430
Index   440

Foreword

While designing the Ambedkar University Delhi (AUD), the imagination behind its School of Human Studies (SHS) was that it would offer a platform for academic and research programmes on various human predicaments such as mental illness, ageing, disability and marginalization on the basis of gender, sexuality, poverty and so on. Some of these are relatively new areas of knowledge and professional practice. It was, therefore, necessary to first of all take stock of how the land lies as regards theoretical and research literature in each of these areas. This was attempted in psychosocial clinical studies, gender studies, psychodynamic psychotherapy as well as in development practice.

I am very happy that in the area of disability studies, Professor Anita Ghai has gone a step further and attempted to bring together scholars and practitioners from this part of the world who have worked in and around disability as a lived reality, as well as a social, political, psychological and an epistemological category to form a multidisciplinary galaxy. Professor Ghai has so effectively brought this rather unusual congregation of scholars to reflect collectively on the contours of disability studies as a praxis and as an area of knowledge. This volume is the result of this intense and protracted exercise.

Having been engaged deeply and intensely in disability studies for many years, for Professor Ghai, this volume is an important step forward and a significant milestone. This is perhaps the first book of its kind published in this part of the world. By bringing out this volume, Professor Ghai is in the process of staking a claim on behalf of disability studies for the status of a university discipline. This is undoubtedly a good beginning. I am hopeful that this book and the related publications that may follow it will provide generations of students and scholars in various disciplines of the social and human sciences and humanities as well as practitioners in disability greater access to the interdisciplinary area of disability studies.

Shyam Menon
Delhi

Acknowledgements

I would like to thank AUD, for promoting equity and social justice with excellence. This has inspired me a lot. The university encouraged me to think of disability as knowledge that would enrich the lives of both disabled and non-disabled in the interdisciplinary academic spaces.

Several people have assisted me and played a decisive role in completing this book. While I would like to thank everyone who has contributed to the process of writing this book, some need a special mention.

First and foremost, I would like to thank the vice-chancellor of AUD, Professor Shyam Menon for encouraging me to reflect on visualizing an anchor text on disability studies and laying down the foundations for the formulation of the reader. This work would not have been possible without Professor Menon's support at every stage of the process.

I would like to express my gratitude to SAGE for giving me the opportunity to share my knowledge of disability with the readers.

This text would not have been possible had the Advisory Committee for Research and Project Management (ACRPM) set up by AUD, not given generous funding to enable the completion of the text. Professor Venita Kaul as chairperson of the ACPRM provided me with the opportunity to initiate the work on this text. I also want to thank Professor Anup Dhar, the present chairperson, for supporting me in procuring the necessary finance for a research assistant. Both of them provided intellectual stimulation, encouragement and reassurance, which put my mind at ease in difficult moments. My special thanks to Dr Sunita Tyagi who because of her patience and unrelenting hard work is a sight for sore eyes.

I would also like to thank Professor Ashok Nagpal, who encouraged me to initiate my work, and the present dean Professor Krishna Menon, who later continually backed me unconditionally to complete this project. I would also like to thank my colleagues Professor Anup Dhar, Professor Rachana Johri, Professor Honey Oberoi Vahali and Dr Rukmini Sen for their ideas and reflections on issues of disability studies.

My thanks to the consultation committee comprising Dr Shanti Auluck, Professor Honey Oberoi Vahali, Professor Krishna Menon and Professor Anup Dhar for their valuable inputs that helped me in evolving the conceptual basis for the forthcoming book.

I would like to appreciate the efforts of my workplace—School of Human Studies (SHS)—for providing a context to understand human predicament through an interdisciplinary approach that has led to the emergence of disability studies as a creative and dynamic field of intellectual inquiry and creative action. Further, the SHS office always provided me with timely and dedicated support in managing the administrative demands involved in developing the book. Thank you Santosh, Minakshi and Sandeep.

My thanks to the Finance Department for their commitment to the effective management of monetary requirements of the book.

My thanks to the AUD library and the librarian Dr Debal Kar, who was always active in getting books, journals and any related information. Many thanks, especially, to Ms Alka Rai for her support in providing articles and reading material for the work.

I also thank Neha Sibal for her diligence and enthusiasm in helping the book become a reality. I would like to thank all the authors without whose contributions this book would have remained a dream—Jagdish, whose work on foregrounding the political agency of people with disabilities (PWD) has strongly challenged stereotypes of passivity and inaction associated with disability; Meenu, whose persistent efforts to develop cross-disability awareness in disability rights have served to expand the epistemological boundaries of disability activism and have brought hitherto subtle aspects of the disability rights movement

(DRM) to the fore; Fiona, whose dedicated efforts to arriving at ever more nuanced conceptions of ableism have decentred the foundations of disability studies from a focus on disabled people to an investigation of the constructions of the concept of disability; Deepa and Valerian Rodrigues for their bold attempt to contextualize liberal notions of justice in Indian realities; Tanmoy for his shrewd and highly reflective cautionary tale about the relationship between disability studies and disability activism; Nandini for her rich and emotional analyses of lived experiences of women with disabilities; Janet and Niluka for a rare, thoroughly intriguing exploration of the historical and cultural crossroads between disability studies and queer studies; Upali for recognizing the immense phenomenological and political potential of the ethics of care and its centrality to disability studies; Nidhi for her nuanced explorations of the notion of intersectionality and its centrality to her life as an activist; Sameer for his thoughtful and moving life story; Asha for sharing a brilliant journey of hope and transformation; Sandeep for his valuable work on the multifaceted nature of disability life-writing; Hem for his brilliant exemplar to disability as an epistemological resource in life narratives; Someshwar for expounding the pervasiveness of disability in the Indian literature; Santosh for a beautiful illustration of the power of metaphor; Shubhangi whose explorations of the cultural nuances of disability across global contexts never cease to amaze; Shilpaa for bringing the historical, the cultural and the medical into dialogues that pave a new direction for disability in the Global South; Ankur for capturing the history of inclusion and its manifestations in real school contexts; Shridevi for her unceasing efforts to bring cultural discourses of disability into inclusive education; Suchaita for reiterating the structural nature of disability; Arun and Nivedita for reminding us of the enduring hold of neoliberalism in disability at the workplace; Amita for a rigorous exploration of legalities of disability; Rukmini for her analysis of changing notions of caregiving within the context of law and Shanti for her inspiring and insightful exploration of disability as an integral component of social diversity.

I would also like to specifically thank Dr Tanmoy Bhattacharya, Dr Jagdish Chander and Dr Rachana Chaudhary for their initial advice in conceptualizing this work; Syamala Gidugu and Divya Jalan in helping edit the chapters on education as well as all the authors for assisting in reviewing the abstracts and articles.

I wish to recognize Sandeep Singh whose advice and support have been crucial in realizing this piece of work. His friendship is both an intellectual support and emotional comfort.

I am deeply indebted to Suchaita, my research assistant, for standing by me throughout this endeavour, both as an assistant and a budding disability studies scholar. Her constructive criticism helped me shape this book in the way it stands today.

Finally, my family members who have supported me unquestioningly and unconditionally in all that I have done. Words can never do justice to their contribution.

Introduction
Epistemological and Academic Concerns of Disability in the Global South

Anita Ghai[1]

> We must leave evidence. Evidence that we were here, that we existed, that we survived and loved and ached. Evidence of the wholeness we never felt and the immense sense of fullness we gave to each other. Evidence of who we were, who we thought we were and who we never should have been. Evidence for each other that there are other ways to live—past survival, past isolation.
>
> —Mia Mingus, *Leaving Evidence*, 2009

> A rhizome has no beginning or end; it is always in the middle, between things, interbeing, *intermezzo*. The tree is filiation, but the rhizome is alliance, uniquely alliance. The tree imposes the verb "to be," but the fabric of the rhizome is the conjunction, and... and... and....
>
> —Gilles Deleuze and Félix Guattari, *A Thousand Plateaus*

Disability studies (DS) as a formal area of academic inquiry has been making significant strides in the Global North since the 1990s with rigorous interdisciplinary scholarship and the emergence of several full-fledged academic programmes. In contrast, DS scholarship in India is in a relatively nascent stage. The epigraphs bring us to the understanding

---

[1] I duly acknowledge my research assistant Suchaita and my colleagues Shad Naved and Sandeep R. Singh for a careful reading of the introduction of the book. Any lapses are mine!

of the Deleuzoguattarian rhizome, which offers a chart and metaphor for the 'field' of DS, as it grows outside the boundaries of a defined discipline or programme. Within the university, we are always confronted with the parlance of connotations such as inquiry in a field, as to that of 'discipline', 'department' or 'programme'. When we think about rhizomatic thinking and growth, we are reminded of Deleuze and Guattari's (1987, 24), 'Don't sow! Grow offshoots! Don't be one or multiple, be multiplicities!'

Kuppers too, musters the rhizome to open up new ways of approaching disabled ways of living, 'disability' as a word and concept, and disability poetry. She offers a 'rhizomatic model of disability that can hold a wide variety of experiences and structured positions in moments of precarious productive imbalance' (2011, 93).

When you think of a new academic programme, the usual pattern is to find out a list of scholars who 'do' whatever they are looking for—sociology, history, psychology, education and so on. It is, however, extremely rare to find someone who 'does' DS because of the historical myopia towards disability within academia. As is the case with women and gender studies, a disability perspective has been considered to be too limiting to be of any epistemological significance.

To reference Raymond Williams, if DS is a 'field', what are our 'keywords' or search words? And if we do not have any, or if we have only insufficient ones, then how can we be found? One of the main concerns with scholarship in keywords in DS is the absence of a lexicon of disability typical of the Global South. If DS is a 'field' or, better still, a 'field of energy', where does it happen, especially in non-Western contexts? The inconspicuousness of DS on some campuses may be a result of the critical ways the field departs from how disability has been treated historically. So much of disability history has entailed the grouping together of disabled people through techniques of surveillance, identification and nomenclature.

Moreover, DS is a 'field without programmes'. We have seen the glimpse of academic understanding of disability, and there is work in Global North that states that 'fields' such as DS have the destabilizing potential of Deleuzoguattarian 'bodies without organs'—that is, 'fields without programmes' might resist the hierarchy and methodical format. Interdisciplinary alliances are one of the ways to address this issue.

DS perspectives, therefore, enlighten how individuals designated 'disabled' are treated in a manner that diminishes their economic, interpersonal, psychological, cultural, political and physical well-being, relegating them to membership in a minority group. The promise of DS can enable academia to think critically not only about disability but also about oppressions that affect all historically marginalized groups. Scholarship in the universities has become enriched through various interdisciplinary and onto-epistemological standpoints of gender, caste and sexuality, urging us to interrogate the very foundations of knowledge itself.

This volume represents both senior and younger scholars who present their writings about DS across and beyond disciplines and from a range of standpoints within the spectrum of disability. The corpus of the book is important as this text might be a forerunner for the DS programme in AUD. This is where we could perhaps insert the previous highlighted section about DS in AUD. The School of Human Studies at AUD is in the process of incorporating DS programmes to establish its own moorings as an area of scholarship and practice. *Disability in South Asia* is intended to be a corpus for the AUD DS programmes. The 'volume' brings multiplicities from various scholars in the newly emerging field of DS.

In the last three decades, these inquiries became critical, as I understood epistemic ignorance as a term used by intellectuals. It became clear that the apolitical stance of academia contains an implicit political ideology; and silence or denial of their involvement is no less a political act than an explicit political action. As Minow (1989, 117) noted, the 'inattention itself does communicate a message of relative disinterest or complacent disregard'. Sometimes, disabled people are 'given' a voice but urged to speak and express their views and perspectives in the name of tokenism. Difference in my way is actualized in such a way so as to render powerless and almost abandoned.

As per the WHO's report on disability (2011), more than 15% of the world's population is affected by disability, including physical and sensory impairments, developmental and intellectual disability and psychosocial disability. For me as an editor, a pertinent question that has been critical is how do we come to know disability? What are the conceptions of the normal? What is autonomy? When exactly is life not worth living? Why does rationality have to be the sole determinant of our humanity? How do we define limit? As an insider, I find that knowledge about disability is all embracing with the most radical re-imagining of new questions. They produce few answers but rather embrace the practice of constantly troubling the questions. As Goodley suggests, 'Disability studies are a broad area of theory, research and practice that are antagonistic to the popular view that disability equates with personal tragedy' (2011, xi). Moreover, 'disability affects us all, transcending class, nation and wealth' (p. 1).

Davis calls for a shift in the focus of DS from the construction of disability to the construction of normalcy. He justifies this approach on the grounds that '...the "problem" is not person with disabilities; the problem is the way that normalcy is constructed to create the "problem" of the disabled person' (2013, 3). As I state elsewhere, 'DS takes up the issues of "Othering", metaphors that guide disability and the need for a paradigm shift.' The idea is to evolve an epistemology of disability through the tool of DS. My aim is to underline DS (neglected in Indian academia) as an interdisciplinary area that utilizes the lenses from the social sciences and humanities to view disability from personal, social, cultural, historical, critical and literary perspectives. In one sense, the development of DS is a corrective endeavour to rectify the misinterpretations of disability. Within India, many scholars have initiated work on DS. Jagdish Chander, for instance, traces the emergence of disability as a political construct through the evolution of the disability rights movement (DRM), particularly through the agitation of the organized blind in India (see Chapter 1 in this volume). Addlakha (2015) observes that the United Nations Convention on the Rights of Persons with Disabilities (UNCRPD) and the people with disabilities (PWD) Acts have initiated a shift in the construction of disability from the welfare, the medical and the charity models to human rights models of disability. However, this shift has not been accompanied by a concomitant emergence of DS as an interdisciplinary area of study that values the experiential realities of disability and the history and culture of people with disabilities (PWD). Hence, there is a need for expanding the limited scholarship in DS in India to capture the heterogeneous and multifaceted nature of disability from various disciplinary and cross-disciplinary standpoints, sociocultural contexts and lived experiences of PWD.

Mehrotra (2011) claims that DS originated from activism across various Western contexts, including India. This has created its own share of opportunities and limitations for DS. On the one hand, DS is grounded in lived realities of disability and emphasizes emancipatory research. But, on the other hand, DS risks inheriting some of the limitations of DS activism, including a limited focus on intersectionality, a problematization of the public/private divide, limited focus on the heterogeneity of disability and so on.

DS has been the academic part of the DRM. The political theorist Michael Walzer seems to have published more than one text in 1987, and I am unable to access them. He has concisely characterized 'social criticism' as 'the educated cousin of the common complaint' (Walzer 1987, 65) to make his argument that effective social theory must never move too far from the very real problems faced by everyday people. Though there is a movement from the medical to the social, framed in cultural contexts, an understanding of disability as legitimate knowledge is still missing. People-oriented movements have highlighted oppressive structures and given voice to marginalized communities; however, these voices do not include the knowledge base of DS. This is critical as knowledge and the study of disability should question not only issues of medical cure or rehabilitation perspectives but also raise an 'academic enquiry' on a par with gender and women's studies, Dalit and tribal studies, race and ethnic studies, and other such areas.

DS has not been privileged within academia, perhaps because the understanding of disability is intimately connected to the study of ignorance, invisibility and identity as academia has not evolved tools for understanding how and why various forms of knowing have 'not come to be', or disappeared, or have been delayed or long neglected, for better or for worse, at various points in history. The absence of disability from the mainstream academia creates and maintains a status quo where the 'disabled' are incorporated within the existing social patterns as 'problems'.

Disability, thus, remains an out-and-out state, both politically and academically—it is the source of its own oppression. Such an understanding suggests that more is at stake than a problematizing discourse of specific categories. By not exploring this relationship, higher education at large has delimited inquiry and pursuit of knowledge of disability. This is perhaps because schools, colleges and universities remain sites where not only knowledge but also a middle-class orientation, with its patriarchal, neoliberal and normative values, is produced and reproduced. So, in my understanding, DS is an interdisciplinary study and representation of the concepts, cultures and personal experiences of disability in all its variations.

DS in the Global North and some universities in India are already tackling the multiplicity of the goals of DS. For instance, the term 'disability studies' cannot be a substitute for special education or rehabilitation sciences. The term cannot be compatible with research into community support and inclusive education either, although research in these areas is in accord with these issues. An academic understanding of disability as a social, cultural and political phenomenon, I believe, externalizes the issue and helps counter the notion of disability as an inherent, unchallengeable trait located in an individual. Such an approach rejects the view that disability is solely a medical problem or a personal tragedy. DS, thus, places the responsibility for re-examining and repositioning the place of disability within society and academics and not on the individual. DS may be many things to many people, but if its full potential is to be realized, then it must avoid being seen as simply a new bottle for old wine.

I am reminded of what Mia Mingus mentioned in her blog about disability being heterogeneous. We cannot ignore the fact that oppression and privilege divulge themselves differently among disabled people. This reality can be damaging to cross-disability understanding. As Mingus says,

> To pretend as though those of us who pass as able bodied or 'don't look like we're disabled', don't receive a totally different reality than those of us who are undeniably and obviously marked as disabled by everyone they meet, would be ridiculous and does not do justice to what we are up against nor how powerful a system ableism. (Talley 2017)

The potential of DS is to understand disability to be as broad as culture itself. For this, the tools and traditions of all our ways of knowing about the world have to be comprehended and perhaps even reconceptualized. The subject matter of DS transforms the understanding of disability from an individual deficit to a complex derivative of social, environmental and biological forces. In academia, disability is an interdisciplinary subject of study within the social sciences and the humanities. The promise of DS can enable academia to think critically not only about disability, but also about oppressions that affect all historically marginalized groups. Scholarship in universities has been enriched through various pieces of work such as gender, caste and sexuality, deepening our understanding of multiple epistemic positions and firms of structural inequalities. The interdisciplinary work in DS, therefore, would initiate and evolve new meanings about disability and examine issues of access, employment, education, sexuality and representation.

The present attempt is to foreground how the inclusion of DS as a field of inquiry within mainstream academia can enrich scholarship and contribute to the understanding of the heterogeneity of disability. My hope is, that the present edited volume can reflect the personal and the political. The interdisciplinary character of DS enables it to incorporate the conceptual frameworks and intellectual tools of various disciplines from history to law, and literature to sociology as well as to enrich these disciplines by questioning their fundamental theoretical and methodological orientations. The works in the present volume are illustrative of this critical reciprocity between DS and other disciplines.

What I am suggesting in the present volume are six themes with an understanding that disability is an epistemology. Notwithstanding a serious reflection on misrepresented public perception, legislations and policy implications for creating a disabled-friendly world, knowledge about disability is equally critical. Such an attempt can only be a microscopic surge in the serious debate on disability.

PART 1: HISTORICAL AND THEORETICAL PERSPECTIVES ON DISABILITY STUDIES

Within the Indian subcontinent, awareness about the issues and concerns of lives touched with disabilities is a fairly recent phenomenon.

It was only in the 49th year of independence that the first legislation advocating equal rights for disabled people became a living reality. At this juncture, it might help to put things into historical perspective. It is reported that the 1880s saw some educational and rehabilitative services being launched (Chauhan 1998, 46); the United Nations (UN), which renewed the efforts to rehabilitate disability, declared the year 1981 as the International Year of Disabled Persons. Largely, their history is predominantly a history of silence. The significance of history reminds us of dichotomies, such as 'Us' versus 'Them', 'Self' versus 'Other' or 'One' versus 'Other', meaning not only difference and opposition, but also superiority and inferiority. All binaries, in psychological parlance, operate in the same way as splitting and projection. Thus, the centre expels its anxieties, ambiguities and irrationalities onto the inferior term, filling it with the converse of its own identity. The other, in its very strangeness, simply mirrors and represents what is deeply familiar to the centre, but projected outside of itself. It is this process of marginality that produces the resentment, enmity and repugnance for the one who is sensed as the other. Framing the argument in this form mandates a justification for the inclusion of disability in the categorization discourse. However, disability provokes fears and anxieties about 'able body' mortality and very easily renders itself as the 'Other'. This process of alterity needs to be understood to comprehend the experience of exclusion. Alterity is a term that has been often used to signify 'Otherness'. The 'Other' in the work of Michel Foucault, for instance, consists of those who are excluded from positions of power and are often victimized within predominantly liberal humanist view of the subject. Mehrotra, in her work on the DRM in India, observes the resistance to institutionalizing DS within the university. 'There is general suspicion of research which challenges or disproves the claims of exclusion, deprivation and discrimination, in short the rhetoric of the movement' (Mehrotra 2011, 70). Mehrotra notes that since DS has its origins in disability activism, it has drawn on many of the redemptory aspects of the DRM such as an emphasis of disabled experiences and recognizing disability as a political category and as an aspect of structural inequality. However, the origins of DS in the DRM run the risk of incorporating many of the shortcomings of activism.

The hierarchy of impairments in the DRM in India is clearly one of the problems which western disability studies scholars have also pointed out. The frequent use of the symbol of the wheel chair often obscures the differences within the movement and the priorities of rights of persons with specific disabilities. This symbol however not only particularly represents persons with loco motor disabilities but also takes its cues from the societal and governmental stereotyping of disability. (Mehrotra 2011, 69)

Thus, cultivating a cross-disability political awareness and recognizing the diversity of lived realities and epistemologies within the heterogeneous category of disability are critical for DS.

The first chapter by Jagdish Chander interrogates the different views regarding time frame of the origin of the DRM in India. He establishes that the movement originated in the year 1989 when the National Federation of the Blind (NFB) began to focus the agenda of its movement on the demand for the enactment of a comprehensive disability rights law, leading to the enactment of the PWD Act in 1995. Crediting the leadership to NFB, there was a sustained movement from 1989 to 1995, which began to use a language encompassing cross-disability issues in 2016.

Meenu Bhambhani traces the historical trajectory of the DRM in India with a thrust on the emergence of cross-disability activism. She analyses the shifts in the composition of disability activists in terms of their structural identities of class and caste. She observes the absence of a large-scale, multilayered and systematic, all-inclusive DRM in India and emphasizes the highly dispersed and often elite nature of disability activism in India. The role of the UNCRPD and the PWD Acts in fostering the movement as well as expanding the base of activities is also explored. Although Jagdish mentions cross-disability activism, his work focuses on a specific kind of disability and blindness, while cross-disability activism is central to Bhambhani's work.

The chapters by Tanmoy Bhattacharya and Deepa Palaniappan and Valerian Rodrigues explore theoretical constructions of DS in India. Historically, the survival issues for disabled people were and are still significant, and theoretical considerations about disability issues have not evolved in the disability discourse in India. The existing literature repeatedly underscores the fact that disability has been long neglected by theorists otherwise fervently committed to exploring and communicating the experiences of marginalization. Undoubtedly, theory has to be envisaged as a critical channel so that disability as an identity category can fulfil the aspirations of PWD. Grech states 'that disability studies, too, has hardly contemplated the subject of disability in the global South' (2015, 11). He then states plainly and powerfully that, 'While many talk about "global disability", there is no such thing as a nuanced "global disability studies" yet' (p. 18). There remains a 'dearth' of empirical research on disability in the Global South as well (p. 13). Any theory is not inherently healing or revolutionary. Theories, in fact, worry us as they can co-opt us in creating a magic world in which we settle down without queries. A good theory has to resonate with people across disabilities, which is directed towards lived realities that comprise void, pain and multiple lacunae. Though a significant connection between academics and activism is critical, the metaphysical aspects of disability deserve equal merit. The purpose was to understand disability as a critical cultural category because disability is part of a fundamental dichotomy, which separates what is deemed to be socially acceptable from what is not and, as such, is a particularly pertinent position from which to better understand the divisions, which exclude certain people from enjoying full and equitable participation in society.

Drawing on the works of Bruno Latour, Fiona Kumari Campbell notes that the project of modernity cannot ever be fully realized, hence foregrounding the centrality of disability to human existence and challenging the normalcy associated with othering people on grounds of disability. Her work creates greater scope for disability's political foundations as an integral part of human existence. Campbell particularly distinguishes between ableism and disablism, a distinction often not clearly made in DS in India. She considers ableism to be a more appropriate concept within DS since it shifts attention away from identity politics to the conditions of possibility typical of modernity that construct disability in the first place.

In the following chapter by Deepa Palaniappan and Valerian Rodrigues, the authors analyse the emergence of the disabled political subject in India. Acknowledging the limitations of disability theory in India in relation to analytical frameworks for caste and gender, the authors seek to develop an analytical framework for disability specifically within the Indian context using Rawls' theory of justice. Their thrust is to explore how disabled people in India construct themselves as subjects rather than rely on the theorizing of their political subjectivity by non-disabled people.

Later, Tanmoy Bhattacharya foregrounds the misunderstanding connected to the spirit of DS in the excitement associated with the birth of a new field and in the context of an uncertain dissociation from the zeal of activism. The author advocates the necessity of the two-way traffic between activism and DS theory building (Bhattacharya 2011). For a specific context like that of India, disability-related activities with its overemphasis on services are alarmingly close to creating a hegemonic discourse that shrinks the space for the emergence of a DS discourse. He reminds us that DS cannot be built on the ashes of activism. Though he does not suggest an either/or existential frame, he focuses on 'estrangement' which is best attempted if we understand the existing practices through the lens of ableism (please see Chapter 3 by Fiona Campbell in this volume) and by engaging in a disability-centric understanding of various themes within the academia. We now move from theorization to a theme that centres on body, sexuality and care.

PART 2: DISABILITY, BODY, CARE AND SEXUALITY

Within the DS discourse, bodies and impairments are not only biological entities but are cultural and social as well. As I state elsewhere (Ghai 1998), I questioned whether a disabled identity could not overlook the material reality of the impaired body. Notwithstanding the social understanding of disability, the exclusion of impairment from the discourse is conceptualized as a medical and psychological problem to be cured or rehabilitated. Considering that disability marks the body as biologically different and thus is a very clear reminder of the materiality of the body, the exclusion has taken some doing. Historically, the neglect probably goes back to Descartes (1979, 97) whose understanding is, 'Although the whole mind seems to be united to the whole body, nevertheless, were a foot or arm or any other part amputated, I know that nothing would be taken away from my mind'. Quoting Siebers, Mitchell asserts that this group of scholars offers approaches that address disability 'as an epistemology that rejects the temptation to value the body as anything other than what it was and that embraces what the body has become and will become relative to the demands on it whether environmental, representational, or corporeal' (2001, 31).

Nandini Ghosh writes about the experiences of the body and reflects on femininity, sexuality and disabled women in India. Using primary case studies of women with disabilities, she underscores that disability is experienced in, on and through the body, just as impairment is experienced in terms of the personal and cultural narratives that help to constitute its meaning. The author reminds us that the bodies that women experience are always mediated by constructions, associations and images which most patriarchal sociocultural formations accept and endorse. Further, she explores the multifarious processes through which disabled women internalize sociocultural constructions of the ideal or 'normal' female body, and how such ideas influence their thoughts about and experiences of their bodies in their daily lives.

Janet Price and Niluka Gunawardena prompt us to ask some epistemological questions in the historical development of the discourses of queerness and disability in South Asia with a focus on India and Sri Lanka. The authors seek to foreground the discussions on the relationship between sexuality and disability in the Global South, which has remained a hitherto limited area of study. They attempt to contextualize this historical and cultural analysis within the context of neoliberalism and globalization and its impact on local and national discourses of disability and queerness. They explore the construction of disabled people as heteronormative and yet de-sexualized and as too dangerous to participate in the processes of reproduction. Thus, queerness and disability are shown to be closely interwoven concepts, which also have a common historical context in India.

Care is a human attribute that is connected to both disabled and non-disabled people. Ubiquity of care needs has to be accentuated as none of us live our lives without relying on care provided by others. The fact that many of us experience the need for care in early and later life cannot be cannot be veiled behind independence and autonomy. Disabled women's caregivers have been primarily mothers who have occupied a complicated, conflicting and marginal position within the discourse of DS. These tensions are compounded when the actions of mothers have been interpreted as constraints on their children's lives, limiting their prospects and ambitions. Within the caring discourse, mothers are constructed as 'special, altruistic self-sacrificing' whose place was absolutely in the home. Though caring, dependency and need are impossible to disentangle, presentations focus mostly on the 'depressive symptoms, anger and resentment that are experienced by caregivers in the caring process'. Disabled people are, therefore, considered as a liability whose agency for defining their own care needs is not prioritized and is, instead, excluded.

Upali Chakravarti problematizes ethics and practice of care and disability, and the gendered nature of caregiving is also implicit. She brings an important issue in developing an ethics of care, which is the view that dependency is created in PWD not because of their functional limitations but because of a variety of economic, political and social forces which produce this dependency. At the same time, Upali recognizes that care is an intrinsic part of the human condition itself and emphasizes the role of the community and kinship structures as well as the state in preventing caregiving from being perceived as a burden by relegating it to the task of individual women. In this chapter, Upali explores caregiving by mothers of children with disability extending into adulthood in comparison with the caregiving provided by the mother only during the course of child rearing and the professional caregiving provided by nurses.

As Puar (2017) writes in her new book's preface, her goal in *The Right to Maim* is to:

> think through how and why bodies are perceived as debilitated, capacitated, or often simultaneously both […] I am arguing that the three vectors, debility, capacity, and disability, exist in a mutually reinforcing constellation, are often overlapping or coexistent, and that debilitation

is a necessary component that both exposes and sutures the disabled/non-disabled binary.

PART 3: KNOWING THE SELF AND WRITING LIFE

No body, no voice; no voice, no body. That's what I know in my bones.

—Mairs (1996a, 96)

Historically, the assumption is that individuals with disabilities did not often write about themselves before the 20th century, specifically before the publication of Helen Keller's classic text, *The Story of My Life* (1903). Recently, some autobiographical work by disabled people, most of whom are also activists, such as Ved Mehta (1957, 2009), Malini Chib (2011), Shivani Gupta (2014) and Firdaus Kanga (1990), have attempted to challenge the historical voicelessness of PWD by constructing their own self-narratives.

The reason for engaging with the memories of self and others is critical to understanding disability as cultural discourses that offer few affirmative resources for disabled people to draw upon in constructing their personal and social identities. The story of the self is critical, more so if the narrative is marked by extended movements back and forth through 'health' and 'illness', and 'ability' and 'disability'. Often, in literature, disability and cancer serve as a metaphor of social breakdown, but in an autobiography, illness is associated with a unique subjectivity because an autobiography serves as a self-reflexive tool that helps to highlight a personal experience. In subtheme 3, I turn to this methodological tool of analysing personal narratives in the hope to offer a solution that is an alternative to the patronizing and marginalizing caricature by others. Autobiography, I believe, enables one to deal with the conscious and unconscious awareness of one's life situations and conditions. In such circumstances, the most critical questions are asked, making it imperative to seek a meaningful existence. Over the years, I have understood that the normative culture carries existential and aesthetic anxieties about difference of any kind, be it caste, class, gender or disability.

People who have lived a peripheral existence on account of their deviation from the societal parameters are considered different and, therefore, marginalized. As mentioned earlier, othering in all cultures symbolically represents a sense of lack, tragic loss, dependency and abnormality. As I state elsewhere (Ghai 2015), I often think of the way Sartre (1956) had described how the look of the other can make one feel objectified, evaluated, embarrassed or ashamed of whom one is. It is true that no actions are experienced as appropriate until another confronts them; then they become improper and awkward when performed before the eyes of the 'other'. As Sartre says, 'by the mere appearance of the Other, I am put in the position of passing judgment on myself as on an object, for it is as an object that appear to the Other' (1956, 189). Whether conscious or not, the self acquires a different identity. Thus, identification of disability losses and gains is never meaningless. This section brings together two authors who share their personal journeys of the disabled self.

Nidhi Goyal wonders whether she is privileged or marginalized. Her narrative is located in the cusp of women's rights and DRMs in India. The author as an activist reflects on her growing up as a bold and stubborn child, the onset of blindness in her teenage years and her advent into disability activism. Within her narrative, one finds a tenuous relationship with marginalization, privilege and its intersections. She raises significant questions about the politics of agency and representation within DRM, the perception of disability as a category of structural inequality by members of other marginalized social groups and the manner in which gender intersects disability in specific contexts of South Asia. Beginning with her own personal experience of turning blind at the age of 15, Goyal narrates how she took all challenges in her stride including the onset of blindness. However, a question that arises in her case is why she feels the need to avoid sharing the possible vulnerability, trauma, confusion and mixed feelings that are likely to have accompanied the onset of her disability. Is it possible that vulnerability is perceived as antithetical to the construction of the self? This is a concern that merits further reflection.

In contrast, Sameer Chaturvedi shares with us a journey of a person who has lived with cerebral palsy. As the author says, he has experienced his physicality as well as societal attitudes towards his personhood. His fascination for cricket, dance and movies did never really allow him to think about his body or the social perception of it. However, the unconscious always revived his fantasy and a desire to normalize. He shares his pain and privileges that constructed his self in family, school and college. Notwithstanding the losses associated with disability, the boundaries between impairment and disability are often blurred as his identity and experiences form a complex narrative. Both Nidhi and Sameer's narratives remind me of Arthur Frank (1995) who calls a 'quest narrative' in which the introduction of disability was accepted and used to derive personal meaning. As Frank (1995, 128) explains,

> [T]he genesis of the quest is some occasion requiring the person to be more than [s/he] has been, and the purpose is becoming one who has risen to the occasion.

I also wonder if both Nidhi and Sameer are articulating a conscious relationship with their own bodies and selves; we do not 'inhabit' an inert object body but we are subjectively embodied in a malleable, developing and crisscrossed process of being. What is the part of the self that we call ourselves as mine, myself or me, divorced from the overall understanding of life?

The next narrative is that of a mother, Asha Singh, who traces the journey of a mother and daughter in the various stages of the course of life. Negotiations, resistances and silences peppered with rebellion form the core of the narrative as a child grows from a baby who reacted to the second dose of DPT immunization to becoming an assistant teacher in a leading private school. One common theme that will weave different narratives will be engagement with an individual person's growing social presence. The ability of the family and individual to take bold decisions and act on impulses as well as reflect on possibilities is analysed in this study. The social spaces inhabited need to encourage all the stakeholders to form collaborations, and show cooperation and consideration.

The following two narratives, written by Sandeep Singh and Hemchandran Karah, move further from self-narratives to analyses of disability life. Kadar (1992) describes life writing 'as genre of documents or fragments of documents written out of life, or unabashedly out of personal experience of the writer' (p. 29). It comprises texts, which are fictional and non-fictional, which are linked by 'a thematic concern of life or self' (p. 29). Sandeep R. Singh traces major assumptions about life writing, particularly on the development and foregrounding of the interiority of the self and the significance of this construction of the self for the development of personal subjectivity. There is then an exploration of the evolution of DS as an area of inquiry and the centrality of the self and personal experience to DS. This claim paves the way for an organic and very important connection between life writing and DS. This chapter uses the works of Oliver Sacks, a neurologist and writer, and his writings about the experiences of his patients. The most essential features of Sacks' work, which are also a major contribution in the field of DS, are his nuanced documentation of the lives and experiences of his patients. This approach to their personal narratives is significantly different from self-narratives. It is also noteworthy in its attribution of agency to ill and disabled people who have hitherto been deprived of the agency of voice.

Hemchandran Karah analyses Ved Mehta's *Continent of Blind* culture. The author analyses the life and works of the prolific blind author, Ved Mehta. The thrust of the author is on the various ways in which Mehta attempts to reconcile his life and experiences with the realities and necessities of blindness while retaining a strong attempt to achieve normality. Central to this writing is the study of the twin cosmologies of the masculine and the feminine represented by Mehta's parents. *Priti vajna* or absolute obeisance to the father and his father's efforts to enable him to get a good education are central to Mehta's attempts to negotiate his masculine identity, while his mother's constant efforts to find a cure for his disability and the relationship between mother and son that ensues are identified as the main narrative anchors of the text. Although not explored substantially, there is an attempt to undertake a psychoanalytic reading of the text with a specific focus on Mehta's own familiarity with psychoanalysis.

PART 4: DISABILITY IN LITERATURE AND CULTURE

Culture is defined as activities and practices—those areas of life in which people are acting together. In sum, through guided participation in cultural practices, the novice becomes 'one of us'. In this quite harmonious picture, both novice and expert are motivated to fulfil their respective functions (learning and guiding) in the joint project of 'doing culture'. In a third approach, the person's subjectivity and experiential world are the places where we meet culture. The person is defined not as a motivated and active participant in mostly harmonious cultural practices, but first and foremost as a homo symbolic us, a meaning-maker (Bruner 1990). The concept of culture is the central feature of several social science disciplines. Though the significance of disability as a culturally produced and negotiated construct is used metaphorically, uniform interpretations through which culture is understood are not clearly stated. Cultural expectations always reflect systems of shared beliefs; values, customs, behaviours and artefacts used by the members of a society to cope with their world and one another. It can refer to language, thought, spirituality, social order and activities, interactive matrix and much more. The term 'culture' has been defined as 'a learned system of meaning and behaviour that is passed from one generation to the next' (Carter and Qureshi 1995, 241), and as all the traditions, ideals and way of life ascertained from the given environment. The continuous use of disability as a source of cultural meaning has been well documented in films, literature, popular culture and folklore and fairy tales. In these contexts, authors' and screenwriters' understanding of disability operates as a form of what Mitchell and Snyder call 'narrative prosthesis' (2003, 15). A review of our cultural forms of expression provides evidence of the metaphoric role of disability, which is deeply ingrained in our social values. Disability, thus, becomes a tool for social, entertaining or political agendas unrelated to disability oppression.

Although DS is considered to emanate from Western activism and academia, several fascinating instances of cultural constructions of disability flourish the world over. However, a nuanced analysis of cultural discourses on disability from the Global South as well as from marginalized populations of the developed world reveals highly evolved and progressive findings that serve to expand and enrich the entire field of DS and various development programmes in the field of disability.

Shubhangi Vaidya attempts to capture and reflect on some of these notable cultural discourses of disability from across the world with a specific focus on the formation of disabled identities and communities. Using the concept of 'biosocialities', the author analyses the formation of disabled solidarities and communities with reference to deaf pride and autistic neurodiversity in the age of globalization and digital networking. Thus, the emergence of transnational communities of disability from across diverse cultures and the significance of these communities for DS shall be explored.

Shilpaa Anand similarly analyses how the notions of corporeality and associated standards cast certain bodies as 'abnormal' in the Indian context. Using the method of cultural history, the author analyses specific examples of disability from India's history including leprosy and dwarfism and compares them to similar narratives from ancient Greece. An attempt is made to foreground the manner in which sociocultural conditions construct the concept of disability. A colonial lens is brought to the fore by the analysis by a British author and an Indian author, which captures the same form of disability experienced differently. There is also a deep exploration of the concept of medicine, healing and treatment that compares Ayurveda to modern medicine. The analysis reveals the centrality of the social context to healing practices in Ayurveda, the individuation of healing in the same tradition and the centrality of patients' narratives to treatment in Ayurveda, which is what crucially distinguishes Ayurveda from Western medicine.

Drawing from postcolonial literature in India, Someshwar Sati interrogates normalcy and explores the various representations of disability in selected prominent texts from the Indian English literature: Anita Desai's *Clear Light of Day* (1980), Salman Rushdie's *Midnight's Children* (1981), Firdaus Kanga's *Trying to Grow* (1990) and Indra Sinha's *Animal's People* (2007). From analyses of general themes in literary DS such as disability as narrative prosthesis and disability as metaphor, there is a thrust on analysing disability as an embodied identity and a lived reality. There is an attempt to analyse the aforesaid texts in the context of transnationalism and global capitalism and the manner in which the local and the global engage in complex interactions as manifested in these texts.

Santosh Kumar explores the manner in which disability is represented in the *Jataka Tales* and the *Panchatantra*. Focusing on the literary device of the metaphor, Santosh attempts to demonstrate how the usefulness of the metaphor in abstracting the particular and enabling ideas to travel needs to be scrutinized adequately because of the reductionist potential of the metaphor. The author suggests that the use of metaphors to describe disabilities in folktales has resulted in extreme injustice and discrimination against disabled people. It is also responsible for the construction and reproduction of stereotypes about disabled people. The fifth subtheme includes the issues of education and employment.

PART 5: DISABILITY, FAMILY, EDUCATION AND EMPLOYMENT IN THE INDIAN CONTEXT

In the philosophy of education, the notion of normalcy tends to demean children with disabilities, as difference is always understood as "special". The understanding leaves out children with disabilities from the mainstream. Since education is closely related to personhood, disabled people however have always existed at the precincts of the society. They have been excluded socially, politically and economically and, more critically, educationally.

In fact, educational issues of disabled children have debates in almost every country. As Lindqvist (1999, 7), former UN Special Rapporteur of the Commission for Social Development on Disability, puts it:

> A dominant problem in the disability field is the lack of access to education for both children and adults with disabilities. As education is a fundamental right for all, enshrined in the Universal Declaration of Human Rights, and protected through various international conventions, this is a very serious problem. In a majority of countries, there is a dramatic difference in the educational opportunities provided for disabled children and those provided for non-disabled children. It will simply not be possible to realize the goal of Education for All if we do not achieve a complete change in this situation. (Emphasis mine)

Within India, the slogan that has been popular is inclusive education as there has been a struggle between integrated and special education. As Corbett and Slee (2000, 136) comment:

Inclusive education is a distinctly political 'in your face' activity that proceeds from larger political, as opposed to technical questions about the nature of society and the status afforded to people in varying forms and structures of social organization. A political movement in the first instance, inclusion is about establishing access for all people. It is not conditional, nor does it speak about partial inclusion. Its impetus emanates from the recipients of professional services rather than from being orchestrated by professional themselves. This subtheme discusses the issues of education with the realm of disability studies.

In the first chapter of this section, Shridevi Rao foregrounds the family epistemologies' resistance of shame that is experienced with children with disabilities. The author draws on the findings of a qualitative study that focused on the perspectives of Bengali families of children with disabilities and their experiences in enhancing the inclusion of their children within their families, neighbourhoods and communities. She focuses on how families use the collective identity of a family to resist pressures to feel 'shame' and relent to the pejorative identities imposed on their child. The families' perception of the child as an integral member of the family, their use of the 'family policy', along with constructions of the child that focus on the humanness of the child, helped not only to resist pejorative labels but also to educate extended family members and the community on ways to accept and include their child.

In the second chapter, Ankur Madan traces the meanings, history and practices of inclusive education in India. She explores the philosophy, vision and implementation of inclusive education in a specific school set-up. The author highlights the constructive lessons as well as challenges that confront the inclusive education. The author laments the failure to ground arguments about inclusive education in the context of specific kinds of disabilities. A contradiction, for instance, is the case of deaf people who regard special education as a marker of social justice that enables them to assert their identity and develop themselves into a community. Complexity of inclusion therefore is not an easy task in a society where differences need to be taken seriously.

In the third and final chapter on education, Suchaita Tenneti underscores the emancipatory potential of a structural understanding of disability and responds to Linda Ware, a well-known DS scholar. In her essay 'Many Possible Futures, Many Different Directions', Ware (2005) explores the contributions that DS could make to critical special education. She observes that the regressive history of special education with its focus on behaviourist and positivist approaches and the preponderance of the medical model of disability have limited the success of critical special education studies. This is primarily because of the persistence of the term 'special education' even in critical appropriations of this body of knowledge. However, DS, she says, can revitalize critical special education by providing an epistemological frame of reference within which fundamental conceptions and assumptions about disability can be questioned. DS carries the potential of transforming disability from a minority discourse to a universal one, thereby countering the reification of disability that takes place within special education. Suchaita mentions different ways in which Ware herself acknowledges the role of the social sciences in constructing disability praxis, especially given the interdisciplinary nature of DS, but ultimately relies on shifting mindsets and diversifying cultural notions about disability as the ultimate means to achieve equality in educational opportunities, which is a flawed approach in the absence of adequate structural and systematic accommodations and changes.

Arun Kumar and Nivedita Kothiyal, in their chapter 'Disability at Work: Media Representations, CSR and Diversity', map and problematize representations in the mainstream media of practices enhancing the employment of persons with disabilities within the private sector in India. Commonly understood as corporate social responsibility and/or diversity management, such practices include, for example, targeted employment schemes, scholarships to individuals working in the private sector for pursuing higher education and livelihood training and skill upgradation programmes for persons with disabilities. They have gained their legitimacy through incentives and promotion by the State; extensive coverage by mainstream media promoting wider adoption and awards and recognitions offered variously and jointly by governments, industrial associations and disability-related organizations.

The next section focuses on legal discourses of disability in India.

PART 6: LEGAL DISCOURSES OF DISABILITY IN INDIA

As understanding of disability evolved in India, many landmark judgments were delivered by the appellate courts between 1996 and 2007 under the Persons with Disabilities (Equal Opportunities, Protection of Rights and Full Participation) Act, which focuses on the central characteristics of disability jurisprudence. The following two chapters provide an insight into the nature of judicial enhancement that can underscore violations faced by disabled persons. Though the Acts have been enacted and judiciary is playing an important role, but for the full implementation of every law, there has to be social consciousness and awareness in the masses. Also, the law in the form of the Justice Verma committee has been changing the notions of disability and personhood in society. As Saptrishi and Addlakha (2009) point out:

> Concerns on the rights of the disabled in India became visible in the public domain in the 1990s when a cluster of legislations was enacted by the Parliament. These were: Rehabilitation Council of India Act, 1992, Persons with Disabilities (Equal Opportunities, Protection of Rights and Full Participation) Act, 1995 and National Trust for Welfare of Persons with Autism, Cerebral Palsy, Mental Retardation and Multiple Disabilities Act, 1999. Earlier, the Indian Lunacy Act, 1912 had been replaced by the Mental Health Act of 1987 which came into effect in 1993. The rise of the disability rights movement and the pro-active role of the United Nations propelled these legislative developments and laid the foundation for nascent disability jurisprudence in the country. The most dramatic development in this regard has been the adoption of the Convention on the Rights of Persons with Disabilities (CRPD) by the United Nations General Assembly on 13 December 2006, which has been ratified by most member states including India.

The fact that legislations were enacted in many countries is a testimony to the changing paradigm of understanding disability from this new perspective.

Amita Dhanda contends that the recognition of the voice of persons with disabilities in the CRPD has made it possible to undertake lawmaking from a DS perspective. The chapter, therefore, firstly elaborates on how the absence of this perspective has impacted upon the making of disability laws in the country and next dwells on what a DS-compliant approach would require from lawmaking in India. The author initiates this inquiry by firstly examining the disability-centric legislations subsisting on the statute book before the CRPD. Further, she examines the processes by which lawmaking on disability was undertaken after the CRPD and how despite wide-ranging consultations the laws were not made in accord with the demands of the sector. Since a DS approach would not brook such a consequence, she concludes the chapter by enunciating what procedures would be needed to be adopted for lawmaking to be informed by the insights of DS.

Rukmini Sen, on the other hand, analyses the concept of care in disability legislation in India. The concept of a caregiver as defined by the PWD Act and the Mental Healthcare Act is itself a new phenomenon in India. It raises questions about the notions of kinship and family and their implications in constructing the disabled legal/social subject. The political economy of care and the construction of women as caregivers are two of the major thrust areas of the chapter as well. She looks at the 'interconnected' threads of care and companionship (within the family), which is now part of the Indian legal landscape for persons with disabilities. She foregrounds the 2007 UNCRPD and its provisions. There is, thus, an inherent connect that the disability movement has with many other social movements in India, and the present legislation which is markedly different from the 1995 one owes its existence to this intersecting manner in which disability has emerged as an issue. It is, therefore, important to locate disability and disability-specific domesticities within the kinship matrix. Further, she explores the politico-legal landscape of care and kin/kin-like companionship keeping persons with disabilities at the centre of this enquiry.

PART 7: CONSTRUCTING DISABILITY AS DIVERSITY

The final two chapters, written by Shanti Auluck and Anita Ghai, reflect on diversity. Drawing on her own experiences, Shanti Auluck writes as a mother of a son with Down syndrome. Auluck underscores the significance of diversity disability with a special reference to cognitive and intellectual disabilities. She argues that disability is inherent to the human condition and is as natural as any of nature's other diversities. She dwells on Indian philosophical traditions and their acceptance of the existence of multiple realities and perspectives. She also reflects on the concept of 'suffering' and the association of disability with suffering. With reference to her own experiences of raising her son and the strong relationship that the two of them share, she asserts that her life as a parent of a child with a disability and that of her son are far from tragedy and suffering. She apparently adheres to the social model's separation of impairment and disability and locates the disadvantages that children such as her son face in oppressive social structures. She reminds us of how eugenics is closely related to PWD. Anita Ghai, on the other hand, writes from a location of a woman with visible mobility impairment. As a DS scholar, she has reflected on the complexity of diversity as an ideology. Diversity is often constructed as a form of restoration and a way of fixing histories of being broken. In the process of unifying people with or without disabilities, this unification is implicated in a biopolitics that purposefully incorporates the ways in which disability is socially, politically and economically produced (in relation to impairment) and which endeavours to erase difference. While diversity incorporates acceptance, respect, empathy and understanding so that each individual is comprehended as unique, the notion of difference gets complicated as there are multiple constituencies that should be recognized with dignity. Logically, we are in accord with the fact that disability can happen to anyone. However, we never encounter the fears that unquestionably operate at the level of the unconscious. While the idea of diversity in theory is enviable, the ground reality is far from desirable.

Writing this volume has been a very productive exercise. I have had to think through the changing issues and theoretical frameworks, trying to guess as to what themes should be underscored. There have been some limitations in dealing with this subject; moreover, it is impossible for a single volume to do justice to the highly multifaceted and heterogeneous nature of disability. Editing this reader had been a tentative yet a critical enterprise in which I had to combine the ability to assess the past, look at the present and think about the future of DS in the Global South. The reader will, thus, come across both the experiential terrain and theoretical nuances of disability. I hope that this book will be of interest to students, faculty, policy makers, activists and lay readers who are touched by the understanding of disability.

REFERENCES

Addlakha, Renu. 2015. *Disability Studies in India: Global Discourses, Local Realities.* New Delhi: Routledge.

Addlakha, Renu and Mandal, Saptarshi. 2009. 'Disability Law in India: Paradigm Shift or Evolving Discourse?', *Economic and Political Weekly* 44 (41/42): 62–68.

Carter, R. T. and Qureshi, A. 1995. 'A Typology of Philosophical Assumptions in Multicultural Counseling and Training.' In *Handbook of Multicultural Counseling*, edited by J. G. Ponterotto, J. M. Casas, L. A. Suzuki and C. M. Alexander, pp. 239–62. Thousand Oaks, CA: SAGE Publications.

Chauhan, R. S. 1998. 'Legislative Support for Education and Economic Rehabilitation of Persons with Disabilities in India.' *Asia Pacific Disability Rehabilitation Journal* 1 (2): 46–52.

Chib, M. 2011. *One Little Finger.* New Delhi: SAGE.

Corbett, Jenny, and R. Slee. 2000. 'An International Conversation on Inclusive Education.' In *Inclusive Education: Policy, Context and Comparative Perspectives*, edited by F. Armstrong, D. Armstrong and L. Burton. London: Davis Fulton Publishers.

Davis, L. 2013. *The Disability Studies Reader.* 4th ed. Abingdon: Routledge.

Deleuze, Gilles, and Guattari, Félix. 1987. *A Thousand Plateaus: Capitalism and Schizophrenia.* Translated by Brian Massumi. Minneapolis, MN: University of Minnesota Press.

Descartes, Rene. 1979. *Meditations on the First Philosophy.* Translated by A. Donald. Indianapolis, IN: Hackett Publishing.

Frank, A. 1995. *The Wounded Storyteller: Body, Illness and Ethics.* Chicago: Chicago University Press.

Bruner, J. S. 1990. *Acts of Meaning.* Cambridge: Harvard University Press.

Ghai, Anita. 1998. 'Living in the Shadow of my Disability', *The Journal* 2 (1): 32–36.

———. 2015. *Rethinking Disability in India.* New Delhi: Routledge.

Goodley, D. 2011. *Disability Studies: An Interdisciplinary Introduction.* Los Angeles, CA and London: SAGE.

Grech, Shaun. 2015. *Disability and Poverty in the Global South: Renegotiating Development in Guatemala.* London: Palgrave Macmillan.

Gupta, S. 2014. *No Looking Back.* New Delhi: Rupa Publications.

Kadar, Marlene. 1992. *Essays on Life Writing: From Genre to Critical Practice.* Toronto: University of Toronto Press.

Kanga, F. 1991. *Trying to Grow.* London: Bloomsbury.

Keller, Helen. 1903. *The Story of My Life.* Available at https://www.questia.com/library/2963624/the-story-of-my-life (last accessed 13 June 2018).

Kuppers, Petra. 2011. *Disability Culture and Community Performance: Find a Strange and Twisted Shape*. New York: Palgrave MacMillan.

Lindqvist, B., M. H. Rioux, and R. M. Samson. 2007. *Moving Forward: Progress in Global Disability Rights Monitoring*. Toronto: Disability Rights Promotion International, 2007.

Mairs, N. 1996. *Carnal Acts*. Boston, MA: Beacon Press.

Mehrotra, Nilika. 'Disability Rights Movement in India: Politics and Practice.' *Economic and Political Weekly* 46 (6): 65–72.

Mehta, Ved. 1957. *Face to Face*. Boston, MA: Atlantic-Little, Brown.

———. 2009. *Mamaji*. New Delhi: Roli Books.

Minow, Martha. 1989. 'Beyond Universality.' University of Chicago Legal Forum 115–38.

Mitchell, David, and Sharon Snyder. 2003. *Narrative Prosthesis: Disability and the Dependence of Discourse*. Ann Arbor, MI: University of Michigan Press.

Mitchell, W. J. T. 2001. 'Seeing Disability.' *Public Culture* 13 (3): 391–97.

Puar, Jasbir. 2017. *The Right to Maim: Debility, Capacity and Disability*. Durham, NC: Duke University Press.

Williams, Raymond. [1976] 2011. *Keywords: A Vocabulary of Culture and Society*. Fontana Communications Series. London: Routledge.

Sartre, Jean Paul. 1956. *Being and Nothingness: An Essay on Phenomenological Ontology*. New York: Philosophical Library.

Talley, Heather Laine. 2013, November 22. 'Feminists We Love: Mia Mingus' (Interview). Available at: http://www.thefeministwire.com/2013/11/feminists-we-love-mia-mingus/ (accessed on 13 December 2017).

PART 1

Historical and Theoretical Perspectives on Disability Studies

Chapter 1

Disability Rights Law and Origin of Disability Rights Movement in India
Contesting Views

Jagdish Chander

Just like other parts of the world, India too underwent many social and political changes in the post-Independence period after gaining independence from the British rule in 1947 (L. I. Rudolph and S. H. Rudolph 1987, 66). The Dalit movement (Omvedt 2001), the socialist movement led by Jai Prakash Narain and Ram Manohar Lohia (Limaye 1984; Mohan 1984), and the Naxalite (radical communist) movement (Vanaik 1990, 182) all led to tremendous political upheavals and social changes. However, it is only recently, beginning in the 1980s and 1990s, that India has witnessed the emergence out of the shadows of previously silent groups such as women and the disabled. The passage of Rights of Persons with Disabilities (Equal Opportunities, Protection of Rights and Full Participation) Act, 1995 (Baquer and Sharma 1997; Bhambhani 2004), popularly known as the 'disability law' or the 'PWD Act', was an example of the success of the disability rights movement. This movement has sustained itself since its origin and has grown richer over a period of time leading to its identifiably greatest accomplishment during the middle of the second decade of the 20th century, resulting in the replacement of the PWD Act with a much more effective and comprehensive disability rights law at the end of the year 2016, that is, the Rights of Persons with Disabilities Act (2016), which was duly passed by the Parliament of India on 16 December 2016.

MOVEMENT FOR THE ENACTMENT OF DISABILITY LAW BY BLIND ACTIVISTS, 1988–95

Like their counterparts in various parts of the world, including the United States, the blind were among the first disability groups in India to wage a vigorous struggle for their rights. The self-advocacy movement of the blind, which is described as the 'movement of the organized blind' in India (Chander 2011), formally began in 1970 with the founding of the National Federation of the Blind (NFB) Graduates, which was renamed in the year 1972 as the NFB, also popularly called the 'Federation'. The Federation launched a sustained focus on the demand for the enactment of the disability law from late 1988 onwards when it changed its focus from the demand for the recruitment of blind in the lower categories of central government jobs to the struggle for the enactment of the disability law. This shift, which led to the focus of the struggle on the enactment of the disability law, marked the origin of the disability rights movement. This chapter makes a brief description of this struggle, and I have attempted to establish my argument that the disability rights movement originated in India in 1988 when the Federation began to focus its struggle for the enactment of the disability law.

A call for the enactment of the disability law was made several times from 1981 onwards, particularly from 1985 to 1987 (*Hindustan* 1985; *The Indian Express* 1985, 1987; *The National Herald* 1985). But the focus of the movement was pressing for the employment of blind people in government jobs. It finally resulted in the employment of 239 blind people during 1987 and early 1988 (Chander 2011, 245), which boosted the morale of the leadership and revitalized its strength. However, the most important development in relation to the introduction of disability law was the formation of a committee under the chairmanship of a former judge of the Supreme Court, Justice Baharul Islam, in 1986 (Bhambhani 2004, 17). The committee submitted its report in early 1988, strongly recommending the enactment of a comprehensive disability law (Abidi 2004). This recommendation proved to be a watershed development leading towards the introduction of such legislation. Similar to the recruitment drive discussed above, the committee's recommendations were a great morale booster for the leadership of the NFB to make this issue a priority. Hence, following these two major developments—the special recruitment drive of 1987 and the submission of the report by the Baharul Islam Committee recommending the need for the introduction of a disability law—it was an ideal time to launch a movement for the enactment of such a law starting from 1988 onwards.

Once the recruitment drive was completed and a good number of qualified blind persons were absorbed in different jobs, the Federation was relatively free to focus its attention on the struggle for the enactment of a disability rights legislation. Santosh Kumar Rungta, who had been the prominent leader of the Federation, was re-elected as the General Secretary of the Federation during its biannual convention in September 1988. The team of leaders who were elected or re-elected made it clear that the demand for enactment of the disability law would be their highest priority and raised this demand through a press statement after they resumed their office.

This group of board members, led by Rungta, organized a rally in early December 1988 (*Jansatta* 1988; *Navbharat Times* 1988). During the rally, they vehemently criticized the government for not making sincere efforts to enact the law by implementing the recommendations of the Justice Baharul Islam Committee, which had submitted its report during the early part of the year (*The Indian Express* 1988; *The Times of India* 1988).

This rally marked the beginning of a series of advocacy activities leading to a strong movement by the Federation in 1989 primarily to lobby for the enactment of the disability law. Hence, starting with this rally, a number of rallies were held with the agenda of demanding the enactment of the law. Finally, a 43-day-long sustained movement was launched beginning on 17 July 1989 to pursue this agenda, and the Federation persistently pressured the government to fulfil this demand for the most part of that year.

The first of the series of activities carried out by the Federation in 1989 was a 24-hour picket in Delhi on January 25, the eve of Republic Day at Raj Ghat, along with picketing of government offices in various state capitals where the Federation had some sort of base (*Jansatta* 1989a). Following this, the activists continued to engage in quiet lobbying through meetings with members of the Parliament in the early part of the year 1989 (*Jansatta* 1989b; *The Indian Express* 1989a). But this did not yield any effective results, and the government once again proved to be apathetic to the interests of blind and other disabled people as the issue of introducing the bill for the disability law was not placed on the agenda of the Budget Session. Nor did the issue concerning the blind receive any government attention in the budgetary allocation for the next financial year. This prompted the Federation to organize a large-scale rally on 6 March. As reported in the press coverage, the one unique feature of this rally was that it was also attended by members of other disability groups:

> More than 500 blind and disabled persons demonstrated at Boats Club here today to press their demand for legislation for the disabled. The rally which was organized by the National Federation of the Blind and the Welfare Society for the Disabled started from the office of the NFB at Paharganj at 9 a.m. (*The Times of India* 1989a)

As also mentioned in another press coverage, the All India Confederation of the Blind (AICB), an organization which was till then confined to service delivery projects in Delhi, also organized a parallel rally the same day: 'The blind held two separate rallies under different banners in the city on Monday to press implementation of the common demand—legislation for the disabled, which would ensure employment for them' (*The Indian Express* 1989b).

Following the two simultaneous rallies, both the NFB and AICB met the minister of social welfare for state, Rajendra Kumari Vajpayee, and delivered the memorandum to her. She assured them that the government would try to enact the disability legislation in that session of the Parliament (*The Hindu* 1989a). But, as usual, the promise was not kept by the government, which forced the Federationists to organize a large-scale rally on 4 May, just before the session was about to come to a close. They insisted on meeting the prime minister to discuss their demands, and a meeting took place on 8 May, during which they were assured of the introduction of the legislation in the ensuing Monsoon Session of the Parliament (*The Patriot* 1989a).

The assurance even by the highest authority too proved to be false, and no progress was made to introduce the legislation in the Monsoon Session of the Parliament. The Federation, therefore, persisted on organizing a 43-day sustained movement to press for its demands from 17 July onwards, soon after the beginning of the Monsoon Session. During this time, the Federationists resorted to various types of contentious politics. These methods ranged from uninterrupted picketing throughout the duration of the movement, to stopping trains, massive rallies, token and indefinite hunger strikes, and even threats of self-immolation.

Within five days of picketing since the beginning of the movement, the minister of social welfare for state, Rajendra Kumari Vajpayee, met the delegation of the Federation. She promised to consider their demands, but did not commit to any immediate, concrete action. She informed the delegation that it would not be possible to introduce the disability law before the new government was formed after the mid-term polls scheduled for the fall of that year. The activists felt betrayed once again, as the prime minister did not uphold his promise to introduce the legislation in the Monsoon Session. Therefore, after the disappointing meeting with the minister of social welfare for state on 21 July, the fifth day of this movement, the Federation announced that the movement would be intensified and radical measures would be adopted, including the stoppage of trains (*Jansatta* 1989c; *The Patriot* 1989b; *Punjab Kesari* 1989e). Consequently, the movement was intensified during the last week of July, and a number of arrests were made in front of the central government offices, in addition to making attempts to stop trains and at times even threatening to commit self-immolations. This time the activists also staged a continuous picket in front of the houses and offices of many government dignitaries, ranging from the social welfare minister to home minister and even the prime minister. This was a unique strategy, as during the earlier advocacy activities, the picketing was organized either in front of the office of the social welfare ministry or at times in front of the prime minister's official residence. But this time, the strategy was to create pressure by picketing the offices or residences of other high-ranking ministers as well.

In order to intensify the movement, the Federation organized a rally at the prime minister's office on 3 August, which was attended by more than 300 activists (*Hindustan* 1989a; *Punjab Kesari* 1989a; *The Times of India* 1989b). This rally was followed by a series of events, including picketing, courting of arrests and hunger strikes.

Following the rally on 3 August, which was the 19th day of the movement, the Federation decided to stage an ongoing picket in front of the prime minister's residence; 30 activists participated on the first day (5 August) (Hindustan 1989b; *The Indian Express* 1989c; *The Patriot* 1989c). This picketing prompted a series of arrests in the next few days, with an average of 20–30 arrests per day (*Jansatta* 1989d; *Punjab Kesari* 1989b, 1989c; *The Hindu* 1989b; *The Patriot* 1989d).

The strategy of picketing did not evoke any notable response from the government. As a result, the activists resorted to the strategy of an indefinite hunger strike starting from 10 August (Evening News 1989; *Jansatta* 1989e).

From the beginning of the hunger strike, the Federation maintained its publicly announced plan of one additional volunteer joining every day. This hunger strike also included a 24-hour-long large-scale hunger strike on the eve of Independence Day, which 300 activists joined (*Hindustan Times* 1989a; *Punjab Kesari* 1989d, 1989e; *The Indian Express* 1989d; *The Times of India* 1989c).

The Federationists were very optimistic regarding the outcome of this movement. But long before anything concrete was accomplished in terms of introducing the disability law, the Monsoon Session of the Parliament came to an end on 18 August, soon after the observation of Independence Day. Almost 50 activists made forceful but unsuccessful attempts to enter the Parliament on the last day of the session (*Jansatta* 1989f; *The Times of India* 1989d). The activists had to finally call off the movement on 29 August after a written agreement was reached with the minister of social welfare for state, Rajendra Kumari Vajpayee, under which the government once again promised to introduce the legislation in the next session of the Parliament, in addition to considering to a few other minor, but pressing, demands made by the activists (*The Indian Express* 1989f).

The next general elections were announced, and hence no advocacy could be carried out for the next few months. The activists, however, did register their protest with the political parties for being apathetic to their interests and criticized them for not including issues concerning the interests of the disabled in their political manifestos and appealed to the fellow disabled to boycott the elections (*Hindustan Times* 1989b; *The Indian Express* 1989g; *Veer Arjun* 1989).

A delegation of the Federation went to meet Prime Minister Vishwanath Pratap Singh in December 1989, soon after he had taken over as the prime minister of the newly formed government (*Hindustan* 1989c). The delegation had requested this meeting to congratulate him on becoming the prime minister and to begin to establish a relationship with him, while the larger purpose was to create a foundation for initiating a dialogue regarding the legislation. The activists then waited patiently for the newly formed government to settle down. During this period, the Federationists engaged in very little public advocacy activity, and they employed a strategy of quiet lobbying with the government to introduce the disability law by July 1990. They were able to obtain a commitment from the then social welfare minister, Ram Vilas Paswan, to get the law introduced in the Budget Session of the Parliament in March 1990 (*The Times of India* 1990).

This little-publicized meeting with Paswan to raise the demand for the introduction of the disability law was an example of a milder form of advocacy that was utilized from time to time. However, since the government did not show any signs of making any serious efforts for the enactment of a law by the summer of 1990, the Federation announced the launch of a rigorous movement by the middle of July

(*Dainik Hindustan* 1990; *Navbharat Times* 1990; *The Times of India* 1990). The Federation had plans to intensify the movement around the time of Independence Day in the middle of August (S. K. Rungta, personal interview, 4 April 2005), but the implementation of the Mandal Commission Report and the subsequent campaign for the construction of temple at the birthplace of Lord Rama in Ayodhya, leading to a situation of political uncertainty, compelled the activists to postpone their plan.

The Federation organized rallies in front of the prime minister's residence in November and again in December (*The Hindu* 1990a; *The Patriot* 1990). They succeeded in obtaining a meeting with the prime minister in the later part of December and, once again, the activists were assured that the desired law would be introduced shortly (*Dainik Jagran* 1990; *The Hindu* 1990b; *Veer Arjun* 1990). However, in fact, no further progress was made towards the introduction of the legislation as this period too was marked by tremendous political uncertainty.

Once the newly formed Congress government led by Prime Minister Narasimha Rao was settled in power, the Federation launched its advocacy activities to lobby for the enactment of the law beginning with a symbolic rally in the middle of March (*Hindustan Times* 1992a; *The Pioneer* 1992). This was followed by another rally and picketing in August after the completion of one year of the Congress government being in power. The leaders met the Minister of State for Personnel, Public Grievances and Pensions, Margaret Alva, who was responsible for recruitment, along with the special officer of the prime minister who assured them that an appointment with the prime minister would be arranged (*Hindustan Times* 1992b; *The National Herald* 1992). Another big rally took place in December, and a memorandum was presented to a representative of the prime minister (*Rashtriya Sahara* 1992; *The Hindu* 1992).

In addition to the quiet lobbying with the government officials, the Federation held a rally in the middle of May 1993 (*Jansatta* 1993; *The Times of India* 1993). Similarly, the Federation again organized a massive rally in the later part of August 1994. During that rally, it threatened to launch a vigorous movement if government officials did not respond positively. But following that rally, it withdrew that plan after receiving a favourable response from the concerned authorities.

During their meeting with the representatives of the Ministry of Personnel, Public Grievances and Pensions as well as the Ministry of Social Welfare, the activists were promised that the government would look into their demands and introduce the proposed legislation in the next session of the Parliament (*Hindustan* 1994; *Hindustan Times* 1994; *Navbharat Times* 1994).

By the middle of 1995, the Congress government led by Prime Minister Narasimha Rao had already been in power for about four years and the next general elections were due in 1996. There was a limit to the extent that the government could continue to get by on false promises. Hence, the demonstrations carried out during 1995 proved to be the catalyst that prompted government officials to introduce the law in December during the Winter Session of the Parliament.

As early as 24 May 1995, the Federation received a convincing response from Sitaram Kesri, the Minister of Social Welfare, regarding the introduction of the disability law in the then current session of Parliament that was going on at that time (*Hindustan Times* 1995a; *The Hindu* 1995; *The Indian Express* 1995). Despite the usual promise of the concerned ministry, the bill for the disability law was not introduced even during the Monsoon Session. Therefore, the Federation again organized a massive rally on 24 July to press for this demand (*Hindustan Times* 1995b; *Jansatta* 1995).

While the sporadic demonstrations led by the organized blind during 1995 finally triggered the enactment of the PWD Act (1995), the foundation for its introduction had already been laid as a result of a long-drawn-out process of lobbying which included various methods of advocacy. At the same time, the disabled were now forming a united front to fight for it, and there were additional conditions that created a conducive atmosphere for the enactment of such a law, in addition to the pressure built by the organized blind. As a result, the government could no longer afford to be oblivious to the demand for the enactment of this law raised by the disabled community, and as Bhambhani (2004, 28) concludes,

> After a prolonged campaign, several rounds of talks, lobbying, sit-ins, protest marches, press-conferences, media mobilization and agitations,

the Persons with Disabilities Act was finally passed by the Indian Parliament on 31st December, 1995 and became a law on 7th February, 1996 with the President, Dr. Shankar Dayal Sharma, giving his assent.

It is, however, worth pointing out that the first broad-based disability rights group (DRG) comprising its members from different categories of disabilities was established in Delhi in 1994, which has made a significant contribution to the enriching of the cross-disability rights movement. Thus, the disability rights movement began to shift from an initiative of blind activists to a cross-disability effort. But the fact cannot be denied that the enactment of the PWD Act (1995) was predominantly the result of a long-drawn-out struggle carried out by the Federation, and the period of the late 1980s must be regarded as the time of origin of the disability rights movement primarily because of the focus of the struggle carried out by the Federation on the demand for the enactment of this law from 1988 to 1995.

ORIGIN OF THE DISABILITY RIGHTS MOVEMENT IN INDIA: CONTESTING VIEWS

There are broadly three identifiable views regarding the origin of the disability rights movement in India. Ghai (2003), one of a few scholars of disability studies in India, is of the opinion that 'the disability rights movement in India got initiated with the declaration of year 1981 as the International Year of Disabled People. Till then, only sporadic attempts were being made to rehabilitate the disabled' (p. 17). On the other hand, in her master's thesis at the University of Illinois at Chicago, Bhambhani (2004, 17) rejects Ghai's argument and argues that the intensification of rehabilitation measures and programmes and policies in the field of disability during the International Year of the Disabled Persons (IYDP) is not associated with the beginning of the disability rights movement. She further argues, until and unless cross-disability is taken into consideration, it cannot be called a disability rights movement. Hence, according to her, the disability rights movement in India began with the formation of DRG in 1994. Likewise, Mehrotra (2011) observes that the disability rights movement essentially began in the early 1990s, as, according to her, the launch of the Asian and

Pacific Decade of Disabled Persons in 1993 provide a definite boost to the movement along with other factors leading to its origin. I would like to challenge Bhambhani's argument that there was a lack of any movement for the rights of the disabled before the formation of DRG in Delhi in 1994. Likewise, I also disagree with Mehrotra that the disability rights movement actually began in the early 1990s primarily as a result of international influence.

Before challenging Bhambhani's and Mehrotra's views, it is worth mentioning that unlike Bhambhani and Mehrotra, Ghai's work is not devoted to the discussion of the disability rights movement. Rather, there is a passing reference to it in the work cited here. Hence, it will not be fair to engage into a detailed analysis or criticism of her views in this context. It is, however, worth mentioning that as discussed in detail in another study, the movement led by NFB had already gained momentum during 1980 (Chander 2011). This year happened to be the most important year in the history of the movement of the organized blind in terms of its vigour and publicity during the initial phase of its growth. It was during 1980 when the issue of *lathi-charge* (beating with sticks) by the police on the peaceful demonstrators on World Disabled Day drew tremendous attention of the general public as well as the parliamentarians and the press (Chander 2011, 204–12). Blind activists from various parts of India had gathered at the time of this incident, and they were engaged in some sort of advocacy for their rights throughout the year. The events of 1980 and the intensification of the movement of the organized blind cannot, therefore, be said to have been influenced by India's involvement in the commemoration of 1981 as the IYDP. Hence, based on the strength of advocacy by the blind activists as well as its radical nature, it is clear that the movement of the organized blind, which happened to be the only movement carried out by any disability-specific group at that time, had been gaining momentum even prior to the commemoration of the IYDP. It is, therefore, wrong to consider the IYDP as a watershed or even a stimulator for launching the disability rights movement.

Rejecting Ghai's theorization of the commemoration of the IYDP as the year of origin of the disability rights movement in India, Bhambhani (2004, 17) opines:

There is no doubt that, with international pressure, advances were made in the government response and some consciousness also developed among disabled people in India. However, this definition of a ['movement'] is a matter of contestation and thorough academic research. Sporadic or desultory attempts at demonstrations by single or impairment-specific groups cannot necessarily be termed a movement.... I believe that the real movement of contentious disability political action in India started in the early 1990s with the formation of the cross-disability advocacy group, Disabled Rights Group.

Based on this statement, two points emerge: first, there is no history of sustained movement even by any impairment-specific group during the 1980s and early 1990s as whatever advocacy activities that took place during this period were basically 'sporadic' or 'desultory' attempts at demonstrations by 'single' or 'impairment-specific groups' (p.17), and second, no history of contentious political action by any impairment-specific group can be regarded as a part of the history of the disability rights movement due to the lack of cross-disability participation prior to the formation of the DRG in 1994. As discussed in detail in the early part of this chapter, the advocacy activities carried out by the blind activists did not remain sporadic and desultory. On the contrary, it is quite evident from the description above that there is a well-documented history of contentious political action resulting into a sustained movement led by the blind activists, particularly from the late 1980s prior to the formation of the DRG.

Bhambhani's argument is right to the extent that the movement led by the organized blind lacked participation of different groups having varying types of disabilities until the formation of the DRG in 1994, but it does not mean that there was no advocacy for the rights of the disabled as a broader category of disability. However, drawing an analogy of the origin of the disability rights movement in the United States, where the Independent Living Movement, as well as the movement for the enactment of the Rehabilitation Act of 1973 and then the implementation of its Section 504 and finally the enactment of Americans with Disabilities Act (1990), was predominantly led by wheelchair users (Barnartt and Scotch 2001; Fleischer and Zames 2001;

Scotch 2001; Shapiro 1993), the period from 1988 to 1995 marks the beginning of the disability rights movement in India. My argument is that even if the movement for the disability law was predominantly led by the organized blind from 1988 onwards, it should be regarded as the beginning of the disability rights movement because of the focus of its agenda, that is, the enactment of a comprehensive disability law dealing with the rights of a broader group of the disabled and not just the blind. The fact, however, can readily be acknowledged that this movement was significantly enhanced by the increasing participation of various disability groups, and there is a coexistence of a cross-disability rights movement as well as an impairment-specific movement in the post-1995 period.

Three key points emerged out of Mehrotra's study (2011): (a) the disability rights movement in India started in the early 1990s, particularly when it received a boost with the launch of the Asian and Pacific Decade of Disabled Persons in 1993; (b) the enactment of the PWD Act was more of a product of impact of women's movement and international push and less of protests or lobbying by disabled persons; and (c) the disability rights movement was led predominantly by the physically impaired and hardly had any representation of those having intellectual or developmental disabilities till the late 1990s. I agree with her as far as the third point is concerned, but disagree with regard to her earlier two arguments relating to the period of the origin of the disability rights movement in India and the factors leading to the enactment of the PWD Act.

It may be right that the launch of the Asian and Pacific Decade of Disabled Persons in 1993 added to the facilitation of the process of enactment of the disability law and a greater recognition of the demand for its enactment pressed hard by blind activists through a vigorous movement carried out primarily since 1988, but it cannot be regarded as the point of origin of the disability rights movement in India. The blind activists were admittedly joined in their endeavour by a relatively broad-based DRG, just before the PWD Act was enacted, which in some ways also provided a boost to the movement already carried out by the blind activists for the enactment of this law. But the fact cannot be denied that the disability rights movement originated in India since 1988 because of the reasons stated above in support of this argument.

Similarly, I agree with Mehrotra that new social movements like the environment movement, Dalit and particularly the women's rights movement in India along with the disability rights movement internationally provided social and political context to the disability rights movement in India. But the passage of the PWD Act was certainly the result of the intense and sustained lobbying with occasional intervals carried out by blind activists to fulfil this objective between 1988 and 1995. Sufficient empirical evidence has been presented in the early part of this chapter to prove this point, and hence, it will be wrong to say that the passing of the PWD Act as argued by her was more of the result of international pressure than lobbying and protests by DRGs. The existence of a vibrant disability rights movement in the West, particularly the United States, during the time preceding the passage of the PWD Act and the resultant pressure by international agencies on the Indian state to introduce more disabled-friendly policies and legislations did help in creating a conducive environment for the passing of this law, but the success resulting in the passage of such a landmark disability rights law would not have been possible without intense lobbying and protests carried out by blind people for at least seven years from 1988 to 1995.

CONCLUSION

With the beginning of the movement of the organized blind in the 1970s, there was a growing consciousness in the minds of the blind activists regarding their rights, and they increasingly adopted a rights-based approach by challenging the traditional charity-based approach towards blindness. By the late 1980s, they realized that their rights can be better protected through a comprehensive disability rights legislation. Also, certain developments in the field of blindness and disability led to an atmosphere conducive to enable them to focus their struggle on the single-point agenda of enactment of such a law since 1988 onwards. This led to a shift from a disability-specific movement confined to advocating for the rights of blind people only to a broader group of different categories of the disabled, thereby leading to the origin of the disability rights movement. Hence, the period between 1988 and 1995, in which the Federation led a long-drawn-out movement focused on the agenda of the enactment of a first comprehensive disability rights law leading to the enactment of the PWD Act (1995), can be regarded to be the period of the origin of the disability rights movement in India.

REFERENCES

Abidi, J. 2004. 'No Pity'. *Health for the millions* (November–December 1995). In M. Bhambhani, *From Charity to Self-advocacy: The Emergence of Disability Rights Movement in India*. Unpublished master's thesis, University of Illinois at Chicago.

Baquer, A., and A. Sharma. 1997. *Disability: Challenges vs Responses*. New Delhi: Concerned Action Now.

Barnartt, S. and R. Scotch. 2001. *Disability Protests: Contentious Politics 1970–1999*. Washington, DC: Gallaudet University.

Bhambhani, M. 2004. *From Charity to Self-advocacy: The Emergence of Disability Rights Movement in India*. Unpublished master's thesis, University of Illinois at Chicago.

Chander, J. 2011. *Movement of the Organized Blind in India: Passive Recipients to Active Advocates of their Rights*. PhD Dissertation submitted at Syracuse University.

Dainik Hindustan. 1990, 12 July. *The Blind Will Agitate for Their Demands*. Delhi.

Dainik Jagran. 1990, 19 December. *Demand of Introducing the Legislation for the Disabled: Assurance by the Prime Minister*. Delhi.

Evening News. 1989, 10 August. *The Blind Began an Indefinite Fast*. Delhi.

Fleischer, D. Z. and F. Zames. 2001. *The Disability Rights Movement: From Charity to Confrontation*. Philadelphia: Temple University Press.

Ghai, A. 2003. *Embodied Form: Issues of Disabled Women*. New Delhi: Shakti Publications.

Hindustan Times. 1989a, 15 August. *Fifth Day Fast by Blind*. Delhi.

———. 1989b, 17 November. *The Disabled May Boycott Polls*. Delhi.

———. 1992a, 16 March. *A Rally by the Sightless*. Delhi.

———. 1992b, 11 August. *Blind Dharna for Law and Job Quota*. Delhi.

———. 1994, 24 August. *Blind Put Off Stir Plan*. Delhi.

———. 1995a, 25 May. *Blind's Rally to Draw Government's Attention*. Delhi.

———. 1995b, 25 July. *NFB Activists Seeking Legislation for Disabled*. Delhi.

Hindustan. 1985, November 19. 'Demonstration of the Blind for Their Demands.' *Hindustan*, Delhi.

———. 1989a, August 4. 'The Blind Gave a Memorandum.' *Hindustan*, Delhi.

———. 1989b, August 6. 'Demonstration on Gol Methi Chauk.' *Hindustan*, Delhi.

Hindustan. 1989c, December 8. 'The Blind Met the Prime Minister.' *Hindustan,* Delhi.

———. 1994, August 24. 'Demonstration of Hundreds of Blind in Support of Their Demands.' *Hindustan,* Delhi.

Jansatta. 1988, September 17. 'The Bill for the Disabled is in Flux.' *Jansatta,* Delhi.

———. 1989a, January 25. 'Blind Staged Dharna.' *Jansatta,* Delhi.

———. 1989b, February 27. 'The Demand for Passing the Legislation for the Disabled.' *Jansatta,* Delhi.

———. 1989c, July 22. 'Disabled Will Stop Trains.' *Jansatta,* Delhi.

———. 1989d, August 9. 'Blind Arrested.' *Jansatta,* Delhi.

———. 1989e, August 11. 'The Federation of the Blind Started Hunger Strike.' *Jansatta,* Delhi.

———. 1989f, August 19. '50 Blind Arrested While Entering in the Parliament.' *Jansatta,* Delhi

———. 1993, May 19. 'Demonstration of the Blind.' *Jansatta,* Delhi.

———. 1995, July 25. 'The Blind Took Out a Rally for the Fulfillment of Their Demands.' *Jansatta,* Delhi.

Limaye, M. 1984. *Socialist Movement in the Early Years of Independence.* In *Fifty years of Socialist Movement in India: Retrospect and prospects,* edited by G. K. C. Reddy, 38–53. New Delhi: Samata Era Publication.

Mehrotra, N. 2011. 'Disability Rights Movements in India: Politics and Practice'. *Economic & Political Weekly* 46 (6): 65–72.

Mohan, S. 1984. 'The Turbulent Years: 1952–55'. In *Fifty Years of Socialist Movement in India: Retrospect and Prospects,* edited by G. K. C. Reddy, 54–60. New Delhi: Samata Era Publication.

Navbharat Times. 1988, September 17. 'Anguish on Delay in Making Law for the Disabled.' *Navbharat Times,* Delhi.

———. 1990, July 12. 'A Demand for a Solid Policy.' *Navbharat Times,* Delhi.

———. 1994, August 24. 'The Blind Took Out a Rally.' *Navbharat Times,* Delhi.

Omvedt, G. 2001. 'Ambedkar and After: The Dalit Movement in India'. In *Dalit Identity and Politics: Cultural Subordination and the Dalit Challenge,* Vol. 2, edited by G. Shah, 143–159. London: SAGE.

Punjab Kesari. 1989a, August 4. 'Memorandum to the Prime Minister by the Blind.' *Punjab Kesari,* Punjab.

———. 1989b, August 8. '20 Blind Detained.' *Punjab Kesari,* Punjab.

———. 1989c, August 9. '25 Blind Arrested While Breaking Prohibitory Orders and Released.' *Punjab Kesari,* Punjab.

———. 1989d, August 17. 'The Hunger Strike of the Blind Continued on 7th Day.' *Punjab Kesari,* Punjab.

———. 1989e, July 22. 'The Blind will Stop Trains on 24'. *Punjab Kesari.* Delhi.

Rashtriya Sahara. 1992, December 3. 'The Blind Demonstrated and Arrested.' *Punjab Kesari,* Delhi.

Rudolph, L. I., and S. H. Rudolph. 1987. *In Pursuit of Lakshmi: The Political Economy of the Indian State.* Chicago, IL: University of Chicago Press.

Scotch, R. K. 2001. *From Good Will to Civil Rights: Transforming Federal Disability Policy*. 2nd ed. Philadelphia, PA: Temple University Press.

Shapiro, J. P. 1993. *No Pity: People with Disabilities Forging a New Civil Rights Movement*. New York, NY: Times Books (Random House).

The Hindu. 1989a, March 7. 'Blind People Demand Law for Job Reservation.' *The Hindu*, Delhi.

———. 1989b, August 7. 'Blind Court Arrest.' *The Hindu*, Delhi.

———. 1990a, December 15. 'Blind Protesters Court Arrest.' *The Hindu*, Delhi.

———. 1990b, December 19. 'P.M.'s Assurance to the Blind.' *The Hindu*, Delhi.

———. 1992, December 3. 'Visually Handicapped Marched for their Rights.' *The Hindu*, Delhi.

———. 1995, May 25. 'The Blind Pressed for their Demands.' *The Hindu*, Delhi.

The Indian Express. 1985, March 18. 'Blind Men Seek Law for Disabled.' *The Indian Express*, Delhi.

———. 1987, July 8. 'Blind to Justice.' *The Indian Express*, Delhi.

———. 1988, December 2. 'Blind Protest Against Govt's Apathy.' *The Indian Express*, Delhi.

———. 1989a, February 28. 'Legislation for the Disabled Urged.' *The Indian Express*, Delhi.

———. 1989b, March 7. 'Blind Hold Rallies.' *The Indian Express*, Delhi.

———. 1989c, August 6. 'Blind Men's Dharna near P.M.'s House.' *The Indian Express*, Delhi.

———. 1989d, August 13. 'Blind Men Begin Indefinite Hunger Strike.' *The Indian Express*, Delhi.

———. 1989e, August 17. 'Condition Deteriorates.' *The Indian Express*, Delhi.

———. 1989f, August 30. 'Federation of Blind Suspends Agitation.' *The Indian Express*, Delhi.

———. 1989g, November 17. 'Disabled Threaten to Boycott Polls.' *The Indian Express*.

———. 1995, May 25. 'Kesari's Assurance to the Blind and Disabled.' *The Indian Express*.

The National Herald. 1985, November 19. 'Rally by Blind Outside P.M. House.' *The National Herald*, Delhi.

———. 1992, August 11. 'Blind for Legislation.' *National Herald*, Delhi.

The Patriot. 1989a, May 9. 'Blind Assured of Legislation.' *The Patriot*, Delhi.

———. 1989b, July 22. 'Blind Threatened Stir.' *The Patriot*, Delhi.

———. 1989c, August 6. 'Blind Dharna.' *The Patriot*, Delhi.

———. 1989d, August 7. 'Blind Detained.' *The Patriot*, Delhi.

———. 1990, November 27. 'Members of the National Federation of the Blind on Their Way to Present a Memorandum to Prime Minister Chandrashekhar to Highlight Their Various Demands on Monday.' *The Patriot*, Delhi.

The Pioneer. 1992, March 16. 'Blind March for Job Reservation.' *The Pioneer*, Delhi.

The Times of India. 1988, December 2. 'Members of National Federation of the Blind Marching Towards Boat Club.' *The Times of India*, Delhi.

The Times of India 1989a, March 6. 'The Disabled Demand Legislation.' *The Times of India*, Delhi.

———. 1989b, August 4. 'Blind Demand Law for the Disabled.' *The Times of India*, Delhi.

———. 1989c, August 15. 'Blind go on Fast.' *The Times of India*, Delhi.

———. 1989d, August 19. 'Blind Marchers Arrested.' *The Times of India*, Delhi.

———. 1990, July 12. 'Blind to Agitate for Law on Disabled.' *The Times of India*, Delhi.

———. 1993, May 19. 'Blind Hold Rally.' *The Times of India*, Delhi.

Vanaik, A. 1990. 'The Painful Transition: Bourgeois Democracy in India.' New York, NY: Verso.

Veer Arjun. 1989, 17 November. 'The Disabled Will Boycott Elections.' *Veer Arjun*, Delhi.

———. 1990, 19 December. Assurance by the Prime Minister to the Blind. *Veer Arjun*, Delhi.

Chapter 2

Emergence of Disability Rights Movement in India
From Charity to Self-advocacy

Meenu Bhambhani

The decade that bridged the 20th and 21st centuries, has witnessed tremendous changes for disabled people in India. This chapter examines the emergence of a self-representing disability rights movement as a crucial factor towards changes in self-perception and group affiliation of disabled persons during 1994–2004. This analysis contributes to the understanding of disability as a social and cultural issue, through a historical review of the nation's past at the cusp of transition from one century to the other.

In 1994, disabled people from diverse disability groups joined hands to form the Disabled Rights Group (DRG). The DRG actively lobbied for the passage of a landmark legislation, called the Persons with Disabilities (Equal Opportunities, Protection of Rights and Full Participation) Act, 1995 (1996; henceforth referred to as the PWD Act). Subsequent to the passage of this federal legislation, disability issues gained visibility across the social and political stages in India. Likewise, disabled persons began to gain recognition collectively as a sector, a movement and significant minority group. Prior to this, self-representing disability movements took a segregated approach (blind for the blind, deaf for the deaf and so on) which forced the community to remain at the receiving end of philanthropic, welfare and charity efforts of both government and non-government agencies. The 1995 legislation established the rights of a large swath of socially disenfranchised persons. In doing so, the Act helped give rise to a visible and vigilant cross-disability movement—a movement that was committed to changing the social situation of disabled persons.

Very little systematic documentation exists of the growing and vibrant disability movement that began to discover itself in the wake of formative legislative commands. Having been a part of this movement, I have personally witnessed and participated in many of the actions and efforts of this time. I have also analysed the movement in retrospect as I personally observed it. The National Centre for Promotion of Employment for Disabled People (NCPEDP) and DRG are two key organizations that led the disability rights movement in India. I can say this with some authority because, as a social actor and participant, I am and have been very much a part of these organizations' activities.

METHODOLOGY

My methodology is a combination of content, event and historical analyses. This methodology has been used by Barnartt and Scotch (2001) in analysing important events of the disability rights movement in the United States in *Disability Protests: Contentious Politics 1970–1999*. I have drawn inspiration from this work in analysing the disability movement in India. The achievements, successes, failures and impact of the NCPEDP and DRG have not been adequately and extensively documented. They are recorded in media reports, conference presentations and advocacy tools such as petitions, press releases, emails and protest letters.

Due to constraints of time and space, it is not possible to discuss in detail the literature that was documented prior to the passage of the PWD Act. However, it would be useful to briefly mention here that since the post-independence era, in every two decades, there has been a paradigmatic shift in perceiving and approaching disability, with particularly significant changes occurring in the 1990s. While the 1950s and 1960s were decades of physical/medical/vocational rehabilitation, the 1970s and 1980s marked the beginning of advocacy by impairment-specific organizations and community-based rehabilitation. With the passage of the PWD Act, there emerged a full-fledged cross-disability movement, which is working within the ideological framework of 'Nothing About Us Without Us'—the philosophy of Disabled Peoples' International (DPI). Although the former periods have been well documented, the literature on disability in India, it seems, has been slow in documenting and analysing the changes of the 1990s.[1]

EMERGENCE OF THE CROSS-DISABILITY MOVEMENT: 1994–2004

The origins of the disability movement in India are contested. Some trace these to the year 1981, and others to the year 1995. I have traced these to the year preceding the passage of the PWD Act. It is beyond the scope of this chapter to critically analyse and enlist all the major events of contentious disability politics that have taken place in India between 1994 and 2004 and the role the PWD Act has played in catalysing the efforts of disability activists. However, my analysis addresses some significant questions as to what the advocacy movement is lacking, its strengths, shortcomings, factors that have facilitated mobilization, tactics that have been used, the framework it has borrowed and followed, the purpose the movement has served and the likely future direction it may take. A critical analysis of the cross-disability movement will also help us understand the kind of advocacy movement it is—a new social movement, a post-materialist movement or part of the transnational movement.

First, I have analysed the factors that have assisted in mobilizing people to join the movement. These factors may be divided into three categories: demands, issues and resources. Next, I have discussed the advocacy tools and tactics utilized and assess whether the success of these strategies in some collective campaigns may be used as a model for similar movements in other countries. In the conclusion, I have reflected upon the current direction and shortcomings of the disability

---

[1] For details on DPI, see www.dpi.org.

movement in India and considered ways in which those shortcomings may be addressed in the future.

MOBILIZING FACTORS

In their examinations of disability protests in the United States, Barnartt and Scotch (2001) have focused on three key factors that help people mobilize for social action and change: demands, issues and resources. In the context of the US disability rights movement, a number of factors have mobilized disabled people for collective action: cross-disability demands, issues of access, implementation of law and demands for services, and resources including media, funding for research and politically sophisticated leaders. In the following sections, I will examine the factors that have facilitated mobilization in India on our way to a social movement.

Cross-disability Demands

A cursory glance at disability protests in India from 1994 onwards demonstrates that the demands of this movement have reflected concerns of a broad spectrum of disability groups. Although the focus of collective action in 1994–95 was the passage of legislation which pertained to only seven categories of disability, in subsequent campaigns, all had, what Barnartt and Scotch (2001, 69) describe as, 'something for everyone'. Truly, cross-disability campaigns have included advocacy on the following issues: inclusion of disability in Census 2001, the annual budget in 2002–03, protest against CII, inaccessibility at WSF 2004 and disabled-friendly polling booths during the general election in May 2004. Barnartt and Scotch argue that success becomes possible and people participate when their 'self-interest is stronger' (2001, 66). Cross-disability demands have a rippling effect and help in 'widening the pool of potential adherents' (p. 69). Prior to 1994, there were protests and collective actions undertaken by impairment-specific groups and also social action initiated by the cross-disability self-help groups in rural south India. However, if one goes by Barnartt and Scotch's contention, such actions cannot be termed a part of the social movement owing to their limited scale and aim. Their demand is limited to their own specific group/interest, and they 'seek to change individuals' rather than 'political process' or policy (2001, xiii). The cross-disability approach to voicing demands has given disabled people more visibility, recognition and also a sense of community and identity.

Issues

There is a need to analyse issues that have motivated people for collective action in India because they reflect the priorities identified by disabled people. On the other hand, they also give an idea of who is setting the agenda and indicate the framework towards which the movement is headed. The primary issues of the disability movement in India can be categorized into two groups: rights-based issues and issues related to services.

Rights-based Issues: Accessibility in Transport and Physical Environment

The process of the implementation of the PWD Act started in 1997, when Javed Abidi sued the Indian Airlines and Union of India for inaccessibility in air transportation. Later, when Professor Stephen Hawking visited India in 2001, the lack of access at the historical monuments was used as a symbol to embarrass the authorities and highlight the fact that 'rights for people with impairments have to include accessibility as a basic demand' (Barnartt and Scotch 2001, 38). NCPEDP's vision includes accessibility as one of the key enablers to employment that, in turn, guarantees a dignified, independent and empowered life to disabled people. In the general elections of 2004, accessibility once again emerged as the rallying point for securing space in the political arena. A comparison of the campaigns for access in 2001 and 2004 shows that, whereas the 2001 campaign highlighted barriers to access for mobility-impaired people, DRG's 2004 campaign for disabled-friendly elections addressed the issue of communication accessibility for people with visual and hearing disability as well.

Whereas accessibility has emerged as a powerful symbol in efforts to demonstrate the denial of rights and to push for a social model of disability, it has also come in for much criticism. Ramanujam (2000) has criticized accessibility as replication of a Western model that is not workable in Indian situations. He says:

> Those who first got interested in the disability issues derived inspiration from the developed western countries, but their models have not yielded much results because the implementation of alien models becomes very expensive and often irrelevant. [...] For example, in the Indian context, especially in villages, without spending much we can ensure mobility and access [...] by removing barriers in public places and paving the floors with rough and non-slippery materials. In all tropical countries walking with crutches is much easier than in the countries with wet, windy and cold climatic conditions, which make wheelchair mobility much easier and less risky. (p. 11)

Without naming anyone in the above passage, Ramanujam alludes to Javed Abidi, who studied in Dayton, Ohio, and also spent considerable time in Chicago (Bornstein 2004, 222). Ramanujam criticizes the Western-centric approach to solutions of local problems of disability in India. In a similar context, Miles and Hossain (1999) have also considered the rhetoric of the social model—which has been widely used by activists in the area of access—as inapplicable in other developing countries. They write:

> There can be no objection to people developing such models and terminology in countries wealthy enough to sustain decades of effort in constructing and adapting public environments to be user-friendly to all sorts and conditions of humanity. But foisting these advanced notions on to an impoverished country where a majority of children are stunted for lack of adequate nutrition (UNICEF 1998) displays some arrogance about the practical realities of development. (p. 80)

If one analyses the issue objectively, it is clear that the efforts of disability activists are not directed at replicating the Western model. The attempt is to sensitize all concerned to come up with local solutions to the problems plaguing disabled people in their own location. Although the movement for access started and spread in urban areas, the policy changes have had some effect in the area of rural accessibility as well. The Government of India, in the year 2001, made provision for the reservation of 3% funds under the Rural Development Project for rural accessibility in the 10th Five-Year Plan. Under the Swarnajayanti Gram Swarozgar Yojana (Golden Jubilee Rural Self-Employment Scheme), six public places in each village were to be made accessible; these included primary health centre, primary school, bus terminus, public toilet, drinking water facility and access at panchayat *ghar* (similar to town hall in cities; Planning Commission, Government of India, 2002–07). One can thus conclude that access has a distinct political advantage and that it has emerged as a powerful symbol that activists have used 'skillfully in entrepreneurial ways to frame issues and consequently policy decisions and policy outcomes' (Scotch 1984, 159).

Issues Pertaining to Inclusion/Integration: Claiming Citizenship Rights

The issues of including disability in the census and the annual budget, opposing a non-disabled person's appointment to the post of CCPD and seeking political participation may be categorized as rights-based issues. In prioritizing such issues, activists are not merely seeking visibility for disability but are claiming citizenship rights that have been denied to disabled people from time immemorial. These issues also symbolize the overall struggle of the disability movement in India and its search for a uniting framework. It is apparent that, in the protest against CCPD or promotion of participation in elections, the movement has tried to articulate 'Nothing About Us Without Us'—the philosophy propounded by Disabled Peoples' International—as the conceptual framework within which it would like to position itself. James Charlton (1998, 16) puts the international disability rights movement as follows:

> [A] 'liberation movement', the essence of which is the demand for 'Nothing About Us Without Us' reflected in its principles of 'independence and integration, empowerment and human rights, self-help and self-determination'. [...] Through its struggle comes a vision that requires a fundamental reordering of priorities and resources. 'Nothing About Us Without Us' suggests such a sea change in the way disability oppression is conceived and resisted.

An adherence to this ideology may lead one to characterize the Indian disability rights movement as a new social or transnational movement because of its international dimension. However, if we look at the issues of service delivery, concessions and facilities, the movement appears more as a post-materialist movement. The issues of integration and inclusion overlap with demands for services. They illustrate the confusion of the movement—does it aim at integration in which the element of choice is restricted or does it aim at getting political power for 'who they want to' integrate with (Crescendo, quoted in Charlton 1998, 127). This ambiguity becomes clearer when we analyse the resources and issues prompting demands for services.

Issues Prompting Demands for Services, Facilities and Concessions

One of the most prolonged campaigns in the recent history of the disability movement in India has been an effort to procure a number of government services and concessions: more financial allocations, the extension of government facilities to all categories of disability, concessions on assistive devices for disabled people and increased employment opportunities. This list of demands suggests the extent to which disability concerns have been immersed in local issues. In a developing country like India, disability is very much an economic issue—what Charlton (1998, 37) terms as a 'political economy informed by class'—and prevention and rehabilitation remain key concerns of the majority of disabled people living in rural areas. Disability activists have achieved some success in addressing the need for rehabilitation and services, not as an act of charity, but as a matter of rights. This, again, may be considered an influence of disability movements in the United States, where 'the frame of rights' has been extended to the demands of independent living, which, in turn, 'is related to social movements such as patients' rights movements, the consumers' rights movements, and the self-help movement, all of which have similar demands' (Barnartt and Scotch 2001, 44). Such demands place disability movements in India within the framework of post-materialism since the issues pertain to the enhancement of quality of life through material resources. The existence of law legitimizes the demand for services and facilities and acts as a handy tool to extend the framework of rights. It confirms what Johnny Crescendo (quoted in Charlton) calls a struggle for 'interdependence rather than integration' (Charlton 1998, 127).

In addition to demands for services and financial allocations, the disability movement in the United States has also taken up issues of assisted suicide, representations, telethons and disability culture (Barnartt and Scotch 2001, 44–49). In India, these issues are debated neither in activist circles nor in academia. The issues of livelihood, education and access to resources and rehabilitation are so pressing that issues of culture, history and media portrayals assume secondary importance in the hierarchy of priorities.

Resources

Any mass movement is largely dependent on resources, both material and human. In India, the DRG initially led the movement for legislation using personal financial and other resources of its founding members. Once the momentum subsided after the passage of the PWD Act, however, the DRG became quiescent. The NCPEDP has given it a fresh lease of life. A combination of the following three resources has helped in reviving the DRG and, simultaneously, the disability rights movement: media, organizational base and young, media-savvy leadership. In the commemorative issue of equity (December 2001), the NCPEDP acknowledges the role of media 'as valuable partners in its campaign to alter the lives of disabled persons for the better.... They have come to appreciate our struggle, and the need for constant pressure on policy makers to ensure that changes happen today rather than tomorrow' (*EQUITY Commemorative Issue* 2001, 21–22). Barnartt and Scotch (2001), in the context of the US disability movement, give credit to media and also offer a reason as to why media report disability protests. According to them, 'the combination of sympathy and stigma and assumptions of incapacity associated with disability in mainstream culture may have made protests by people with disabilities (PWD) appear more remarkable to the media, and their protests more newsworthy' (p. 63). The NCPEDP and DRG have been only partially successful in mobilizing the media. A study of media reports on disability protests in the year 2003 demonstrates that out of 45 published newspaper reports, only 10 were published in Hindi, a language spoken and understood by a vast majority in North India. The remaining print media coverage was all in the English language media—read, understood and spoken only by the elite upper class in major urban centres. From my own personal experience, I can say that even in other forms of electronic media such as TV and radio, English language news channels have been more responsive in reporting disability issues. The mobilization of English media has definitely embarrassed the bureaucratic authorities and also led to some policy changes, but it has failed to facilitate mass movement beyond urban centres.

NCPEDP's own strong organizational base has facilitated the DRG and the advocacy movement. The NCPEDP, through its membership base—comprising of disability organizations across India, disabled people, corporate organizations and so on—communication network and results of research activities, has provided crucial resources upon which the movement is built. McAdam, McCarthy and Zald (1996, 13) confirm that 'for a movement to survive, insurgents must be able to create a more enduring organizational structure to sustain collective action'. Further, they also write that 'it is the formal organizations who purport to speak for the movement, who increasingly dictate the course, content, and outcomes of the struggle' (p. 15). The DRG, and indeed the movement as a whole, owes its revival to the NCPEDP's provision of a structure from which to sustain itself and grow.

The third necessity of a movement is strong leadership. In the US disability movement, 'politically sophisticated', articulate and educated disabled people such as Judy Heumann and Justin Dart led the movement of protests in the 1970s (Scotch and Barnartt 2001, 62). In India, people like Javed Abidi—young, dynamic, articulate, educated in the United States, a communications graduate—have played a major role in creating situations of contentious politics and thus initiating cross-disability activism in the 1990s. The disability movement in India owes visibility and recognition to the creative genius and entrepreneurship of people like Abidi who have successfully 'invented social problems' and 'marketed' them with 'ideology laden-symbols' (Scotch 1984, 160). The spate of successes in public interest litigations, the outcomes of which were influenced by media mobilization and organized protests, can be attributed to his activist politics.

While charismatic leadership has been in many ways a strength of the movement up to now, it has its limits as well. No new leadership has emerged since the 1990s. Abidi's dominant position in the movement has drawn criticism from within the Indian disability community, albeit in an oblique way. While it is crucial to have what Phil Lee (2002, 148) describes as 'articulate, organized and effective disability activists' who could put 'politics into disability', this form of leadership can also be very limiting since it focuses 'too exclusively on the political activists, their actions and desires'. In the light of this statement, one can say that the movement has a top-down approach and that the agenda for the movement is not decided in a democratic way. There is little participation in agenda-setting from members of the disability community, and this has prevented the movement from trickling down to rural areas. The issues addressed pertain to higher education, employment in government and corporate sectors and accessibility in public places. These issues concern largely urban and educated disabled people, whose number is much smaller than that of disabled people in rural India. According to the latest National Sample Survey (NSS) Report(2003), the prevalence of disability in rural in India was 1.85% as against 1.50% in urban India.

TACTICS AND TOOLS

Barnartt and Scotch (2001) have divided the tactics of disability protests into two approaches: traditional, non-contentious tactics and disruptive tactics. Petitioning, lawsuits, lobbying, conferences, letter-writing and signature campaigns constitute non-contentious tactics of advocacy. Protests, sit-ins, marches, takeovers and strikes are described as disruptive tactics of non-violent resistance. In fact, the origin of non-violent disruptive tactics lies in the Gandhian techniques of civil disobedience, which influenced the US civil rights movement in the 1960s. The US disability movement drew inspiration from the tactics of civil rights activists. To some extent, the legacy of the civil rights movement continues to provide a framework for its own political efforts. The disability movement in India is hardly any different since the disability activists use the same tactics used by disability activists in the United States, which seem to inform the movement through a civil rights frame. Scotch and Barnartt (2001, 18) suggest that 'if a culturally appropriate frame does not exist or cannot be created, the social movement is unlikely to succeed in having its demands met. Leaders of social movements are unlikely to invent new frames if they can avoid it'. The tactics used by the disability activists in India suggest that there is no definite frame within which the movement is operating. On the one hand, it uses the civil rights frame, and on the other, the movement employs Gandhian techniques too—both of which provide models for action.

The tactics employed by the disability movement follow a systematic pattern. The movement operates within campaigns which sometimes are launched in response to emergent situations of strategic importance, and at other times are initiated in response to situations which have been strategically created. The Decennial Census of 2001 and elections of 2004 may be considered events of strategic importance. In contrast, the campaign for inclusion of disability in the annual budget was launched around the anniversary of the PWD Act (7 February). Another campaign in which an opportunity was seized upon and an issue essentially created was the access advocacy campaign raised around the visit of Professor Stephen Hawking. Some campaigns require filing of lawsuits while others do not. In almost all the protests, the target of attack is the government. Most of the campaigns start with writing a letter to the authorities concerned. A failure on the part of authorities to respond leads the campaign to its second stage: that of signature campaigns, mobilizing the disability community and media coverage. If this also fails to yield results, then it is followed by intensified protest in the form of *dharna* (sit-ins) and protest marches. The ultimate tactic is resorting to hunger strikes or fast-unto-death protests. The campaigns thus begin with non-contentious tactics and move to increasingly disruptive, yet non-violent, tactics. The purpose of disruptive tactics is 'to elicit support from the public, and that support may affect the outcomes of lawsuits or other type of institutionalized actions that occur at the same time' (Barnartt and Scotch 2001, xxii).

As far as tools are concerned, the PWD Act has been the most convenient tool for disability activists. All contentious issues are taken up as rights issues, the framework for which is provided by law. Just as 'the adoption and implementation of Section 504 contributed to the growth of advocacy organizations representing disabled people and helped to orient them toward civil rights issues' in the United States (Scotch 1984, 150), the PWD Act in India and its implementation have catalysed the self-advocacy movement.

CONCLUSION

> Is there a huge, popular movement across Asia.... No. Frankly, no. There is no popular mass movement concerned with disability.... Is there a strong Asian professional movement for more appropriate services and support to the ordinary, everyday lives of disabled people and carers? No. Frankly, no. In the 1990s, the buzz has been Inclusion, Social Model, Leadership by Disabled People, and elimination (maybe) of polio. None of these offers or ideologies came with even the slightest recognition that South Asia might have some interesting indigenous experiences with which to contribute to its own future.... Very few of their advocates ever stop to enquire whether or how they [western priorities] might fit with the vastly varied and intricate patterns of South Asian rural or urban communities that have been evolving over several millennia. (Miles 2004)

In the above quote, Miles aptly sums up the stage at which the 'disability movement' was in South Asia in the year 2000. He claims that there is no disability movement in South Asia—which includes India as well. He criticizes the Western-centric approach of struggles initiated by the 'disability activists' and their indulgence in using catchphrases such as 'social model', 'leadership by disabled people' and 'inclusion' imposed by funding agencies of the developed countries. On the other hand, disability activists like Javed Abidi observe 'the emergence of several advocacy and self-help groups in different parts of the country [...] as an indicator of the "impending change" [...] led by disabled people themselves' (Abidi 2000). From 2000 to 2004, India witnessed some aggressive disability rights campaigns, which I have analysed in detail. Throughout my chapter, I have not only attempted to contest what Miles suggests (non-existence of a popular disability movement), but I have also critiqued the way movement is progressing. In the period between the promulgation of the PWD Act in 1996 and the year 2000, activists worked towards creating awareness about the law and developing a basic machinery to enforce the act's provisions. Once this was done, the movement started picking up immediately. The opportunities have been seized and created to get disability addressed in the area of policy making.

As we have discussed, the Indian disability movement has had its detractors. Scholars such as Miles dismiss the existence of disability movements in South Asia—including India. Karna (1999, 147) considers the movement 'circumspect' in nature. Ghai (2003, 113) describes the disability movement in India as 'male-centric' and thus patriarchal. Ramanujam (2000, 14) endorses 'positive developments in some metropolitan cities of India, particularly in Delhi; which show the way to bring together the disabled advocacy groups'. He also says that disability does not enjoy 'political clout' because disabled people 'are scattered geographically, socially, educationally and economically' (p. 14). He calls for the development of a mechanism to coordinate and unify disabled people.

There is no doubt that there are shortcomings in the movement. There are several issues and groups that have remained either unaddressed or only partially touched and forgotten. These include people with mental disabilities, learning disabilities, women with disabilities and a vast majority of disabled people in rural areas. Visibility has been attained for the educated, politically aware disabled urban residents with physical and sensory impairments. The movement is also accused of Western-centred approaches to local issues of disabled people and failure to attend to the development of new leadership to carry the movement forward. By participating in the general elections, the DRG attempted to 'engage with the wider, conventional political system' (Lee 2002, 144). However, putting a single independent candidate forward to contest without forging coalitions was clearly not a strategically successful move. The candidate was forced to depend solely on the support of the disability community and its sympathizers. This made disability appear to be an isolated category.

Many times, the fault does not lie solely with the people or organizations that are 'supposedly' leading the movement. There are many other reasons which are out of the purview of activists. Charlton (1998, 79–80) beautifully sums up the reasons in the following words:

> First, self-identification with disability is difficult because there is no history of disability—it has not been written and it is not known—nor is it acknowledged. Second, one cannot 'imagine' something that does not exist—a disabled community. Our community is isolated, scattered, and without a positive signification (who would want to self-identify as a cripple, an invalid?). Third, there has never been a disability culture passed down in families or by other means through stories, customs, and language. Fourth, people with disabilities have not had a 'web of affiliations' to relate to and get support from. Finally, it needs to be emphasized that as an amalgam of similar and divergent characteristics, people with disabilities have multiple, partially overlapping and semi contradictory identities.

To address the issues of disability history, identity, culture, community and the creation of a mass movement, the movement in India needs to learn from, adapt to, engage and forge alliances with other movements in which 'identities may be supplanted by issues, as substantive campaigns around housing, health, welfare, education, employment, immigration, reproduction and media representations combat the multidimensional oppression matrix' (Humphrey, quoted in Lee 2002, 158). As Miles argues, the movement will transform into a burgeoning one if, instead of working in isolation, it tries to 'find a place somewhere amidst the throng of Women, Dalits, Religious Minorities, Greens, regional language advocates, environmental protesters, etc.' (Miles 2000). I agree with Miles that unless it does that, it may not go very far. Finally, like other minority identity movements—the women's movement, gay, lesbian, bisexual, transgendered movements and civil rights struggles—which have responded intellectually to their efforts and consolidated their position through tackling and infiltrating mainstream academia, the disability movement in India will also have to secure a strong position and consolidate it further.

REFERENCES

Abidi, Javed. 2000, March. 'India: Home to 70 Million Disabled Persons.' *RANAP Newsletter*, 1–2.

Barnartt, Sharon, and Richard Scotch. 2001. *Disability Protests: Contentious Politics 1970–1999*. Washington, DC: Gallaudet University Press.

Bornstein, David. 2004. *How to Change the World: Social Entrepreneurs and the Power of New Ideas*. Oxford: Oxford University Press.

Charlton, James I. 1998. *Nothing About Us Without Us: Disability, Oppression and Empowerment*. Berkeley, CA: University of California Press.

EQUITY Commemorative Issue 3.4. 2001, December. (Unpublished). National Centre for Promotion of Employment for Disabled People, New Delhi.

Iyer, V. R. Krishna. 1978. *V.R. Krishan Menon Law Lectures: Social Justice and the Handicapped Humans*. Trivandrum: The Academy of Legal Publications.

Karna, G. N. 1999. *United Nations and Rights of Disabled Persons: A Study in Indian Perspective*. New Delhi: A.P.H. Publishing Corporation.

Lee, Phil. 2002. 'Shooting for the Moon: Politics and Disability at the Beginning of the Twenty-First Century.' In *Disability Studies Today*, edited by Colin Barnes, Mike Oliver and Len Barton. Cambridge, MA: Polity Press.

McAdam, Doug, John D. McCarthy, and Mayer N. Zald. 1996. *Comparative Perspectives on Social Movements: Political Opportunities, Mobilizing Structures, and Cultural Framings*. Cambridge, NY: Cambridge University Press.

Miles, M. 2004, June 11. 'Disability in South Asia: From Millennium to Millennium.' *Asia Pacific Disability Rehabilitation Journal* 11(1). Available at: http://www.dinf.ne.jp/doc/english/asia/resource/apdrj/z13jo0500/z13jo0504.html (accessed April 25, 2018).

Miles, M., and Farhad Hossain. 1999. 'Rights and Disabilities in Educational Provision in Pakistan and Bangladesh.' In *Disability, Human Rights and Education: Cross-cultural Perspectives*, edited by Felicity Armstrong and Len Barton. Buckingham and Philadelphia, PA: Open University Press.

Ministry of Law, Justice and Company Affairs. 1996. *Persons with Disabilities (Equal Opportunities, Protection of Rights and Full Participation) Act, 1995*. New Delhi: Universal Publishing Company.

NSSO. 2003, December. *Disabled Persons in India: National Sample Survey 58th Round Report* No. 485 (58/26/1). New Delhi: NSSO.

Ramanujam, P. R. 2000. 'Social Policies on Disability in India: Some Reflections.' *International Journal of Disability Studies* 1 (October–December): 3–15.

Scotch, Richard. 1984. *From Good Will to Civil Rights: Transforming Federal Disability Policy*. Philadelphia, PA: Temple University Press.

Other Online Sources

IndiaSocial.Org. 2004, March 13. 'India's 40-Million-Odd Disabled Face Disenfranchisement.' Available at: http://www.indiasocial.org/cgi/news.asp?id=3096&sel=1 (accessed on April 25, 2018).

Tribune News Service. 2002, May 7. '200 Disabled Activists Court Arrest.' Available at: http://www.tribuneindia.com/2002/20020507/ncr1.htm#14 (accessed April 25, 2018).

Ministry of Social Justice and Empowerment. 2004, June 10. 'Scheme of National Scholarship for Persons with Disabilities.' *socialjustice.nic.in* Available at: http://socialjustice.nic.in/disabled/scholar.htm#sch5 (accessed April 25, 2018).

engineerstudies.com. 2004, June 12. 'Schemes for Disadvantaged Sections.' Available at: http://www.engineerstudies.com/info/UGC.htm (accessed April 25, 2018).

AsiaNews.It. 2004, May 5. 'The Political Fight for India's Disabled Voters: Enabling the Disabled.' Available at: http://www.asianews.it/view.php?l=en&art=733 (accessed April 25, 2018).

Planning Commission, Government of India. 2002–2007. *Social Development Chapter 5 Tenth Five Year Plan.* Available at: http://planningcommission.nic.in/plans/planrel/fiveyr/10th/volume2/v2_ch5_3.pdf p.495 (accessed April 25, 2018).

ncpedp.org. 2004, May 16. 'National Centre for Promotion of Employment for Disabled People.' Available at: http://www.ncpedp.org (accessed April 25, 2018).

wsfindia.org. 2004, June 16. 'The World Social Forum.' Available at: http://www.wsfindia.org/whoweare.php (accessed April 25, 2018).

Chapter 3

Refocusing and the Paradigm Shift
From Disability to Studies in Ableism[1]

Fiona Kumari Campbell

Feminist Rosemary Tong (1999) long ago alluded to the profound possibilities of using a critical disability studies theory to recomprehend and respatialize the landscape of thinking about race and gender as sites of signification. This chapter presents a conversation in the emergent field of Studies in Ableism (SiA) and desires to not only problematize but also refuse the notion of able(ness). Our attention is on ableism's production and performance. Such an exploratory work is indebted to conversations already commenced by Campbell (1999, 2001, 2005, 2008a, 2009, 2011, 2013, 2014, 2015a, 2015b, 2017b), Hughes (2008) and Overboe (1999, 2007).

My approach is three-pronged. First, I explore the problem of speaking/thinking/feeling—about the Other (in this case, persons referred to as 'disabled people') and the 'extraordinary' Other, the 'Abled'. This conversation is captured under the banner of 'The Ableist

---

[1] This revised chapter is a composite of F. K. Campbell (2008b, 2017a), and as such some citations have not been updated or added. For access to my papers, visit https://dundee.academia.edu/FionaKumariCampbell, accessed 1 May 2018.

Project'. Here, I argue that it is necessary to shift the gaze of contemporary scholarship away from the spotlight on disability to a more nuanced exploration of epistemologies and ontologies of ableism. As part of this project of exposure, my second task then will be to tease out the strands of what can be called 'Ableist Relations', including the effects of the compulsion to emulate ableist regulatory norms. Finally, as part of a commitment to make the necessary connections between theory and practice, I look at the tasks ahead in the refusal of ability and the commitment to a disability/not-abled imaginary.

SHIFTING THE GAZE: 'THE ABLEIST PROJECT'

Typically, the literature within disability and cultural studies has concentrated on the practices and production of disableism, specifically by examining those attitudes and barriers that contribute to the subordination of PWD in liberal society. 'Disableism' is a set of assumptions (conscious or unconscious) and practices that promote the differential or unequal treatment of people because of actual or presumed disabilities. On this basis, the strategic positions adopted to facilitate emancipatory social change, whilst diverse essentially relates to reforming those negative attitudes, assimilating people with disabilities into normative civil society and providing compensatory initiatives and safety nets in cases of enduring vulnerability. In other words, the site of reformation has been at the intermediate level of function, structure and institution in civil society and shifting values in the cultural arena. Such an emphasis produces scholarship that contains serious distortions, gaps and omissions regarding the production of disability and reinscribes an able-bodied voice/lens towards disability. Disability, often quite unconsciously, continues to be examined and taught from the perspective of the Other. The challenge then is to reverse, to invert this traditional approach, to shift our gaze and concentrate on what the study of disability tells us about the production, operation and maintenance of ableism.

The earlier work of Tom Shakespeare concludes, '… perhaps the maintenance of a non-disabled identity… is a more useful problem with which to be concerned; rather than interrogating the Other, let us de-construct the normality-which-is-to-be-assumed' (1996, 28). Bill Hughes captures this project forcefully by calling for a study of the 'pathologies of non-disablement' (2007, 683). Lest we believe that people who fail to meet the ableist imaginary might think otherwise about human ontology and corporealities, Overboe (1999, 2007) and Campbell (2008a, 2009) point to the compulsion to emulate the norm through the internalization of ableism. Ableist normativity results in compulsive passing, wherein there is a failure to ask about difference, to imagine human beingness differently. 'An abled imaginary' relies upon the existence of an unacknowledged imagined shared community of able-bodied/minded people, held together by a common ableist homosocial world view that asserts the 'preferability' of the norms of ableism. Such ableist trajectories erase differences in the ways humans express our emotions, use our thinking and bodies in different cultures and in different situations. Corporeal Otherness is rendered sometimes as the 'disabled', 'perverted' or 'abnormal body', instead of the more neutral designation 'variable' bodies.

A critical feature of an ableist orientation is a belief that impairment or disability is 'inherently' negative and at its essence is a form of harm in need of amelioration, cure or indeed exculpation. SiA inverts traditional approaches, by shifting the gaze and concentration to what the study of disability tells us about the production, operation and maintenance of ableism inclusive of morphologies of 'difference' in sentient life forms as well as the terms of theoretical engagement from 'Object' relations to 'Process' relations.

What is meant by the concept of ableism? The literature suggests that the term is often used fluidly with 'limited definitional or conceptual specificity' (Clear 1999; Iwasaki and Mactavish 2005). Ableism is deeply seeded at the level of epistemological systems of life, personhood and liveability. Ableism is not just a matter of ignorance or negative attitudes towards disabled people, it is a trajectory of perfection, a deep way of thinking about bodies, wholeness and permeability. Bluntly, ableism functions to 'inaugurat[e] the norm' (Campbell 2009, 5). As such integrating SiA into social research represents a significant challenge to practice as ableism moves beyond the more familiar territory of social inclusion and usual indices of exclusion and the very divisions of life (species/ism). Ability and the corresponding notion of ableism are intertwined. Although ableist relations purport to operate out of a binary modality, this interpenetration is more complex and multifaceted than mere binary relations would imply. 'Compulsory ablebodiedness' (cf., McRuer 2006) is implicated in the very foundations of social theory,[2] religious systems, medicine and law, be it in terms of a jurisprudence of deliberative capacity or in cartographical mappings of human anatomy.

In terms of pedigree, 1981 appears to be ableism's groundhog day, with the signifier first used to delineate negative stereotypes towards disabled people in a themed 'women with disabilities' issue of the journal *Off Our Backs* (volume 11, issue 5) written by disabled women activists in the United States who championed ableism as the source of social exclusion (Aldrich 1981; House 1981). In the following decade, work referring to ableism emerged within the fields of black and feminist studies. From around 1998, the concept of ableism remained underdeveloped within disability studies research. A first definitional attempt by Rauscher and McClintock (1997) postulated ableism as a system of discrimination and exclusion. What was missing were any nuances about processes and predilections of such 'systems'. In 2001, I provided a crude attempt to locate ableism as an epistemology:

> A network of beliefs, processes and practices that produces a particular kind of self and body (the corporeal standard) that is projected as

---

[2] Rising star of critical sociology, the cognitive justice movement, Boaventura De Sousa Santos is a case in point. He, in *Epistemologies of the South: Justice against Epistemicide* (Santos 2014), acquiesces to ableist thinking. Not only does his book display a remarkable absence of women authors and scholars reflecting an 'Asian standpoint', this work is littered with ableist metaphors denigrating 'blindness' and 'disability', in such as phrases as 'disabled global North' (p. 19); or 'mutual blindness- the blindness of practice [and] .. the blindness of theory' (p. 35), to cite a few. Moving beyond the metaphysical to an episteme of a 'characterological' nature; Chapter 5 is titled 'Towards an Epistemology of Blindness' (p. 136) and a later subheading reads as 'From the Epistemology of Blindness to the Epistemology of Seeing' (p. 154) establishing the localization of Santos' thought within the realm of ableism reasoning. A cursory reading of Santos' reference list indicates that he has not engaged with critical disability studies, let alone studies in ableism. This is unacceptable.

the perfect, species typical and therefore essential and fully human. Disability then is cast as a diminished state of being human. (Campbell 2001, 44)

In a similar vein, Chouinard defines ableism as 'ideas, practices, institutions and social relations that presume ablebodiedness, and by so doing, construct persons with disabilities as marginalised... and largely invisible "others"' (1997, 380). In contrast, Amundson and Taira attribute a doctrinal posture to ableism in their suggestion that 'Ableism is a doctrine that falsely treats impairments as inherently and naturally horrible and blames the impairments themselves for the problems experienced by the people who have them' (2005, 54). Whilst there is little argument with this presupposition, what is absent from the definition is any mention of ableism's function in inaugurating the norm. Campbell and Chouinard's approach is less about the coherency and intentionalities of ableism, rather their emphasis is on a conception of ableism as a hub network functioning around shifting interest convergences. Linton (1998, 9) defines ableism as 'includ[ing] the idea that a person's abilities or characteristics are determined by disability or that PWD as a group are inferior to non-disabled people'. There are problems with simply endorsing a schema that posits a particular world view that either favours or disfavours dis/able-bodied people as if each category is discrete, self-evident and fixed. As I will argue later, ableism sets up a binary dynamic which is not simply comparative but rather co-relationally constitutive. Campbell's (2001) initial formulation of ableism not only problematizes the signifier disability but also points to the fact that the essential core of ableism is the formation of a naturalized understanding of being fully human, and this, as Chouinard (1997) notes, is articulated on a basis of an enforced presumption that erases difference. Since the publication of *Contours of Ableism: The Production of Disability and Abledness* (Campbell 2009), there has been a plethora of journal articles, an occasional book and an abundance of blogs that purport to extend and apply various conceptualizations of ableism.

Compulsory ableness and its conviction to and seduction of sameness as the basis to equality claims result in a resistance to consider ontologically peripheral lives as distinct ways of being human least they produce a heightened devaluation. Ontological reframing poses different preoccupations: what does the study of the politics of 'deafness' tell us about what it means to be 'hearing'? Indeed, how is the very conceptualization of 'hearing' framed in the light of discourses of 'deafness'? By decentring abledness, it is possible to 'to look at the world from the inside out)' (Linton 1998, 13) and unveil the 'non-disabled/ableist' stance. In a different context, Haraway (1989, 152) exclaims '… [this] cannot be said quite out loud, or it loses its crucial position as a precondition of vision and becomes the object of scrutiny'. The utility of ableism to interrogate new sites of subordination has occurred in management studies, counselling, law, racism, immigration studies and political theory. In attempting to develop conceptual clarity and work on developing SiA as a research methodology, after much discernment, I 'revised' my definition of ableism as a:

> system of causal relations about the order of life that produces processes and systems of entitlement and exclusion. This causality fosters conditions of microaggression, internalized ableism and, in their jostling, notions of (un)encumbrance. A system of dividing practices, ableism institutes the reification and classification of populations. Ableist systems involve the *differentiation, ranking, negation, notification* and *prioritization* of sentient life. (Campbell 2017b, 287–88)

SiA is at a crossroads, slippery and imprecise delimitations, and deployment of the concept has meant that an analysis of implications of theorization for praxis has become hamstrung and vexed mainly due to a lack of conceptual rigour; hence, there are ensuing difficulties in addressing critical questions of our time.

Whether it be the 'species typical body' (in science), the 'normative citizen' (in political theory) or the 'reasonable man' (in law), all these signifiers point to a fabrication that reaches into the very soul that sweeps us into life and as such is the outcome and instrument of a political constitution: a hostage of the body (Foucault 1977). The creation of such regimes of ontological separation appears disassociated from power. Bodies in this way become elements that may be moved, used, transformed, demarcated, improved and articulated with others. The identities of 'disabled' and 'abled' are performed repeatedly, daily. An ethos of compulsory abled-bodiedness, as McRuer (2006, 93) puts it, 'showcase[d] for able-bodied performance' pursuant to the incessant consuming of objects of health, beauty, strength and capability. In the next section, the dividing practices of ableism are considered in more detail.

'ABLEIST RELATIONS'

Although it is hard to pin systems of ableism down because these systems are a series of permeable practices, it is possible to argue that a characteristic of ableist systems is that they create the illusion or fabricate a world view that is unidirectional, reifying 'cause' and 'effect', where the uncertainties and leakiness of the body disappear within a teleological narrative of 'progress'.

The Divisions

The formation of an ableist epistemology occurs on the basis of relationships shaped by binaries that are mutually constitutive. For example, I propose that it is not possible to have a fully inclusive notion of 'health' without a carefully contained understanding of not-health (we call this disability or sometimes chronic illness and refigure health as harmony). Central to a system of ableism are two elements, namely, the notion of the normative (and normal individual) and the enforcement of a constitutional divide between a so-called perfected or developed humanity (how humans are supposedly meant to be) and the aberrant, the unthinkable, underdeveloped and therefore not really human. Many religious systems posture that the divine or enlightened one is characterized by certain marks of perfection with anomalous bodies being deemed less holy or impure (Appleton 2014; Campbell 2014; Faure 2003; Mrozik 2007; Powers 2009; Sangari and Vaid 1990). The ableist divide can also capture asymmetrical relations based on differences of sex, (not white) race and animality, which in different ways, in epistemology and social practices, has been constituted as sites of aberrancy or disability. This constitution provides the layout, the blueprint for the scaling and marking of bodies and the ordering of their terms of relation. It is not possible to have a concept of 'difference' without ableism. Let us take each of these two elements separately and explore them more closely.

It is necessary to establish and enforce a constitutional divide. The divide is at the levels of ontology, materiality and sentiency. I wish to focus on the constitutionality of that divide between the normal and the pathological and mechanisms of ordering. This analysis is influenced by the proposals advanced by Latour in *We Have Never been Modern* (1993).

Latour speaks of the practices of 'translation' and 'purification':

> '[T]ranslation' creates mixtures between entirely new types of being, hybrids of nature and culture. The second, by 'purification,' creates two entirely distinct ontological zones: that of human beings on the one hand, that of nonhumans on the other. (1993, 10–11)

The devices of translation and purification can assist us to grapple with that which seems 'unholdable' and elusive, the uncontainability of the disabled body. 'Translation' is based on the notion that structures or networks are not obvious or self-contained. Latour uses the example of a chain flowing from the upper atmosphere, industrial strategies and onto the concerns of government and greenies. Constitutions are concerned with jurisdiction and boundaries between persons, things and actions (typical of Roman civil law) and the ways in which each of these elements assembles and interpenetrates (Mussawir 2011). As such, constitutionality is linked to cosmography and order the terms of relations. Constitutions (rule matrices) establish the terrain, the ground rules for governance, processes for clearance and right relation (*samma ditthi* [Pali] literally 'view'), and how things are or how they are meant to be. Whilst constitutionality and codification are the default inferences of jurisdiction, an alternative rendering is to conceive of jurisdiction and constitutional divides as a 'relation that is immanent, practical and "lived"' and hence shifting (Mussawir 2011, 6).

Divisions of constitutionality require people to identify with a category—'Are you disabled or not?' 'Oh, no I am not disabled, I am ill or depressed!' or 'I am able-bodied'. For the ease of conversation, we often feel the need to minimize any confusion. The carrying of an 'Enumerative' or 'Diagnostic Passport' is a blatant propaganda that supports the argument developed by Philosopher Latour (1993, 10–11), who states '… these two independent practices of normalising and pathologising]… must remain distinct in order for them to work/

function'. If the definitions of abled-bodied and disabled become unclear or slippery, the business of legal and governmental administration would have problems in functioning. Alarm would arise due to uncertainty as to how to classify certain people and in which category.

'Purification', in contrast, engages in the creation of divides of ontological distinctions, which espouse a foundational (almost first cause) self-evidence. Here, Latour (1993) cites the partition between nature (as self-contained), non-humans and culture (created and driven by humans). This 'modern critical stance', as Latour calls it, acts as the ethos or template of modernity. Social differentiation produces difference: the abled and disabled, which in turn are products of our ways of looking and sensing, that is, it is not merely comparative 'but rather co-relationally constitutive' (Campbell 2009, 6). People are made different by a process of being seen and treated as disabled, as outlawed disability or abled (Lawson 2008, 517). Western political theory attests to constitutionality divides. As Campbell (2013) notes:

> The political concept of people enshrined in the documents of the French Revolution and subsequent human rights instruments foreground two different conceptions—people as a whole, the social body cast against multiple excluded bodies (the aberrant) or in the alternative, an inclusive whole without outsiders.

Already embedded within these divisions are 'fundamental bio-political fracture[s] [In other words]... what cannot be included in the whole of which it is a part as well as what cannot belong to the whole in which it is always already included' (Agamben 2000).

In the context of ableism, Latour's schema proves helpful. The processes and practices of translation cannot be separated from the creation of that ordering category termed 'disability'. For many people deemed disabled, in the world of technoscience, their relationship with non-human actants has been profoundly cyborgical and hybridizable (e.g., the use of communication and adaptive devices, implants and transplants). As such, the networks of association between human and non-human (sentient beings and machines) have always been and are increasingly pushing the boundaries of the practices of purification. The disabled body induces a fear as being a body out of control because of its appearance of uncontainability. The practices of purification insist on this being the case. Ableism's constitutional divide posits two distinct and entirely clear ontological zones: disabled and abled (normate). Latour (1993, 11) explains:

> [W]ithout the first set, the practices of purification would be fruitless or pointless. Without the second, the work of translation would be slowed down, limited, or even ruled out.... So long as we consider these two practices of translation and purification separately, we are truly modern—that is we willingly subscribe to the critical project, even though that project is developed only through the proliferation of hybrids down below. As soon as we direct our attention simultaneously to the work of purification and the work of hybridization [translation], we immediately stop being wholly modern, and our future begins to change.

The challenge then is to look 'beyond' social context, at the interactivity between the processes and techniques of purification and translation, in particular to investigate what this interactivity clarifies and obfuscates. Even though Latour claims that purification is not an ideology in disguise, I would assert that the existence of processes of purification creates a simulation, if you like, of the conditions of naturalism. Latour's discussion of whether relations are conscious and unconscious or are illusion and reality is an important one. He concludes that moderns are not unaware of what they do; rather it is the holding steadfast to dichotomies, the divides, that makes possible the processes of translation. We can, by analogy, argue that matters of intentionality or discourse and so forth are not critical to the emerging technologies of ableism, but rather it is the act of holding stoically to the distinction between ableness and disabledness.

In contemporary developments in high-tech and biotechnologies, it is occasionally possible to witness the glitches from the purview of purification, whether that is in the debates over transhumanism, xenotransplantation or the emergence of new 'life' in the form of artificial intelligences (AI's, robotics, cloning). The confusion about where human life begins and ends harks back to the Enlightenment era, where philosophers such as Locke inquired 'What is It?' in trying to make sense of the humanness of changelings (Campbell 1999; Locke [1689]1979). In addition, these questions also problematize the dominant Western notion of an atomistic stable Self, a perspective long challenged within Buddhism and other South Asian philosophical systems (cf., Duerlinger 2005). The fortunes of technoscience continue to disrupt the fixity of defining disability and normalcy, especially within the arenas of law and bioethics. Whilst anomalous bodies are 'undecidable' in being open to endless and differing interpretations, an essentialized disabled body is subjected to constant deferral—standing in reserve, awaiting and escaping able(edness) through morphing technologies and as such exists in an ontologically 'tentative' or 'provisional' state.

Latour points out the ultimate paradox of this modern constitutional divide is that whilst the proliferation of hybrids is allowed for, at the same time, this constitution continues to deny the very existence of hybrid entities within its formulation (Latour 1993). Contemporary conditions suggest that it is not the event of denial that is operational; rather it is the 'place' or significance given to such ambiguous entities that disrupts the rather neat demarcation zones. Practices of purification continue to rein in (successfully or otherwise) the chaos created by increasing 'grey zones' along the continuum of human/non-human difference. In the governing of prostitution, Razack (1998) points to the creation of 'anomalous zone' to contain and tolerate the deviance. In dealing with political prisoners, the despised, those interned in concentration camps and institutions, Agamben (1998, 2005) indicates the manufacturing of states of exception that exist beyond the law and spatiality to enable 'treatments' of those existing in the realm a 'bare life'. The significance of the enforcement of a constitutional divide, for the practices of ableism, is that such orderings are not just repressive, but they are ultimately productive; they tell us stories, they contain narratives as to 'who' we are and how we 'should be'.

In the closing pages of *We Have Never Been Modern*, Latour (1993) argues that as science creates new definitions of being human, these new formations do not displace the older versions, rather humanism is redistributed. I am not entirely convinced of this emergent multiplicity and expansion of ontologies of humanness. Contradicting Latour, Hayles

(1999) argues that should sentiency be conceptualized on the basis of informationalcy, this new rendering would amount to a profound shift in the theoretical markers used to categorize all life (or what is 'life'). In this moment, there is a rallying of networks scurrying to squeeze new ontological formations of dis/ability into 'old' systems of ordering and thus attempt to avoid recognizing an abundance of (postmarginal, postperipheral) morphisms. Anthropomorphism becomes the catch cry of ableism. As Latour (1993, 137) rejoices:

> Morphism is the place where technomorphisms, zoomorphisms, phusimorphisms, ideomorphisms, theomorphisms, sociomorphisms, psyomorphisms, all come together. These alliances and their exchanges, taken together, are what define the anthropos. A weaver of morphisms—isn't that enough of a definition?

What Normate... Ableist Normativity?

Canguilhem (1978, 69) states 'every generality is the sign of an essence, and every perfection the realization of the essence... a common characteristic, the value of an ideal type'. If this is the case, what then is the essence of normative abled(ness)? Such a question poses significant conceptual challenges, including the dangers of bifurcation. It is reasonably easy to speculate about the knowingness of life forms deemed disabled in spite of the neologism disability's catachresis orientation. In contrast, able-bodied, corporeal perfectedness has an elusive core (other than being posed as transparently average or normal). Charting a criterion of abled to gain definitional clarity can result in a game of circular reductionism—saying what it 'is' in relation to what it 'isn't' that which falls away. Disability performances are invoked to mean 'anybody capable of being narrated as outside the norm' (Mitchell 2002, 17). Such an analysis belies the issue whether at their core, women's, black and queer bodies are ultimately ontologically and materially disabled?

Inscribing certain bodies in terms of deficiency and essential inadequacy privileges a particular understanding of normalcy that is commensurate with the interests of dominant groups (and the assumed interests of subordinated groups). Indeed, the formation of ableist relations requires the normate individual to depend upon the self of 'disabled' bodies being rendered beyond the realm of civility, thus becoming an unthinkable object of apprehension. The unruly, uncivil, disabled body is necessary for the reiteration of the 'truth' of the 'real/ essential' human self who is endowed with masculinist attributes of certainty, mastery and autonomy.

The discursive practices that mark out bodies of preferability are vindicated by abject life forms that populate the constitutive outside of the thinkable (that which can be imagined and re-presented) and those forms of existence that are unimaginable and therefore unspeakable. The emptying (*kenosis*) of normalcy occurs through the purging of those beings that confuse, are misrecognizable or, as Mitchell (2002, 17) describes, are 'recalcitrant corporeal matter' into a 'bare life' (see Agamben 1998) residing in a zone of exceptionality. This foreclosure depends on necessary unspeakability to maintain the continued operation of hegemonic power (cf. Butler 1997). For every outside there is an inside that demands differentiation and consolidation as a unity. To borrow from Heidegger ([1953]1977), in every *aletheia* (unveiling or revealedness) of representation, there lies a concealedness. The visibility of the ableist project is therefore possible only through the interrogation of the revealedness of disability/not-health and abled(ness). Detienne summarizes this system of thought aptly:

> [Such a]... system is founded on a series of acts of partition whose ambiguity, here as elsewhere, is to open up the terrain of their transgression at the very moment when they mark off a limit. To discover the complete horizon of a society's symbolic values, it is also necessary to map out its transgressions, its deviants. (1979, ix)

Viewing the disabled body as simply 'matter out of place' that needs to be dispensed with or at least cleaned up is erroneous. The disabled body 'has' a place, a place in liminality to secure the performative enactment of the normal. Detienne's summation points to what we may call the double bind of ableism when performed within Western neoliberal polities. The double bind folds in on itself—for whilst claiming 'inclusion', ableism simultaneously always restates and enshrines itself. On the one hand, discourses of equality promote 'inclusion' by way of promoting positive attitudes (sometimes legislated in mission statements, marketing campaigns and equal opportunity protections), and yet, on the other hand, ableist discourses proclaim quite emphatically that disability is inherently negative, ontologically intolerable and, in the end, a dispensable remnant (Campbell 2017b). This casting results in an ontological foreclosure wherein positive signification of disability becomes unspeakable. Disability cannot be thought of/spoken about on any other basis than the negative, and to do so, to invoke oppositional discourses, is to run the risk of further pathologization. An example of this is an attempt at desiring or celebrating disability which is reduced to a fetish or facticity disorder. Therefore, to explicate ourselves out of this double bind, we need to persistently and continually return to the matter of disability as negative ontology, as a malignancy, that is, as the property of a body constituted by what Oliver (1996, 32) refers to as 'the personal tragedy theory of disability'.

We now return to the matter of definitional clarity around abled(ness). McRuer (2002, 2006) is one of the few scholars to journey into ableism's non-axiomatic life. He argues that ableism (McRuer refers to compulsory abled-bodiedness) emanates from everywhere and nowhere and can only be deduced by crafty reductionisms. In contrast to the assertions about the uncontainability of disabled bodies which are (re)contained by the hyper-prescription and enumeration, the abled body mediated through its assumption of compulsion is absent in its presence—it just is—but resists being fully deducible. Drawing on Butler's work, McRuer writes:

> [E]veryone is virtually disabled, both in the sense that able-bodied norms are 'intrinsically impossible to embody' fully and in the sense that able-bodied status is always temporary, disability being the one identity category that all people will embody if they live long enough. What we might call a critically disability position, however, would differ from such a virtually disabled positions [to engagements that have] resisted the demands of compulsory able-bodiedness…. (2006, 95–96)

My argument is that insofar as this conception of disability is assumed within discourses of ableism, the presence of disability upsets the modernist craving for ontological security. The conundrum disability is neither a mere fear of the unknown nor an apprehensiveness towards that which is foreign or strange. Rather, disability and disabled bodies are effectively positioned in the nether regions of 'unthought'. For the ongoing stability of ableism, a diffuse network of thought depends upon the capacity of that network to 'shut away', to exteriorize and to unthink disability and its resemblance to the essential (ableist) human self. This unthought has been given much consideration through the systematization and classification of knowledge about pathology, aberration and deviance. That which is thought about (the 'abled' norm) rather ironically in its delimitation becomes vacuous and elusive. In order for the notion of ableness to exist and to transmogrify into the sovereign subject, the normate individual of liberalism, it must have a constitutive outside—that is, it must participate in a logic of supplementarity. When looking at relations of disability and ableism, we can expand on this idea of symbiosis, an 'unavoidable duality' by putting forward another metaphor, that of the mirror. Here, I argue that people deemed disabled take on the performative act of mirroring in the lives of normative subjects:

> To be a Mirror is different from being a Face that looks back... with a range of expression and responsiveness that are responses of a Subject-in-Its-Own-Right. To be positioned as a Mirror is to be Put Out of Countenance, to Lose Face. (Narayan 1997, 141)

In this respect, we can speak in ontological terms of the history of disability as a history of that which is unthought, to be put out of countenance; this figuring should not be confused with erasure that occurs due to mere absence or exclusion. On the contrary, disability is always present (despite its seeming absence) in the ableist talk of normalcy, normalization and humanness (Overboe 2007 on the idea of 'normative shadows'). Disability's truth-claims are dependent upon discourses of ableism for their very legitimization.

DISABILITY IMAGINARIES: RECONCEPTUALIZING THE HUMAN?

Phenomenological studies have long recognized the importance of focusing on the 'experience' of the 'animated living body' (*der Leib*), in recognition that we dwell in our bodies and live so fundamentally 'through' them. This intensity is captured by Kalekin-Fishman as follows:

> Before every action, there is a pause... and a beginning again. The pause is for description, for mulling over the requirements of balance, for comparing the proposed action with movements that are familiar, and for explaining to myself why I can or cannot do what is at hand.... In the course of daily living, the thinking is not observable; the behavior just happens, part of what this person does naturally. The physiology of 'a slight limp' is part of the unmediated expression of what my 'I' is.... (2001, 136)

In short, we cannot 'know' existence without being rooted to our bodies. To this extent, it is problematic to speak of bodies in their materiality in a way that distinguishes between emotions and cognition. This generative body is shaped by relations of power and complex histories and interpreted through a bricolage of complex interwoven subjectivities. This approach to perceiving the body in terms of *geist* or animation can be applied to rethinking peripheral bodies deemed disabled. It is this body that infuses the discourses and animates representations. Refusing able(ness) necessitates a letting go of the strategy of using the sameness for equality arguments as the basis of liberal freedom. Instead of wasting time on the violence of normalization, theoretical and cultural producers could more meaningfully concentrate on developing a semiotics of exchange, an ontological decoder to recover and apprehend the lifeworlds of humans living peripherally. Ontological differences, be that on the basis of problematical signifiers of race, caste, sex, sexuality or dis/ability, need to be unhinged from evaluative ranking and be re-cognized in their various nuances and complexities without being re-presented in fixed absolute terms. It is only then, in this release, that we can find possibilities in ambiguity and resistance in marginality (cf., Hooks 1990).

Instead of asking 'how do you manage not being like (the non-stated) *us*?' (the negation argument), disability imaginaries think/speak/gesture and feel different landscapes not just for being in the world, but also on the conduction of perception, mobilities and temporalities. Linton (1998, 530) points out that the 'kinaesthetic, proprioceptive, sensory and cognitive experiences' of disabled people as they go about their daily lives have received limited attention. Mairs (1996) notes a disability gaze is imbricated in every aspect of action, perception, occurrence and knowing.

In order to return bodies back to difference in the human, a reconceptualization of knowing (episteme) is paramount. Only this knowledge is of a carnal kind, where thinking, sensing and understanding mutually enfold. Whilst ever present in ableist normalizing dialogue, disability's veracity is undeniably contingent upon conversations of ableism, its production and performance, to confer validity.

REFERENCES

Agamben, G. 1998. *Homo Sacer: Sovereign Power and Bare Life*. Standford, CA: Standford University Press.

———. 2000. *Potentialities: Collected Essays in Philosophy*. Vol. 31, No. 2. Stanford, CA: Stanford University Press.

———. 2005. *State of Exception*. Chicago, IL: The University of Chicago.

Aldrich, M. 1981. 'Beginning Bibliography.' *Off Our Backs* 11 (5): 39–39.

Amundson, R., and G. Taira. 2005. 'Our Lives and Ideologies: The Effects of Life Experience on the Perceived Morality of the Policy of Physician-assisted Suicide'. *Journal of Policy Studies* 16 (1): 53–57.

Appleton, N. 2014. *Narrating Karma and Rebirth: Buddhist and Jain Multi-life Narratives*. New York, NY: Cambridge University Press.

Butler, J. 1997. *Excitable Speech: A Politics of the Performative*. New York, NY: Routledge.

Campbell, Fiona Kumari. 1999. '"Refleshingly Disabled": Interrogations into the Corporeality of "Disablised" Bodies.' *Australian Feminist Law Journal* 12 (March): 57–80.

———. 2001. 'Inciting Legal Fictions: Disability's Date with Ontology and the Ableist Body of the Law.' *Griffith Law Review* 10 (1): 42–62.

———. 2005. 'Legislating Disability: Negative Ontologies and the Government of Legal Identities.' In *Foucault and the Government of Disability*, edited by S. Tremain, 108–30. Ann Arbor, MI: The University of Michigan Press.

———. 2008a. 'Exploring Internalised Ableism Using Critical Race Theory.' *Disability and Society* 23 (2): 151–62.

———. 2008b 'Refusing Able(ness): A Preliminary Conversation about Ableism.' *M/C—Media and Culture* 11. Available at: http://journal.media-culture.org.au/index.php/mcjournal/article/view/46 (accessed on 1 May 2018).

———. 2009. *Contours of Ableism: The Production of Disability and Abledness*. Basingstoke: Palgrave Macmillan.

Campbell, Fiona Kumari. 2011. 'Geodisability Knowledge Production and International Norms: A Sri Lankan Case Study.' *Third World Quarterly* 32 (8): 1425–44.

———. 2013, August. 'Re-cognising Disability: Cross-examining Social Inclusion Through the Prism of Queer Anti-sociality.' *Jindal Global Law Review*, Special Double Issue: *Rethinking Queer Sexualities, Law and Cultural Economies of Desire* 4 (2): 209–38.

———. 2014. 'Ableism as Transformative Practice.' In *Rethinking Anti-Discriminatory and Anti-Oppressive Theories for Social Work Practice*, edited by C. Cocker and T. Hafford Letchfield, 78–92. Basingstoke: Palgrave.

———. 2015a. 'Disability, Law and Mobilization in Sri Lanka: Barriers and Possibilities.' In *South Asia and Disability Studies: Redefining Boundaries and Extending Horizons*, edited by S. Rao and M. Kalyanpuram, 73–98. New York, NY: Peter Lang Publishers.

———. 2015b. 'Ability.' In *Keywords for Disability Studies*, edited by R. Adams, B. Reiss and D. Serlin, 46–51. New York, NY: New York University Press.

———. 2017a, June 19. 'Answering Our Detractors—Argument in Support of Studies in Ableism as an Approach to Negotiating Human Differences and Tackling Social Exclusion.' Keynote for Conference on Studies in Ableism (Unpublished), University of Manchester.

———. 2017b. 'Queer Anti-Sociality and Disability Unbecoming: An Ableist Relations Project?' In *New Intimacies/Old Desires: Law, Culture and Queer Politics in Neoliberal Times*, edited by O. Sircar and D. Jain. New Delhi: Zubaan Books.

Canguilhem, G. 1978. *On the Normal and the Pathological*. London: D. Reidel Publishing.

Chouinard, V. 1997. 'Making Space for Disabling Difference: Challenges Ableist Geographies.' *Environment and Planning D: Society and Space* 15 (4), 379–87.

Clear, M. 1999. 'The "Normal" and the Monstrous in Disability Research.' *Disability & Society* 14 (4): 435–48.

Detienne, M. 1979. *Dionysos Slain*. Baltimore, MD: John Hopkins University Press.

Duerlinger, J. 2005. *Indian Buddhist Theories of Persons*. London: Routledge.

Faure, B. 2003. *The Power of Denial: Buddhism, Purity and Gender*. Princeton, NJ: Princeton University Press.

Foucault, M. 1977. *Discipline & Punish: The Birth of the Prison*. New York, NY: Vintage Books.

Haraway, D. 1989. *Primate Visions: Gender, Race, and Nature in the World of Modern Science*. New York, NY: Routledge.

Hayles, K. 1999. *How We Became Posthuman: Virtual Bodies in Cybernetics, Literature, and Informatics*. Chicago, IL: The University of Chicago Press.

Heidegger, M. (1953)1977. 'The Question Concerning Technology.' In *Martin Heidegger Basic Writings*, edited by D. Krell, 284–317. New York, NY: Harper & Row.

Hooks, B. 1990. *Yearning: Race, Gender and Cultural Politics*. Boston, MA: South End Press.

House, S. 1981. 'A Radical Feminist Model of Psychological Disability.' *Off Our Backs* 11 (5): 34–35.
Hughes, B. 2007. 'Being Disabled: Toward a Critical Social Ontology for Disability Studies.' *Disability & Society* 22 (7): 673–84.
Iwasaki, Y., and J. Mactavish. 2005. 'Ubiquitous Yet Unique: Perspectives of People with Disabilities on Stress.' *Rehabilitation Counselling Bulletin* 48 (4): 194–208.
Kalekin-Fishman, D. 2001. 'The Hidden Injuries of a "Slight Limp".' In *Disability and the Life Course: Global Perspectives*, edited by M. Priestley, 136–48. Cambridge: Cambridge University Press.
Latour, B. 1993. *We Have Never Been Modern*. New York, NY: Harvester Wheatsheaf.
Lawson, A. 2008. *Disability and Equality Law in Britain: The Role of Reasonable Adjustment*. Oxford: Hart Publishing.
Linton, S. 1998. *Claiming Disability: Knowledge and Identity*. New York, NY: New York University Press.
Locke, J. (1689) 1979. *An Essay Concerning Human Understanding*. Oxford: Clarendon Press.
Mairs, N. 1996. *Waist-High in the World: A Life Among the Nondisabled*. Boston, MA: Beacon Press.
McRuer, R. 2002. 'Compulsory Able-Bodiedness and Queer/Disabled Existence.' In *Disability Studies: Enabling the Humanities*, edited by S. Snyder, B. J. Brueggemann and R. Garland-Thomson, 88–90. New York, NY: Modern Language Association.
———. 2006. *Crip Theory: Cultural Signs of Queerness and Disability*. New York, NY: New York University Press.
Mitchell, D. 2002. 'Narrative Prosthesis and the Materiality of Metaphor.' In S. Snyder, B. J. Brueggemann and R. Garland-Thomson, 15–30. *Disability Studies: Enabling the Humanities*. New York: Modern Language Association.
Mrozik, S. 2007. *Virtuous Bodies: The Physical Dimensions of Morality in Buddhist Ethics*. Oxford: Oxford University Press.
Mussawir, E. 2011. *Jurisdiction in Deleuze: The Expression and Representation of Law*. Abingdon: Routledge-Cavendish.
Narayan, U. 1997. *Dislocating Cultures: Identities, Traditions and Third World Feminism*. New York, NY: Routledge.
Oliver, M. 1996. *Understanding Disability: From Theory to Practice*. Basingstoke: Macmillan.
———. 1999. 'Difference in Itself: Validating Disabled People's Lived Experience.' *Body and Society* 5 (4): 17–29.
Overboe, J. 2007. 'Vitalism: Subjectivity Exceeding Racism, Sexism and (Psychiatric) Ableism.' *Wag.a.du: A Journal of Trasnational Women's & Gender Studies* 4 (Summer): 23–34.
Powers, J. 2009. *A Bull of a Man: Images of Masculinity, Sex, and the Body in Indian Buddhism*. Cambridge: Harvard University Press.

Rauscher, L., and McClintock, N. 1997. 'Ableism Curriculum Design.' In *Teaching for Diversity and Social Justice: A Sourcebook*, edited by M. Adams, L. A. Bell and P. Griffin, 198–229. New York, NY: Routledge.

Razack, S. 1998. 'Race, Space and Prostitution: The Making of the Bourgeois Subject.' *Canadian Journal of Women & Law* 10 (2): 338–76.

Sangari, K., and S. Vaid. 1990. *Recasting Women: Essays in Indian Colonial History*. New Brunswick, NJ: Rutgers University Press.

Santos, B. 2014. *Epistemologies of the South: Justice against Epistemicide*. Abingdon: Routledge.

Shakespeare, T. 1996. 'Disability, Identity and Difference.' In *Exploring the Divide*, edited by C. Barnes and G. Mercer, 94–113. Leeds: The Disability Press.

Tong, R. 1999. 'Dealing with Difference Justly: Perspectives on Disability.' *Social Theory and Practice* 25 (3): 519–530.

Chapter 4

Disability within Rawlsian Framework of Justice
Challenging the Injustice Rationale

Deepa Palaniappan and Valerian Rodrigues

POLITICAL THEORY AND THE 'DISABLED SUBJECT'

Contemporary critical political theorizing in India is heavily influenced by both Dalit and feminist methodological frameworks of exclusion, discrimination and social justice. To analyse and research disability within the public policy framework in India is by default assumed to be a study of discriminatory and exclusionary practices and injustices faced by people with disabilities. While an emancipatory research paradigm espoused by disability researchers does call for such a politically empowering perspective for analysis and research, there are undoubtedly some dangers to the discrimination–exclusion reading of disability, including (but not limited to) the fact that non-disability is taken for granted as a fixed, constant self for the disabled 'other'. Political theorizing on disability should focus on the conceptual roots that contribute to visualizing people with impairments as pitiable caricatures of undesirable, unhealthy bodies.

The analytical tools that political theory yields for disability research contribute in further constituting the disabled individual as a suffering, excluded, victimized 'other'. Disciplinary understanding of what we can research on disability is already shaped by what we assume to be the 'problems faced' by disabled people. In such a scenario, the worst affected and most neglected within political theory, is disability research because Dalit and feminist studies have completed their trial runs with their respective methodological frameworks, whereas disability research in India still has no critical methodological framework to call its own, much less a framework specific to Indian political theory since disability researchers continue to rely upon both feminist and Dalit perspectives as tools of analysis. Even at a seemingly early stage of research development, disability research in India has rejected empirical research based on a positivist framework. For instance, Ghai (2002) had not only followed critical feminist framework but also had the courage to talk back to the mainstream feminists, educating them of their own ableist assumptions about gender-related discrimination. Addlakha (2013) had critically analysed sociological assumptions about mental illness and psychiatric disabilities. Anand (2016) has subjected to scrutiny the existing model-based definitional approach of disability studies, especially from a South Asian perspective. Ghosh (2012, 2016) has opened up discussion on sociopolitical nuances of interrogating disability from an Indian perspective. Jagdish Chander (2011) and Shilpaa Anand (2009) have critically reviewed the historiography of Indian disability studies. Nilika Mehrotra (2012) has sought to methodologically revamp disability studies from India. Michele Friedner (2015) has critically analysed the experiences of deaf people under changing socio-economic conditions of contemporary India. We have attempted here to take forward the task set by Indian disability studies' scholars in creating unique methodological frameworks for disability research from an Indian perspective. This chapter is an attempt to build a dialogue between political theory and the key critical conceptual developments arising from an Indian disability movement's perspective. There is a huge disconnect between the everyday realities dealt by disability movement practitioners in India and the theoretical tools of analysis available for creating a disability critique from an Indian public policy perspective.

THE INJUSTICE IN JUSTICE THEORIES: FRAMING AN ENTRY POINT FOR DISABILITY PERSPECTIVE

How disability is defined and perceived within a justice paradigm is more important than to judge whether the justice theories meet the demands of disabled by offering the correct 'solutions'. It is important to understand how justice theories perceive and evaluate disability, and to explore whether their 'just' societies would also be inclusive societies. We find that in contemporary societies, the contention of the disability movement is still against the disabling attitudes and perceptions that invariably result in evoking feelings of shock, pity, guilt and patronizing charity. Disabled people the world over have to face these, and no amount of improved policies could aid in solving these dilemmas unless our critical, reflective tools of analysis begin to strongly question the internalized categories and binaries that are eventually normalized. It is generally deemed as a 'humane obligation' and 'morally binding' for our social institutions to take into consideration the 'plight' of disabled people in our society. All the policies and interventions therefore emerge from such an obligation. They are clearly 'from' the non-disabled 'to' the disabled. Impairments are common in human lives, and everyone sooner or later falls into the category one way or other. Impairment in itself could be understood as a fact of life for not a few disabled, but all people in this world. Yet, we should be careful not to reduce the lived experiences of people with disabilities by carelessly universalizing the impairment/disability experience by opening it up as 'everyone's experience'. It is important to retain the marginalized identity and political strength of the disabled as political subject.

The policy initiatives revolve around the perception that disability is pitiable and abnormal; hence, the solution is found in piecemeal gestures (such as travel concession, bus pass and 'correction'-oriented interventions aimed at 'normalizing' the ab-normal bodies).

Where disability is seen as an 'individual problem', the injustice too is seen from a medical/individual perspective (the 'karma' of the individual) as if nothing else could be done about it. In the second case, if lack of resources owing to these impairments is deemed as the injustice, it could be compensated by reallocation of the resources, whereas in the third and more complicated injustice that pertains to prejudice and attitudinal barriers, a mere reallocation of resources is clearly of no help. In the case of marriage allowance, the state providing ₹0.1 million to ₹0.3 million for those 'willing' to marry a person with disability is in no way a linear solution to the issue of marriage hurdle faced by persons with disabilities in India. Neither a general appeal to a sense of justice on society's part nor a consideration of justice to be primary virtue of social institutions would be of help to the disabled, if the injustice that surrounds them is more to do with the attitudes, perceptions and the categorization that evolve out of these. Hence, as to the question of injustice, there is a need to juxtapose the disability movement with the justice theories to assess if both see eye to eye as to what constitutes 'injustice' for a person who is disabled. Only then the solutions offered could convince the disability movement practitioners.

It is vital to locate and critically analyse moral values that dictate society's sense of justice. What is it in a sense of justice, that makes us so proud and patronizing on having been just, fair and fulfilled the moral obligations? And how we can locate critical disability rights perspective from within this prism of Justice and Moral Obligation?

The focus here is not to juxtapose the theories of justice vis-à-vis the demands of disability movement to see whether they are compatible—on the grounds of understanding disability. This is an attempt to seek how disability is understood and defined within these moral, justice theories. And extend the argument further to pose the question, what is it deemed to be 'unjust' within a disability scenario? What is the 'injustice' that surrounds disability—is it the mere inability to walk, talk or see; is it the lack of resources on account of these impairments; or is it the aesthetic conclusions that are drawn upon these impairments together with the disabling social prejudices that operate on those conclusions? In the first case, it is clearly a medical/individual approach to injustice (the 'karma' of the individual) as if nothing else could be done about it. In the second case, if lack of resources owing to these impairments is deemed as the injustice, it could be compensated by reallocation of the resources whereas in the third and more complicated injustice, clearly a mere reallocation of resources is of no help. Neither a general appeal to a sense of justice on society's part nor a consideration of justice to be the primary virtue of social institutions, would be of any help to the disabled, if the injustice that surrounds them are more to do with the attitudes, perceptions and the categorization that evolve out of these. Hence, as to the question of injustice, there is an urgent need to juxtapose the disability movement with the justice theories to assess if both see eye to eye as to what constitutes 'injustice' for a person who is disabled. Only then the solutions offered could convince the disability movement and the scholars who have criticized these theories. Here we are restricting our focus to Rawlsian approach to Justice and reclaiming the approach for critical disability rights perspective.

In studying state policies towards the disabled, to merely blame bad policies and lack of implementation should not be the only public policy route to build a disability critique. To hold the state as solely responsible for the existing conditions of the disabled people is to be as apathetic as the state itself, by not searching for more explanations on why the situation is what it is today. Disability movement in India is now abounding with fresh questions on the attitudes and cultural imagery (both visible/invisible) that re-establishes and strengthens disabling binaries. The focus is to unravel those attitudes and prejudices that are inherent (and mostly invisible) behind the policy scenario. How disability is viewed, defined and sought to be evaluated means a lot for building inclusive policies, more than an abrupt change in the built scenario, educational and employment opportunities could possibly achieve.

TOWARDS A CRITICAL METHODOLOGY FOR DISABILITY IN INDIAN POLITICAL THEORIZING

There are many reasons for which the critical disability framework ought to be unique for India. For instance, the question of category and identity is not so clearly defined in the disability context. There are invisible disabilities, spectrum disorders, those who do not like to be identified or referred as 'disabled' and those who consider disability as a political identity. There are also parents of children with psychosocial disabilities and CODA (children of deaf adults) who take part in the disability movement. Furthermore, the identity issue gets further muddled by a legal framework where those who possess 40% and above are considered as 'disabled persons' by law. This makes those self-identifying as disabled outside the scope of disability policy but still within the framework of the disability rights movement. Who ought to be counted as a disabled person is a question that befuddles not only census and policy makers but also active participants of the disability movement as well as researchers. Issues pertaining to a disability certificate that essentially legally defines a person with disability, and the challenges and issues in accessing this certificate, the social welfare model of pension allocation for poor disabled and the importance of percentage in the Indian disability certificate are hardly common knowledge, even among public policy experts studying social exclusion in general. The injustices surrounding disability are always taken for granted to be arising from the impairment itself but not from the political and social spheres that operate upon those impairments. Disability scholars have long been discussing about medical and social models of disability which highlight the difference between understanding disability from a personal tragedy/individual perspective and socially created barriers that create disability, not the impairment in itself.

We are at that moment of disciplinary history in India where disability research has possibly come of age, building within itself the tools that could possibly realign existing boundaries around which social science disciplines have been rigidly built in India. The disability framework is so elaborately diverse and fluid that it gives a definite possibility for us to tweak with vital research questions such as 'Who is the research subject?', 'What is the objective of the study?', 'What comprises field?' and so on. This chapter is therefore an attempt to begin this reassembling process within political theory by focusing on justice theories, especially the liberal egalitarian frameworks and their Indian critiques.

DISABILITY CRITIQUE AND POLITICAL THEORY: DEFINITIONAL ISSUES

If the inescapability of old age, illness and mortality of human life is understood by everyone, then disability would no longer be a 'tragedy' of a select few, but a common human reality that need not be pitied but merely taken into consideration in our everyday acts, be it in the way we design our built environment or the way we design our policies and implement them. The binaries—normal/abnormal, beauty/ugly and perfect/imperfect—entrenched within our minds, are what perpetuate disability, making it a 'problem' for the person living with it.

What Strengthens the Binaries that Perpetuate Disability?

1. The justification that such binaries receive from norms and values (justice, pity, charity).
2. The normalized everyday practices and 'solutions' that permeate the space and time of disabled individuals. In fact, the policies shaped

by distorted attitudes manifest in the everyday experiences of the disabled people (and those who are not [yet]), thereby (re)producing the cultural, philosophical norms.
3. Language has an intrinsic ability to produce and maintain binaries. Language is in fact so powerful that it manages to successfully parade as a harmless tool with no biased assumptions.

How to Undermine These Factors That Strengthen Binaries?

Interjecting the 'knowledge' space with powerful questions would undermine the power that such knowledge yields. No assumption based on any given knowledge or truth can be taken for granted. Everything has to be questioned, and every question has to be made part of the existing discourse. In effect, constant questioning of the roots (assumptions of knowledge and truth) has the potential to undermine and subvert those very roots. Power relations are produced/sustained by discourse and can therefore be altered by discourse.

Theoretically, Indian disability scholars have maintained that disability is a cultural/social construction which is 'created' and skewed out of established notions of normality. Now for the sake of entering into philosophical debate on justice, which revolves around resources, opportunities, luck and so on, we need to develop an alternate model which conforms to the parameters of disability being a social construct, but still uses the language of political philosophers. Instead of asking a direct question as 'what is disability' (because 'disability is naught' would then be our answer), we start with a first question.

What Expectations Does One Have in Life (from Oneself, State, Society, Family)?

From Oneself	To act/perform to the maximum of her ability and stretch her limits further on.
State	To pave way for the individual collectivities to meet their expectations and remove all obstacles.

Society	- To appreciate and accept one for what one is, rather than for what one ought to be. - Recognition of 'achievement' of her efforts and a space for self-expression.
Family	Mutual support and care (given as well as expected).

How many of one's expectations are met 'do not always depend' on the bundle of resources she has or is given (by society, State or family). Meeting her expectations on all counts would directly depend upon how her resources interact with the facilities, opportunities available in the external environment. For instance, a girl might have learnt pottery as a hobby. She would expect herself to be able to make the best and beautiful pots. Whether she achieves this depends not merely on her skills but on how the external environment interacts with her skill. For instance, if she is residing in a very conservative society, she might neither be able to travel to learn or practice her skill from men nor be able to travel far and wide to learn from women. She might accept the situation posed by her family, State and society as 'reality' and blame herself entirely for not meeting her expectation. A 'dynamic' interaction between an individual's resources and the externalities is a key criterion to achieve the level of one's ability. The individual's expectations and ability are not fixed and rigid. They are to be understood as a dynamic and vibrant life-long evolution. Moreover, there are some expectations which the individual is not aware of herself but which can be classified as rightful expectation from all three—for example—basic rights, liberties, access to health, food and education, good infrastructure and so on. These are a constant and need to be met no matter whether an individual knows enough to expect from the State or not.

DISABILITY FROM POLITICAL THEORY PERSPECTIVE

Disability can be seen as the stagnant point in a continuum that starts from an individual's range of expectations to meeting her ability. It can be explained as shown in Figure 4.1.

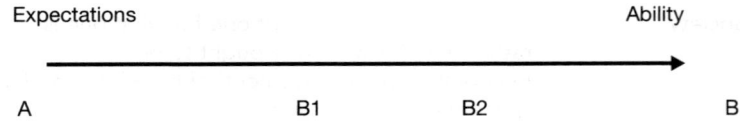

Figure 4.1 *Disability Continuum*
Source: Author.

I expect myself to act/perform to meet my own ability (whether it is at B1, B2 or B) and move forward thence. In this continuum, if the individual is at point A, it means she has not met any of her expectations and has not performed up to her own ability. At this point, if the society, State or family has not fulfilled her expectations, there is a huge chance that she will be blamed for where she is, because now the focus would be turned on 'her' failure to achieve. Her inability will be the focus rather than the inaction of society and State. This is the personal tragedy model in disability theorization. Here, she is a disabled individual unable to meet her ability and move beyond it.

If she is at point 'A' and at least has knowledge about her ability, then she could initiate the interaction of her resources with the external environment. This is where the individual wins against all odds. But if she is unaware of her own potentialities (similar to the 'tamed housewife' problem raised by Sen, 1985), then it 'is' the responsibility of all the other three externalities (State, society and family) to initiate the interaction of her expectations and resources with the opportunities and facilities available.

In this model, an individual who is still at A is the disabled individual (disabled by her externalities and being blamed for her situation).

As long as the individual has reached or is moving towards her own B point, then she is as normal as anybody else. The journey is what that counts. Disability is her condition, only when she is on the stagnant A, without the adequate resources or opportunities to move forward, slowly losing the will to do so. As long as she is moving towards her goal of meeting her maximum ability, there is no disability, provided the society does not pose obstacles for her and the State has taken care to provide her with adequate opportunities, infrastructure, education and so on along with basic liberties. It is a collective responsibility and has to be recognized as such.

DISABILITY AND RAWLSIAN THEORY OF JUSTICE

John Rawls ties his idea of justice to an equal consideration extended to all, so long as we treat people as equals not by removing all inequalities but only those which disadvantage someone.

He puts forward two principles arranged according to a principle of lexical priority:

1. Each person is to have an equal right to the most extensive total system of equal basic liberties compatible with a similar system of liberty for all.
2. Social and economic inequalities are to be arranged so that they are both:
   a. To the greatest benefit of the least advantaged, and
   b. Attached to offices and positions open to all under condition of fair equality of opportunity.

First priority rule (the priority of Liberty)—The principles of justice are to be ranked in lexical order and therefore liberty can be restricted only for the sake of liberty.

The second priority rule (The priority of justice over efficiency and welfare)—The second principle of justice is lexically prior to the principle of maximizing the sum of advantages. (Rawls 1971)

Rawls argues that his principles of justice are superior because they are the outcome of a hypothetical social contract. In what he calls as an Original Position,

> no one knows his place in society, his class position or social status, nor does anyone know his fortune in the distribution of natural assets and abilities, his intelligence, strength and the like. I shall assume that the parties do not know their conceptions of the good or their special psychological propensities. The principles of justice are chosen behind a veil of ignorance. This ensures that no one is advantaged or disadvantaged in the choice of principles by the outcome of natural chance or

the contingency of social circumstances. Since all are similarly situated and no one is able to design principles to favor his particular condition, the principles of justice are the result of a fair agreement or bargain. (Rawls 1971, 12 in Kymlicka 2002)

Here, the rational agents have no way of knowing beforehand their respective position in the society or the prejudices that operate on any positions. So even if they get to know they are going be in one category or other, they have no idea about which would be the more favoured category or which would be discriminated the most. Rawls believes that people in this original position would rationally choose the principles of justice, at least out of self-interest, because they have no way of knowing whether they would be better off or well off in the future turn of events. The principles of justice to which all are to be bound are chosen in the absence of any information about their advantageous/disadvantageous positioning in the future. All parties in his original position are equal and rational. The veil prevents anyone from being biased against social class and positioning other than their own.

A 'rational man' would not accept an institution if there is a considerable chance that it would affect his own interests. Feminists such as Susan Okin have already criticized the 'man' in original position, claiming that the social structure that arises out of this would have the institutions modelled in men's understanding of justice (impartial and abstract). For the disability movement, the 'rational' man would be an unsettling qualification to fulfil. Who is rational? Anyone who is sane enough to decide about his welfare? Then what about those who have psychosocial disabilities or are 'afflicted' with a simple case of irrationality?

Dworkin (1978) and Kymlicka (2002), among others, take exception to the fact that natural disabilities are not being compensated in the Rawlsian justice framework. The parties in Rawls' original position have knowledge beforehand about an index of social primary goods: rights and liberties, opportunities and powers, self-respect, income and wealth. Being rational agents, they would select the two principles of justice acting on self-interest. That the parties discuss about only social primary goods is a general disableist critique of original position, but one feels that it could be a blessing in disguise for the cause of creating awareness on disability to be mostly a social/cultural construct. In the original position, by not confining to disabilities that could be damned as 'natural', Rawls inadvertently leads us to a much wider scope for disability debate.

The reason there was no 'compensation' for natural disabilities is that there would have been felt no need for this (where agents are totally unprejudiced about being born with deformities, because they do not know the possibility of social construction on normality/abnormality operating on individual bodies). In addition, because they do not know about such binaries, neither will they subscribe to nor create any on their own in the future. Therefore, those entering the original position have no reason to consider a bodily impairment (like loss of a limb or vision or speech) as a disaster that needs to be compensated. If the social and political environment does not accommodate the impairments and provide mobility and accessibility, then the same impairments would, of course, be 'social' inequalities, and if agents choose the principles of justice, this problem would not arise in the first place. Environmental, political and educational infrastructure would accommodate everyone equally. Problems of cultural prejudice do not come into the picture because agents chose rationally to protect themselves against any disadvantageous position they could have been born into. If they did not consider bodily deformities as any special disadvantage that needs extra resource—just for being a deformity—then so be it. The question of extra resource burden for prosthetic leg would not arise because loss of a limb (or speech) would be shrugged off as a natural body occurrence and 'normality' would be everything that is, rather than everything that ought to be.

This is a very optimistic reading of Rawls' original position, which he himself surely did not intend. (He fails to mention disability because he simply thought of it as a distraction from the most important task at hand.[1]) But the possibility of going back to a time and place, where everything as is now, could be erased and rewritten, is the stuff that

---

[1] Four years after *Theory of Justice* was published, he replied to critics that he did suppose,

disableist dreams are made of. Anyone who strongly feels against the situation as it is has surely at one time or other wished to be able to go back and erase it all and neutralize (for reversing would be too mean indeed) the appeal of the aesthetic, normal and the rational. Elaborating on his original position is not to try and apply the same in practical situation, but it serves more of a symbolic purpose, as a tool to envisage an alternate paradigm. Such visualization is important because the 'abnormality' of disabled is so entrenched in our minds that there are far and few opportunities to even question why it could be otherwise. Furthermore, being born with any (de)formity would count as a misfortune only if the environment is designed against them in totality. But since the agents are already choosing to allocate the social primary goods equally to all, then the design of the external environment would be to the suitability and convenience of all parties, taking all their variations into consideration.

The above arguments have such far-fetched, yet far-reaching, assumptions about the rational 'self' choosing to ignore (or inherently ignorant of) the natural inequalities and their probable consequences in well-being. In this section, we analyse the Rawlsian idea of self if it is compatible with the assumptions made above. Because communitarians would have shrugged off all the above-mentioned claims of re-evaluation, on the ground that self is always 'embedded' or 'situated' in existing social practices, and it is difficult for us to 'stand back and opt out of them'. 'For them, self-determination is exercised *within* these social roles rather than by standing outside them'. (Kymlicka 2002, 221; emphasis added)

> ...that everyone has physical needs and psychological capacities within the normal range, so that problems of special health care and how to treat the mentally defective do not arise. Besides, prematurely introducing difficult questions that may take us beyond the theory of justice, the consideration of these hard cases can distract our moral perception by leading us to think of people distant from us whose fate arouses pity and anxiety. Whereas the first problem of justice concerns the relations among those in the normal course of things are full and active participants in society and directly or indirectly associated together over the course of a whole life. (Rawls 1975)

This needs immediate attention, and to sustain the sanguine disableist reading of Rawls, we need to justify the possibility of a self that so rationally unencumbered itself from the realities that are entwined with it. This dilemma of the self needs to be resolved in order to defend the disableist reading of Rawls.

It needs to be mentioned here that Rawls was not always favourably read from a disableist perspective. While the obvious criticisms were around the absence of compensation for natural inequalities, there are a few whose defence in itself does little justice to both Rawls and the disability movement. For instance, Brighouse (2001) though is open about his attempt to reclaim an appreciation for a Rawlsian approach to disability, he is problematic in his own views on disability. In a misguided attempt to evoke support for Rawls, he ends up misconstruing the disability movement in its entirety. Few instances are as follows:

1. What counts as a disability for our purposes? It is a chronic departure from normal human functioning, with its source in some medical or biological problem (ibid., 539).[2]
2. Many disabilities also have a social component to them, which exacerbates the departure from normal human functioning (ibid.).[3]

His views on disability totally stand in contradiction with what disability scholars themselves have written about disability since the 1970s. Therefore, a support of the Rawlsian framework that arises out of such weak understanding of disability (as a medical 'problem') only serves to juxtapose Rawls and the disability movement in conflicting platforms.

RAWLSIAN VEIL OF IGNORANCE AS A TOOL TO EXPOSE ABLEIST ARROGANCE

Not only could Rawls be made available to fit into a radical disableist perspective to deconstruct the normal/abnormal binary, there is also

---

[2] Right from the 1970s, disability scholars, especially in the West, have consistently criticized against such tragic, 'medical' view of disability (Charlton 1998).

[3] Note the unmistakable (arrogant) assumption about 'normal' human functioning.

a parallel relevance in Rawlsian veil of ignorance. From Rawls' later work, particularly *Political Liberalism* (1993), we can reinforce the above reading of fair consideration. People might be located in distinct cultural settings or entertain diverse comprehensive visions of what is good and bad for them. Such settings and visions often are informed by values deferential towards the disadvantaged. These values can surely be tapped to strengthen the radical disableist perspective.

As mentioned in the introduction to this chapter, everyone is moving towards old age and illness, and everyone will eventually cross the ability/disability boundary line. A perfect/able body is a temporary status, if not a resounding illusion. In today's scenario, deep within, we all feel unsettled by corporeal insecurities (which explains the success of 'health and accident' insurance policies). A perfect body and sound mind is as temporary as a clear sky in a stormy weather. All it takes is one road accident, a breast cancer or a simple display of 'abnormal' behaviour to cross the line right away. Yet, we choose to ignore such imminent future possibility and willingly subscribe to those norms and derivatives which would eventually alienate us when we cross the line and move over to attain disabled status. This is a question which could throw critical light on the Rawlsian veil of ignorance. Rawls assumes that when agents are behind a veil of ignorance, they would choose a difference principle that would benefit the least well off, because they do not know their future positioning in the society. If such a scenario is a possibility, then why are we not choosing our words, actions, policies and norms keeping in mind where we ourselves are moving towards? What could explain the 'blissful ignorance' which blinds us from acknowledging the inevitable fatality of alterable/temporariness of our 'perfect' body?

Anyway, this question is raised 'not' with an intention to undermine Rawlsian veil of ignorance but to ponder over the deep-rooted nature of the binaries we are attempting to shatter. Moreover, this question serves to prove our earlier appreciation of tremendous possibilities arising out of an alternate reading of Rawls. At least for the kind of questions we are able to pose, the Rawlsian framework is increasingly valid for a contemporary disability movement.

Another dilemma that disability critique poses for Indian political theorizing would be that we cannot afford to go too far into the philosophical ruminations on what disability is/is not, nor can we afford to deny the real worldly political implications of living with impairments in India. In Jharkhand's Jadugoda district, uranium mining is causing whole villages to be inflicted with impairments. In Kerala's Kasargod, endosulfan has resulted in heavy impairments. There is documented evidence of skeletal fluorosis in Karnataka, Assam, Bihar and several other states[4] caused by fluorosis in water. These issues are in addition to the widespread poverty and malnutrition that are already resulting in a skewed number of people with disabilities, with heavier concentration in rural and remote areas of India. The interconnections between poverty and disability as well as the issues faced specifically by women with disabilities in India make disability critique an imminent necessity for political theory in India.

Taking disability studies seriously will do more good to political theorizing because the questions (as well as the answers) that disability perspective will bring to the discipline will surely realign the boundaries of existing limits of theorization. Furthermore, a re-reading of the entire normative system and justice framework is the point of departure for which further study need to be focused on.

REFERENCES

Addlakha, R. 2013. *Disability Studies in India: Global Discourses, Local Realities.* New Delhi: Routledge.

Anand, S. 2009. *Delusive Disclosure: Tracing the Conceptual History of Disability in India.* Chicago, IL: University of Illinois.

———. 2016. The Models Approach in Disability Scholarship: An Assessment of Its Failings. In *Interrogating Disability in India*, edited by N. Ghosh, 23–38. New Delhi: Springer.

Brighouse, Harry. 2001. 'Can Justice as Fairness Accommodate the Disabled?' *Social Theory and Practice*, 27(4): 537–60.

Chander, J. 2011. 'Movement of the Organized Blind in India: From Passive Recipients of Services to Active Advocates of Their Rights.' Doctoral Thesis, Cultural Foundations of Education, Syracuse University, Syracuse, New York.

---

[4] https://www.thethirdpole.net/2017/05/10/fluoride-contamination-cripples-a-thousand-children-in-assam/ (accessed May 2, 2018).

Charlton, J. 1998. *Nothing about us Without Us: Disability, Oppression and Empowerment*. Berkeley: University of California Press.

Dworkin, R. 1978. *Taking Rights Seriously*. Cambridge Massachusetts: Belknap Press of Harvard University Press.

Friedner, Michele. 2015. *Valuing Deaf Worlds in Urban India*. New Brunswick, NJ: Rutgers University Press.

Ghai, A. 2002. 'Disability in the Indian Context: Post-colonial Perspectives'. In *Disability/Postmodernity: Embodying Disability Theory*, 88–100. London: Bloomsbury.

Ghosh, N. 2012. *Disabled Definitions, Impaired Policies: Reflections on Limits of Dominant Concepts of Disability*. Kolkata: Institute of Development Studies.

———. 2016. *Interrogating Disability in India: Theory and Practice*. New Delhi: Springer.

Kymlicka, W. 2002. *Contemporary Political Philosophy: An Introduction*. Oxford: Oxford University Press.

Mehrotra, N. 2012. Methodological Issues in Disability Research: An Introduction. *Indian Anthropologist* 42 (1): 1–10.

Rawls, John. 1971. *A Theory of Justice*. Cambridge Massachusetts: Belknap Press of Harvard University Press.

———. 1993. *Political Liberalism*. New York, NY: Columbia University Press.

Sen, Amartya. 1985. *Commodities and Capabilities*. Amsterdam: North-Holland.

Chapter 5

Disability Studies as Resistance
The Politics of Estrangement

Tanmoy Bhattacharya

The spirit of disability studies (DS) is often misunderstood in the excitement associated with the birth of a new field and in the context of an uncertain dissociation from the zeal of activism. I will make a strong point here with respect to the latter. Although, in earlier work, I have advocated the necessity of the two-way traffic between activism and DS theory building (Bhattacharya 2011), I now believe that disability-related activities in India, with their overemphasis on services, are alarmingly close to creating a hegemonic discourse that shrinks the space for the emergence of a DS discourse even further. In fact, what feeds each other within the Indian context is not DS and activism but activism and service, the former accentuating the latter. This association is threatening to develop into a nexus that will steadfastly keep DS out forever. Therefore, it is time now to move away for a while from the excitement of sloganeering and to build a tradition of true scholarship in DS that in fact feeds activism back in various new ways. The formality of this estrangement is best attempted, I suggest, by looking at existing practices through the lens of ableism and by engaging in exposing, strategizing and acting against disability injustice through a disability-centric understanding of various themes within the academia.

INTRODUCTION: WHY 'ESTRANGEMENT'?

This chapter proposes a controversial position that DS scholars working within India must take in order to first bring about recognition for the field and then 'save' it from being neglected and finally pushed towards ossification in the form of library archives. The idea proposed emanates from stray experiences with disability activism associated with both policymaking and scholarship since the beginning of the last decade, that is, 2001.

Before elaborating the stance in detail, let us look at its simplified version in a graphical form (Figure 5.1) that summarizes the underlying thesis of this chapter.

That is, it is services that disability activism is naturally geared towards, as shown in the first box. However, it is the blocking off of any connection between the first and the second box that must sound as a warning bell for DS scholars. In fact, the underlying thesis of the chapter, hinted as above, is a stronger one, which states that the very fact that disability activism is 'solely' geared towards services threatens to strategically keep DS out of the scene altogether. Although it is quite clear from considering social contexts and history elsewhere that it need not be so, that is, it is quite possible for activism to be geared towards 'both' services and DS. In fact, the general tenet assumed by DS scholars in the West is that there is no essential disconnect between activism and DS.

However, I will claim that the situation as in Figure 5.1 obtains as an expected consequence of strategic prioritization of the so-called practical things as opposed to the so-called theoretical things in the context of a struggling economy, where anything that smacks of 'studies' is perceived with suspicion, and the logic of a consumerist culture feeds

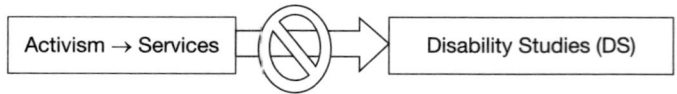

Figure 5.1 *The status quo*
Source: Author.

this. Thus, this is in no way a unique situation limited to DS alone but is true of other branches of knowledge. However, what is ironic with regard to DS meeting the same fate is that this specific branch of knowledge, similarly to gender studies, is by definition moves hand-in-hand with activism. Ideally, activism is supposed to derive further fuel from DS and vice versa.[1] I will rather claim that in the context of extreme and/or uncertain economic situations, the definitional 'purity' of a particular form of knowledge is sacrificed at the altar of activism that is geared towards services (or sectorial benefits), although the latter is the manifestation of the former.

And that is where the danger lurks. In this chapter, therefore, I suggest a way out by keeping activism at abeyance—by constructing a politics of estrangement or abeyance. I will specifically suggest to incorporate the process of construction of knowledge as knowledge itself is a formal device representing the politics of abeyance. I will consider the unalienated examination of the self as an act of 'small liberation' within oneself from the perspective of disability research; this, I would suggest, is the closest one can come to the concept of 'activism' in the framework of DS I am suggesting. Further, I will elaborate this interpretation of 'activism' in the last section of the Chapter, titled 'Formalising Estrangement'. I present the following genesis as an exemplar of this strategy.

GENESIS OF THE IDEA: WHY 'RESISTANCE'

In my work first as the member of the Equal Opportunity Cell, University of Delhi, and then its coordinator, I have had to wage a series of struggles from the very beginning to evolve policies and run activities that are not solely service-oriented. The University Grants Commission's (UGC) mandate in this respect is about services to students, staff and teachers with disabilities. These struggles were waged against not only authorities and administrators but also sympathizers. Many of the scholars were invited to teach in the 'Disability and Human Rights' course there, but to even suggest it, to draw up the syllabus, the

---

[1] Although see Bhattacharya (2015) for problematizing the traffic from activism to DS.

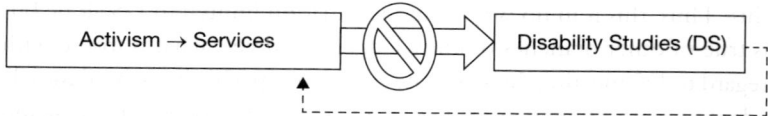

Figure 5.2 *DS back-feeding activism*
Source: Author.

ways it was to be run and many more issues had to be fought over. This situation prevailed not only in an academic event such as courses but also in other events, workshops and facilities, including the day-to-day running of the centre. The inclusion of a DS component in the various courses and organization of a conference with a broad DS perspective (in 2011) were pieces of resistance against this prevailing reality. With such a strategy as the basis, I suggest a new picture (Figure 5.2), though much like Figure, with an additional back-traffic from DS to activism (shown here in dotted lines):

Figure 5.2 claims that even if there is no traffic from activism/services to DS, the latter through 'small acts of resistance'—to be elaborated further in the last section of the chapter—can inform and invigorate activism/services. I will now discuss briefly the need for this resistance.

THE VAGARIES OF THE PRESENT CONDITION

Due to a variety of reasons, we have seen the resurrection of the dominant discourse, a value system, around us based on various shades of empiricism—that all knowledge is derived from/reducible to aspects of experience, that is, reality cannot be knowable from reason or rationality alone. Policies, funding, sympathies and 'knowledge' are all geared towards what is 'visible' or visibly effective. Devaluing of DS because it is perceived as unnecessary is a sacrifice that awaits the fate of many other knowledge spheres. 'The Death of a Rationalist' need not be a recent newspaper headline but a process (and an operation) that was triggered much earlier. Further support for this status quo, namely, that empiricism is de rigueur of our existence, can be gleaned from the results of the PhilSurvey as given in Table 5.1.

Table 5.1 *Knowledge: Empiricism or rationalism?*

Other	1,158/3,226 (35.9%)
Accept or lean towards: empiricism	1,254/3,226 (38.9%)
Accept or lean towards: rationalism	814/3,226 (25.2%)

Source: http://philpapers.org/surveys/results.pl (31 March 2017).

In fact, if we go by the various groups of respondents, the highest leaning towards empiricism obtains for (philosophy) undergraduates (42.4%) and the lowest leaning towards rationalism obtains for the group not affiliated to philosophy (22.9%) at all. Although this is a small survey restricted mostly to philosophy students and faculty, it, nonetheless, shows the trend clearly; the trend being, for every person who leans towards rationalism, there are almost two persons who lean towards empiricism. If this is the result of a survey conducted among philosophy-affiliated students and faculty, a similar survey in the context of an economically poorer region of the world will surely widen this gap considerably; and when such a survey is made open to the general public, the gap will be even wider.

There is, of course, one aspect of an empiricist view of knowledge that has a direct bearing on representations in a discipline like DS that cannot be ignored—the role of personal experience of disability. For its own good, a discipline like DS cannot deny the importance of the disability experience in DS discourse. I will come back to this issue in the next (and the last) section, where I outline the strategy/methodology for a renewed DS framework. This framework is based on an ecology of understanding that emphasizes the living body or *leib* or, in other words, it values knowledge that is situated or contextualized.

FAILURE OF PHENOMENOLOGICAL RESEARCH

In fact, the mutually feeding dyad of activism and DS has failed to produce any meaningful dialogue in the Indian context. So, the advice that DS should act as the theoretical arm of the disability rights movement has not taken off, as the two parties do not meaningfully interact with

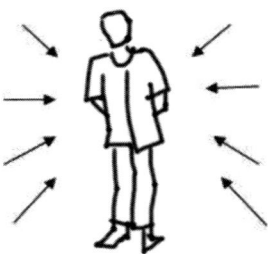

Figure 5.3 *Receiver of services*
Source: Author.

each other. In fact, all that a phenomenological consideration (i.e., the disability experience of individuals) produced was sucked wholly into activism, and it did not result in any research.

Both these points seem to directly clash with the other major theme that must also be considered, namely, the notion of subjectivity. If activism based on a rights movement cannot highlight the phenomenology of disability (i.e., disability experience of the individual or collective), how and where does subjectivity find a place? How can the disabled person be foregrounded? The present scenario can be aptly summarized in Figure 5.3.

Figure 5.3 shows that the disabled body of the individual acts only as the receiver of various services, the latter being a result of activism. But the individual experience of the body does not find an expression in this unidirectional flow since services are never reinforced or informed by individual experiences of the disabled body. In short, the disabled subject is never foregrounded in its recipient-only role.

AGENCIES AND SERVICES

I will very briefly touch upon some instances, in this section, of governmental policies (international and national) and non-governmental organizations (NGOs) to highlight the connection of these agencies with providing services for disabled persons. In other words, this section further highlights the deep connection of disability with services as a prevailing status quo. It should, however, be noted that there are many NGOs that do not place such a premium on services. A related issue is the inevitability of the component of services with anything that is related to disability; this, I believe, is due largely to the charity view of disability that continues to rule large parts of the disability experience in India. In short, the services component cannot be avoided and should not be either. However, my point here is about the over-insistence on services that now threaten to take over and engulf all that is there to do with disability. How can DS remain unaffected in such a scenario?

In the rest of the chapter, I will discuss how the following two aspects emerge as possible pieces of resistance for the *en passé* that ensues once activism is divorced from DS:

1. Reorienting the politics of DS: dislodgement of the ableist stance and embracing a critical DS approach.
2. Reorienting the politics of activism: challenging ableism in every sphere based on a disability justice approach.

With respect to these, I will offer some examples, but first note that both the approaches assume challenging ableism as the foundational basis of resistance. With respect to the first point, an examination of the fragment of the discursive constructions at respite centres reveals that the normalization model of disability has inherent ableist posturing. With respect to the second point, the position I wish to emphasize has to do with resisting a certain normalization of services as a privative engagement.

Non-governmental Agencies

As per the tenets of the proposal advocated here, the back-traffic from DS to activism/services is the only hope to prevent the complete disconnect between the two. Although the last section identified the disabled body being subjected to a recipient-only state, in a four-year time gap between the presentation of the present chapter and its written-up version, a surprising change in the NGOs has taken place in relation to their commitments to services. I would like to read this change as a result of the pockets of research that have been going on in DS in this country.

With a search string such as 'India NGO disability', the first non-commercial and unbroken link obtained in August 2013 was that of the NGO Astha. And the very next one is Give India, both of which clearly showed the connection between NGOs and services, as services is the main theme in their mission statements. The snapshots of the home URL from 2013 are shown in Figures 5.4 and 5.5.

The home page of Astha has the following mission statement as the first point: 'To provide *services* to children/persons with disability and their families'. Similarly, the Give India home page declares that it has seven pages on 'services' for the disabled. Both of these, thus, clearly show the connection between NGOs and service, and providing services is clearly the very raison d'être of these organizations.

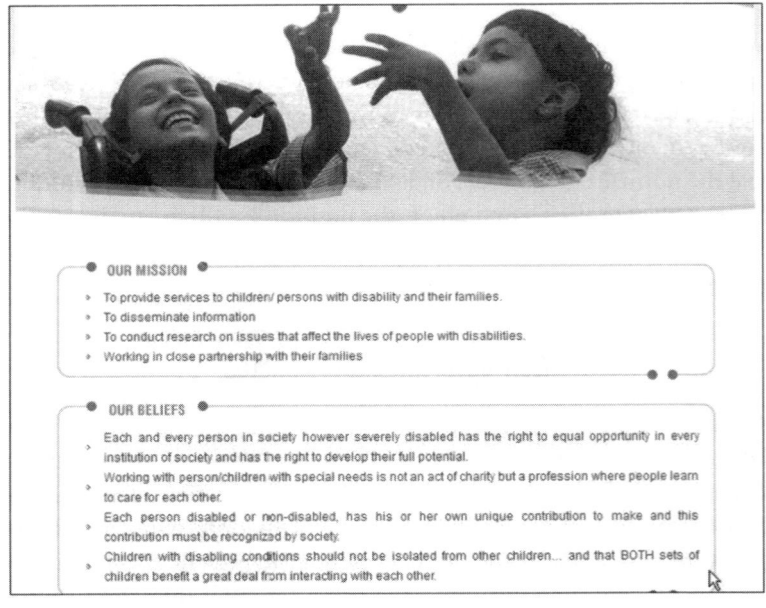

Figure 5.4 *The home page of the NGO Astha from 2013*

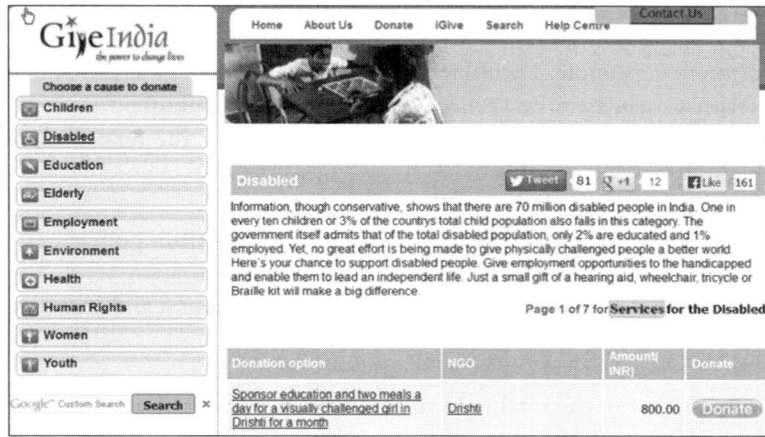

Figure 5.5 The home page of the NGO Give India from 2013

However, when one uses the same search string now after five years (in 2018), the scenario has altered considerably. For Astha, their mission statement no longer mentions the word 'services' and instead states two points:

1. To work in partnership with children and persons with disabilities and their families.
2. To uphold rights and work with all stakeholders to build an inclusive society.[2]

Give India, on the other hand, has completely focussed on 'giving' as a concept and wants to 'promote efficient and effective giving that provides greater opportunities to the poor in India' as their mission.[3]

How did this change happen? The change from a service-oriented NGO to an organization that is focussed on inclusion is the result of the DS discourse the world over, and, I believe, due to pockets of 'resistance' in the form of DS in India that has begun to take effect.

---

[2] http://www.asthaindia.in/home.php (accessed August 25, 2013).
[3] http://www.giveindia.org/t-abtus_mission.aspx (accessed May 9, 2018).

Governmental Policies

In the first example, I will highlight the role of services in the World Health Organization's *World Report on Disability* published in 2011. The first two recommendations made at the end of the report reveal the insistence on services:

1. Recommendation 1: Enable access to all mainstream policies, systems and 'services'.
2. Recommendation 2: Invest in specific programmes and 'services' for people with disabilities.

Only the last of the total nine recommendations talks about research:

Recommendation 9: Strengthen and support research on disability

However, within this recommendation, we find the following as one of the suggestive areas of research, 'barriers to mainstream and specific *services*, and what works in overcoming them in different contexts', thus bringing services back even in research.

As for translating the recommendations into actions, the roles of different agencies and their function are outlined as follows:

Government

1. Barriers to mainstream and specific 'services', and what works in overcoming them in different contexts.
2. Regulate 'service' provision by introducing 'service' standards and by monitoring and enforcing compliance.
3. Allocate adequate resources to existing publicly funded 'services' and appropriately fund the implementation of the national disability strategy and plan of action.
4. Provide technical assistance to countries to build capacity and strengthen existing policies, systems and 'services'—for example, by sharing good and promising practices.

Disabled Persons' Organizations

1. Represent the views of their constituency to international, national and local decision makers and 'service' providers, and advocate for their rights.
2. Contribute to the evaluation and monitoring of 'services' and collaborate with researchers to support applied research that can contribute to 'service' development.
3. Conduct audits of environments, transport and other systems and 'services' to promote barrier removal.

'Service' Providers

1. Ensure that staff are adequately trained about disability, implementing training as required and including 'service' users in developing and delivering training.
2. Develop individual 'service' plans in consultation with disabled people and their families where necessary.
3. Introduce case management, referral systems and electronic record-keeping to coordinate and integrate 'service' provision.

Private Sector

1. Develop a range of quality support 'services' for persons with disabilities and their families at different stages of the life cycle.
2. Ensure that ICT products, systems and 'services' are accessible to persons with disabilities.

Quite surprisingly, out of the 12 action points, the words 'service' and 'services' appear 14 times, and there is not a single action point that is not devoted to services. Thus, even at the international level, governmental-level policies establish an undeniable link between services and disability.

Let us now briefly look at the Persons with Disabilities Act (PwD Act) and the RPwD Bill and Act in this light to gauge the situation at the national level.

In the chapter on Education in the PWD Act, 1995, Article 28 deals with research for designing and developing new assistive devices, teaching aids and so on, which has been partly revised in the RPD Bill of September 2014 by getting rid of assistive devices (in the section on research and development) and instead it mentions 'issues which would enhance habilitation and rehabilitation of persons with disabilities' (Article 27). The 2012 version of the Bill, though, had an article (28) on assistive devices. In the 1995 Act, within the same chapter, Article 30 deals with providing transport facilities, supply of books and so on. These provisions have been retained since the 2012 version of the Bill and in new RPD Act of 2016 as well (Article 179(g)).

In the chapter on Affirmative Action, Article 42 of the older Act deals with aids and appliances to persons with disabilities. The new Bill of 2012, through the suggested Articles 50, 52 and 53, talks about accessibility of services, access to goods and services and provision of service animals for PwDs, and the later versions and the Act of 2016 do not have these provisions. In the 2012 version of the Bill, the emphasis in general had been about accessibility of services. In its Article 57 (human resource development), it clearly talks about the development of human resources in appropriate numbers to make services to disabled persons available (see Articles 57(1)a and 57(1)c). It should be noted that there is no article in the UNCRPD, the motherboard for the RPwD, equivalent to Article 57; therefore, it is only expected that the later versions as well as the final Act do not have these provisions.

Thus within the context of the governmental policies, although we see encoded within the policies a deep connection between services and disability at the international level, at the national level, there have been various correctives to not encode them in a similar fashion within the polices and the acts. Similar to the examples in the case of NGOs, we thus find a change in the framing of policies in the governmental documents that can also be attributed to pockets of resistance emanating from a reimagined version DS outlined here.

DISABILITY STUDIES

In this section, in order to understand how best to reimagine a DS project sans services and also to return to the promise of Figure 5.2,

I will outline, very briefly and partially, some of the major ideas on DS that, nonetheless, provide a window to a possible characterization of DS programmes anywhere. The review below will also show that, structurally, services do no figure anywhere in a DS programme and therefore cannot be the central concern of DS.

Linton (1998) is one of the foremost in advocating the discipline of DS and laid out the characters of such a discipline. She advocates DS as an interdisciplinary field of inquiry, which is nevertheless grounded in the liberal arts, structured and designed to study disability as a social, political and cultural phenomenon. However, she advocates DS theorists to deal more directly with 'impairment' and recognize its significance in the complex characterization of 'disability'.

Furthermore, she also advises revised applied approaches, especially teaching in the applied fields, need to be based on ideas of inclusion, self-determination and self-definition, though they should be called 'Not Disability Studies'. DS should also have a say in the curriculum of rehabilitation education.

The research by Cushing and Smith (2009) was an interesting survey of the growth of DS, where they identified three key dimensions of growth: independent, hybridized and integrated. They reported that the Society for Disability Studies developed and adopted a set of 'Guidelines for DS programmes', and the common threads between those and other approaches are listed as follows:

1. Challenges the dominance of medical, individual, deficit-based models of disability (while not dismissing their contributions).
2. Considers disability part of the continuum of human experience (Linton disagrees with this).
3. Examines the environmental and social barriers to greater participation.
4. Interdisciplinary approach.
5. Inclusive: participation of disabled people and their families is essential.
6. Accessibility in DS courses, conferences, journals, websites and buildings.
7. Geographical specificity and diversity: accounts for cultural and historical contexts.

These guidelines are based clearly on the achievements of the rights-based movements launched by disabled people the world over, especially an equality-based model like the social model (Oliver 1983, 1990; Oliver and Barnes 2012; UPIAS 1976). Note also that except the issue of accessibility in the sixth point, to some extent, nothing remotely smacks of service; with regard to accessibility, we will elaborate further its current conceptualization within the notion of disability justice, in the section 'Formalizing Estrangement', and claim, in fact, that this reconceptualization leads to resistance and activism, respecting the back-traffic from DS, as in Figure 5.2.

During their research, Cushing and Smith (2009) also faced the following issues from observers, which provide us with further characterization of a field like DS:

1. Does being located within the medical sciences automatically discredit you from being DS?
2. Should a module be called DS even if only a course or two deals with DS theory directly?
3. Do applied courses that deal with progressive themes like social inclusion, autonomy and human rights (but not critical theory) count as DS?
4. Can a degree that primarily trains people to work in the interventionist services be DS?
5. What difference can be achieved in applied professionals' outlook via a DS course or two?
6. Is a little DS better than no DS or more harmful because of the dilution?

These are subtle and advanced findings that any worthwhile DS programme must grapple with at some stage. Their findings with regard to growth of DS in hybrid and integrated settings are of importance from the point of view of deciding the 'location' issue of a DS programme, namely, the question of where does DS belong.

In an important work, Campbell (2009) shifts the spotlight on disability to a more nuanced exploration of epistemologies and ontologies of ableism. Instead of the prevailing practice of examining disability from the perspective of disableism, she suggests that we concentrate on what the study of disability tells us about the production, operation and maintenance of ableism.

Wolbring (2012) is another step in the right direction. He suggests an extended form of ableism which can become a seed for new discourses, perspectives and paradigms that focus on ability favouritism as a basis for analysing existing and future cultural dynamics. He contends that DS scholars face numerous impact challenges such as (a) who to serve (academia, disabled people or both); (b) which field of academics to impact; (c) which problems to tackle; (d) which space to influence and (e) the ghettoization of the DS field and its impact.

With respect to the last issue, he raises the question: How can they convince others, not directly related to their area, of the utility their work has for 'others'? DS-based research, especially the work around the concept of ableism, has strong utility outside DS.

SUMMARY

In summary, let me just point out that apart from the obvious overlaps, the two salient points that emerge from studying carefully the above literature on DS are the following:

1. The politics of DS: dislodgement of the ableist agenda/stance
2. Epistemological question: positioning of DS.

For any DS programme to sustain itself, these pillars must be first established. In conceptualizing DS within such a strategy, we can see that there is no scope of overemphasizing a services component. As for activism, as long as it keeps to the politics of DS as in point 1 intact as its goal, then it is least likely to become merely a fodder to producing services.

EPISTEMOLOGICAL RE-VISIONING

With respect to the two tenets discussed in the previous section, I will offer some examples in this section to consolidate the point that not only is there no place for services in a DS programme, but any DS approach must also adhere to the two principles. For the 'politics of DS', a look at the concept of respite centres reveals that the normalization model of disability (Wolfensberger 1998) has inherent ableist posturings. In one study, Rhoades and Browning (1982) point out that certain respite group homes consider inappropriate appearance, poor eating habits and bad manners, poor cooking and shopping skills, inadequate skills for managing money, inadequate skills to use public transportation, inability to make and keep appointments, poor work habits and inappropriate sex behaviour as highly undesirable. Principles of normalization are applied to suppress these behaviours so that the 'retardation' will be invisible to others or go unnoticed; the 'retarded' person goes from the point of visibility to invisibility, thereby learning to blend.

However, interestingly in this study, the programme coordinator's voice (Rhoades and Browning 1982) is without ellipses or hesitation, pause or even fast speech phenomenon like 'wanna' for 'want + to' or 'gettin' for 'getting' and so on to make it look more standardized and therefore in opposition to the residents (with 'mental retardation' or MR) voices elsewhere; similar are the voices of the home staff and staff members. Here is a random sample:

Resident:

See my mom lives by herself now since my dad died and she's gettin' pretty old. I wanna get married when the time is right .... I wanna learn how to shop and cook and keep my budget and things like that.

Programme Coordinator:

It is here that the cooking skills, housekeeping skills and budgeting skills are truly probed. Up to now, the resident did not have to purchase food and had to cook only one evening meal a week. Once in the independent kitchen, the resident is monitored on a diminishing basis until it is shown that he or she can indeed function independently in this area. When a resident is able to purchase food, prepare meals, maintain the kitchen, pay rent and live within a budget, he or she is ready.

Although the coordinator's statement is admittedly a report or summary, the 'voice' that is constructed in this manner is, nevertheless, contrasted with the 'speech' of the resident. A careful DS perspective would be more sensitive to this portrayal and would instead try to look at the work in respite centres from the point of view of the person with MR rather than the other way round.

I may also point out that 'picking' on the discourses of this nature is quite in line with a postconventional theoretical approach like that of the Critical Disability Studies (CDS; Meekosha and Shuttleworth 2009), which, apart from looking for social justice—based as it is on a modernist paradigm like the social model—extends the disability paradigm beyond the social, political and economical planes to several other planes, including the discursive.

With respect to 'Positioning of DS', I will briefly discuss two examples from sign language from my previous work.

The multimodal property of sign languages opens up dimensions otherwise invisible in spoken languages. Centring sign language in language studies can thus enable us to look at language—the pure representation of the human mind—in a new light (Bhattacharya and Hidam 2011). In terms of practice, this implies that if adequate services are provided in the classroom with deaf students in terms of teaching through sign language, acquisition of this medium of communication will open up an enriching experience for the hearing student such that it may radically alter their understanding of the world around them. In this perspective, an inclusive education will transform the lives of the so-called non-disabled majority students in immeasurable ways.

Bauman's (2008) example of iconicity discussed in Bhattacharya (2014) is a fine example that clearly shows that the metaphoric performance is bigger than just a generation of proposition as derived from quantifying terms and variables:

> [H]ow one of my students at Gallaudet University explained the process of reading Foucault. He first signed that it was difficult to read, with his left hand representing the book, open and facing him, and his right hand was in a V shape, the two finger tips representing his practice of reading, re-reading, and then finally, his fingers got closer to the book, and finally, made contact; at this point, the eyes of the V shape then became a digging apparatus, digging deeper into the text. He then reached in between the lines of the page, now signified by the open fingers of the left hand, and began to pull ideas and new meanings from underneath the text. The notion of reading between the lines gained flesh, as the hands literally grasped for buried meanings. The result of reading Foucault, he said, changed his thinking forever, inspiring him to

invent a name-sign for Foucault. The sign he invented began with the signed letter 'F' at the side of the forehead, and then twisting outward, showing the brain undergoing a radical reorientation.

POSSIBILITY OF DS IN INDIA

If we are to look for a possible framework to introduce a DS programme that does not get overshadowed by the practice of activism that is geared only towards services, the governmental machinery does not provide a good guide. Inequity in higher education has been a concern, and UGC and the Planning Commission have had specific recommendations to improve the situation. Among the various recommendations that were made, a few of them were directed towards improving the quality in higher education. There are at least three other existing UGC schemes that offer this opportunity: (a) Centre for Study of Social Exclusion and Inclusion Policy, (b) Centre for Human Rights and (c) Centre for Potential for Excellence in a Particular Area.

By looking at the first one, an analysis of the current situation (Bhattacharya 2015, forthcoming) with respect to a representative sample of the 35 currently existing centres, set up under the 11th Plan, reveals the state of affairs. If it is a representative sample, although 30% of them have a disability-related objective, none of them have any research output, activity (seminar, conferences, workshops and special lectures) or degrees in disability. Only one of them has a research associate specializing in a disability-related field. We can only conclude from this fact that although disability falls within the ambit of social exclusion in almost exactly the same lines as other forms of exclusion, disability as a sector/oppressed group is simply forgotten/bypassed in this context of higher education.

INVERSION OF THE PRESENT CONDITION

I present here one example, although there are many, that inverts the situation encountered earlier (see Figure 5.3) in the context of searching for a disability perspective for disaster mitigation and resilience (Bhattacharya 2013). I wish to present a case for turning our gaze towards a strong form of sustainability, which involves a social critical view of the dominant value system, and trace it to Hunt (1966). The effect of any human tragedy is pronounced manifold due to impairment and special needs. The severity of the effect demands measures in terms of preparedness at a heightened level, involving quick egress, accessibility in sheltering and appropriate rehabilitation. Such lessons, I suggest, when incorporated in disability services become more effective and meaningful. In fact, a DS perspective, suitably fortified by this aspect of disaster mitigation and resilience, can act as an essential tool in planning for disasters. Policies may benefit from a reassessment by considering disability as a construct and eliminate the ableist bias in existing policies and agendas.

This epistemological inversion is afforded by reimagining a different centre than prevailing practices and turning disaster mitigation of disabled persons to mitigation by them; the inversion that I wish to emphasize is shown in Figure 5.6.

This way of questioning a culture, biased as it is to engender inaccessibility in the first place, is based on a politics of dislodgement of the ableist agenda, and yet, at the same time, it finds echoes in the notion

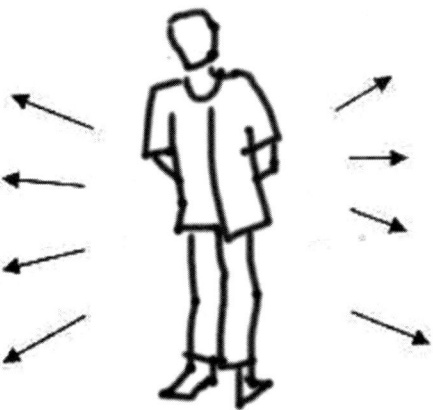

Figure 5.6 *Provider of services*
Source: Author.

of disability justice that increasingly incorporates differences and challenges normativity in every sphere.

This inversion lies at the centre of the estrangement politics that I am trying to outline. In this inversion, the notion of accessibility is viewed differently from an equality-based approach like the social model. It is instead based on the premise of questioning normativity—one of the pillars in any DS programme mentioned in the summary of the section on DS.

FORMALIZING ESTRANGEMENT: AN ECOLOGY OF UNDERSTANDING

At the heart of this inversion proposed above lies the underlying determining factor of the true nature of human ecology, where a person is not understood in abstraction detached from their environments and inter-connections but is rather understood in totality. This is a familiar theme—knowledge being contextually specific. However, I would like to read it from an even older tradition of Husserl's (1913/1982) concept of *Lebenswelt* or Life-World: We experience objects as not something that occupies space–time and is made of some material but as objects we deal with in kitchen, streets, gardens and so on or in practical or social activities such as dinning or playing together. Each of us experiences his/her own body not as a physical system of bones, organs and so on, but as 'my body'. He uses two expressions to distinguish these aspects of one's body: my physical body (*körper*) and my living body (*leib*), and it is through empathy (*Einfühlung*) that we experience 'other I's'.

I return now to the methodological question of how to practice the politics of estrangement/abeyance and to the strategy of how to incorporate experience (and therefore subjectivity) within our studies on the face of a new DS vision that is removed from concerns for services. In fact, the answer lies in our understanding of ecology envisioned above. More specifically, I suggest that we adopt within this renewed vision of DS a 'fractured foundationalism' perspective of Stanley and Wise (1990), which, among other things, advocates strategies for a feminist sociology which treats 'knowledge' as situated, indexical and elliptical, as small slices of reality confronting each and engages in unalienated research where the act of knowing determines what is known (Morris 1993).

> If we are to resist oppression, then we need the *means* to do so. The means to resist oppression, we believe, are to be found where all of our oppressions are themselves to be found. Without knowing *how* oppression occurs we cannot possibly know *why* it occurs; and without knowing how and why it occurs we cannot find out how to avoid its occurrence, how it is that liberation might be achieved. (Stanley and Wise 1990, 165; emphasis in original)

In order to know how oppression occurs, we need to find out the minute details of mechanisms, experiences, behaviours and conversations of such occurrences; in other words, we need an ecology of understanding.

One of the abiding characteristics of the critical conceptualization of disability that gives rise to the very recent current of 'disability justice' is its desire to understand through its various ways of challenging the equality-based notions of access, the ways of organizing and building community spaces based on mixed-ability and cultivating solidarity between people with different disabilities (Mingus 2010).

This is the so-called second wave of the disability rights movement and is being waged most prominently in the underbelly of Canadian disability quarters in Toronto and other cities. Here, values are based on interdependence and a new politicized notion of care. Interdependence is an antidote to the capitalist social construct of independence. As Eddie Ndopu says:

> [A]ny attempt to politicize care in relation to organizing calls for something different. It calls for new ways of negotiating liberation. It calls for a new praxis and a new kind of activism. (Hande and Mire 2013, 11)

I would like to claim that this new way of organizing resistance can be seen through a disability justice lens emanated from a reconceptualization of DS as we understand it from a purely sociopolitical and predominantly Marxian perspective. Rather this reimagining is achieved through a quest of knowledge that is not rooted in knowledge alone but first and foremost in disability injustice. If this is not done, then the injustice will remain invisible and therefore unrecognized. So, the primary 'act' of DS must be to expose injustice and then to outline a strategy. Only then can activism begin.

This has to be the sequence in every act of DS; no act of DS can assume that injustice is already exposed—one has to engage in it anew every time, and not just in terms of statistics, but in acts of obvious neglect and ableism. Thus, the steps in DS that is proposed here are as follows: step 1: expose; step 2: strategize; step 3: act.

In step 2, we have all the concerns of organizing spaces and critical membership. This step of strategizing must also lay down all the previous knowledge gained in this domain, that is, it must rely on a network of knowledge and not pretend it to be an isolated case of injustice calling for right-based action strategies.

Note that if one engages in all that that have been laid down as part of step 2, one would realize that this is nothing but DS. In addition, 'emancipatory' research will be an automatic consequence of this framework that constantly conceptualizes and reconceptualizes strategies based on feedback cycles from field actions.

CONCLUSION

Having elaborated in detail the prevailing situation that this chapter began with, namely, the blocking of traffic form activism to DS, by looking at existing national and international policies and governmental frameworks for possible DS programmes, I have argued for a renewed notion of 'activism' by reconceptualizing DS through the lens of disability justice; this form of 'activism' is aided by an epistemological inversion of the perception of what service for a disabled person means. This back-traffic from DS to activism is at the centre of a politics of estrangement proposed in this chapter.

REFERENCES

Bauman, H-Dirksen. 2008. 'Listening to Phonocentrism with Deaf Eyes: Derrida's Mute Philosophy of (Sign) Language.' *Essays in Philosophy,* 9 (1, Article 2). Available at see https://commons.pacificu.edu/cgi/viewcontent.cgi?article=1288&context=eip

Bhattacharya, Tanmoy. 2011, March 3–5. 'Methods in Disability Studies.' Paper presented at the National Annual Conference on Disability, Delhi University.

Bhattacharya, Tanmoy. 2013, December 9. 'Disaster Resistance and Care: A Disability Studies Perspective.' Paper presented at the NAPSIPAG's (Network of Asia Pacific Schools and Institutes of Public Administration and Governance) 10th International Conference, JNU, New Delhi.

———. 2014. 'Sign Iconicity and New Epistemologies.' In *The Sign Language(s) of India*, edited by Tanmoy Bhattacharya, Nisha Grover and Surinder Randhawa. Delhi: Orient BlackSwan.

———. 2015, February 6–7. 'Service and Knowledge: The Role of Disability in Higher Education.' Paper presented at the 'Disability Studies in India: Reflections on Future' Conference, Jawaharlal Nehru University, New Delhi.

———. 2016. 'Diversity and Workplace and in Education.' In *Interrogating Disability in India*, edited by N. Ghosh. India: Springer.

———. (Forthcoming). 'Service and Knowledge: The Emergence of Disability Studies Extension.' In *Doing Disability Research in India: Methodological Issues*, edited by N. Malhotra. India: Springer.

Bhattacharya, Tanmoy, and Gaurshyam Singh Hidam. 2011. 'Space-Machine.' In *Proceedings of Episteme 4: International Conference to Review Research on Science, Technology and Mathematics Education*. Mumbai: Homi Bhaba Centre for Science, Mumbai.

Campbell, Fiona Kumari. 2009. *Contours of Ableism*. Hampshire: Palgrave MacMillan.

Cushing, Pamela, and Tyler Smith. 2009. A Multinational Review of English-language Disability Studies Degrees and Courses. *Disability Studies Quarterly* 29 (3). Available at: http://dsq-sds.org/article/view/940/1121 (accessed May 1, 2018).

Hande, Mary Jean, and Muna Mire. 2013. '"The Pace We Need to Go": Creating Care Culture.' *Action Speaks Louder* (Fall): 10–11.

Hunt, Paul. 1966. *A Critical Condition*. In *Stigma: The Experience of Disability*, edited by Paul Hunt, 145–59. London: Geoffrey Chapman.

Husserl, Edmund. 1913. *Ideas Pertaining to a Pure Phenomenology and to a Phenomenological Philosophy—First Book: General Introduction to a Pure Phenomenology*. Translated by F. Kersten in 1982. The Hague: Nijhoff.

Linton, Simi. 1998. Disability Studies/Not Disability Studies. *Disability & Society* 13 (4): 525–40.

Meekosha, Helen, and Russell Shuttleworth. 2009. What's So 'Critical' About Critical Disability Studies? *Australian Journal of Human Rights* 15 (1): 47–75.

Mingus, Mia. 2010. 'Changing the Framework: Disability Justice: How Our Communities Can Move beyond Access to Wholeness.' *Resist Newsletter* November/December. Available at: https://leavingevidence.wordpress.com/2011/02/12/changing-the-framework-disability-justice/ (last accessed November 8, 2017).

Morris, Jenny. 1993. Feminism and Disability. *Feminist Review*, 43 (Spring): 57–70.

Oliver, Mike. 1983. *Social Work with Disabled People*. Basingstoke: Macmillan.

———. 1990. *The Politics of Disablement*. Basingstoke: Macmillan.

Oliver, Mike, and Colin Barnes. 2012. *The New Politics of Disablement*. Basingstoke: Palgrave.
Rhoades Cindy, and Philip Browning. 1982. Normalization of a Deviant Subculture: Implications of the Movement to Re-socialize Mildly Retarded People. *Mid-American Review of Sociology* 7 (1): 139–70.
Stanley, Liz, and Sue Wise. 1990. 'Method, Methodology and Epistemology in Feminist Research Processes.' In *Feminist Praxis: Research, Theory and Epistemology in Feminist Sociology*, edited by Liz Stanley, 20–60. London: Routledge.
Wolbring, Gregor. 2012. Expanding Ableism: Taking Down the Ghettoization of Impact of Disability Studies Scholars. *Societies,* 2(3): 75–83.
Wolfensberger, W. 1998. *A Brief Introduction to Social Role Valorization: A High-order Concept for Addressing the Plight of Societally Devalued People and for Structuring Human Services*. 3rd ed. Syracuse, NY: Training Institute for Human Service Planning, Leadership & Change Agentry, Syracuse University.
UPIAS. 1976. *Fundamental Principles of Disability*. London: Union of the Physically Impaired Against Segregation.

PART 2

Body, Care and Sexuality

Chapter 6

Experiencing the Body
Femininity, Sexuality and Disabled Women in India

Nandini Ghosh

INTRODUCTION

Disability Studies has historically emphasized disability politics, by highlighting that individuals with bodily impairments are oppressed by disabling social arrangements, which are a result of the twin processes of discrimination (Barnes 1992) and prejudice (Shakespeare 1994). This structural analysis of oppression treats disablement as a collective experience, wherein disability is seen as a part of a historically constructed discourse and practices of dominant, ableist culture, an ideology of thinking about the body under certain historical circumstances. Davis (1996) says the body is a way of organizing through the realm of the senses, the variations and modalities of physical existence as they are embodied into being through a larger social/political matrix. Disability has profound significance for the self and its embodiment as the day-to-day difficulties of impairment and autonomy actually constitute selfhood by transforming the complex relationships between the self, body image and environment. Impairment emerges only at the intersection of bodies, minds and cultures, and is both an experience and a discursive construction. Impairment enters into the experience and the politics of disability as forms of resistance and the struggle for bodily control, independence and emancipation are embodied. Narratives of lived experience are always partial, locatable, critical knowledges (Harraway 1997), but they are cognitive sites that help us to understand the complexities of the world and how we are constructed in it. The impaired body is a lived body as disabled people experience impairment, as well as disability, as part of a complex interpenetration of oppression and affliction. Disability is experienced in, on and through the body, just as impairment is experienced in terms of the personal and cultural narratives that help to constitute its meaning.

Feminist Disability Studies attempt to understand the ways in which the representational systems of gender, race, ethnicity, ability, sexuality and class mutually construct, inflect and contradict one another and intersect to produce and sustain ascribed, achieved and acquired identities. The simultaneous experience of gender and disability highlights the ways in which bodies interact with socially engineered environments, which includes the natural environment, the built environment, culture, the economic system, the political system and psychological factors and conform to social expectations (Garland-Thomson 1997). The bodies that women experience are always mediated by constructions, associations and images, which most patriarchal sociocultural formations accept and endorse. Patriarchal power and the gaze construct the female body within different sociocultural contexts and power/knowledge discourses by representing female embodiment as inferior to male embodiment (Bordo 1993, 1996). Women come to discipline and survey their own bodies by engaging in practices which produce their own bodies according to the dictates of idealized normative construction of feminine embodiment. As ideal embodied femininity is linked with social acceptability, to have a feminine body—a body socially constructed through the appropriate practices—is most crucial to a woman's sense of herself as a female sexually desiring and desirable subject (Bartky 1992).

As a cultural statement of gender/power relations, a multiplicity of cultural meanings is attributed to the gendered disabled body, which becomes a medium through which the oppressive cultural norms of femininity and ableism are expressed. This chapter explores the multifarious processes through which disabled women internalize social–cultural constructions of the ideal or 'normal' female body, and how such ideas influence their thoughts about and experiences of their bodies in their daily lives. The chapter also seeks to elaborate the ways in which disabled women come to accept and negotiate the demands of an impaired body with the imperatives of a normative femininity, thereby adapting and redefining notions of femininity. The chapter uses primary case studies from India to reflect on the gendered practices used by disabled girls to accommodate the imperatives of their impaired bodies to the prescribed behaviour patterns, which become increasingly important to all girls as they grow up.

CONTEXTUALIZING THE EXPERIENCE OF FEMININITY

Feminist theorists have explored difference, domination and agency in order to understand women's bodily experiences and embodied practices as well to problematize the ways in which different cultures and social contexts construct the female body. Differences between bodies assume great importance in the construction of identities, as the body is historically inscribed with sociocultural meanings derived from cultural values, and for the classification into social groups (Thapan 1995). Dube (1989) and Bagchi (1995) have argued that differences between bodies are culturally produced, inscribed and interpreted through social practices that differentiate between bodies marked by gender, caste, religion and so on. Certain images of gendered bodies in different sociocultural contexts are put forward as the norm and as desirable (Castelnuovo and Guthrie 1998), which is legitimized and reinforced by social institutions like family, and community and State mechanisms such as education, medicine and popular media. These norms associated with issues of power and control become established as the goal towards which multiple and heterogeneous bodies of men and women must aspire (Bordo 1993).

As a cultural statement of gender/power relations, a multiplicity of cultural meanings is attributed to the gendered body, which becomes a medium through which the oppressive cultural norms of femininity are expressed. The imposition of normative femininity upon the female body requires modes of training through disciplinary practices that operate in systems of micro-power that are fundamentally in egalitarian and asymmetrical (Bartky 1992). Thus, disciplinary regimes produce and maintain socially appropriate 'docile' female bodies through constant and repeated inscriptions to conform to the norm (Foucault 1979). The cultural meanings attributed to the female body are concretized through subtle, pervasive and ambiguous processes of discipline and normalization through cultural representations. The female body has been regarded as the primary object through which masculinist power operated as women are oppressed in and through their bodies. In India, the patriarchal cultural discourses impose control over female bodies as a symbol for the community's expression of caste, class and communal honour (Sarkar 1995).

The social and historical settings in which women are located affect the nature of their embodied experience as well as their articulation of it. The female body is, therefore, produced not only through the cultural practices that shape and manipulate the physical body but also through the women's lived experiences of their bodies. All girls internalize, from a young age, this notion of the normal body, the preferred body and the valued body—imbued with particular physical qualities, acceptable attitudes and modes of behaviour and social expectations. Women become conscious of their bodies in terms of size, shape, weight, skin colour and associated characteristics. As the ideal female body is linked with social acceptability, to have an appropriate feminine body is most crucial to a woman's sense of herself as a female sexually desiring and desirable subject (Bartky 1992). Women are forced to be aware of the form and appearance of their bodies and are responsible for creating the surface in accordance with cultural ideals and images dictated by class, race and other cultural iconography (Bordo 1993). Within gendered discourses of femininity, women internalize the cultural constructions of the fashion–beauty complex that glorifies and depreciates the female body simultaneously (Thapan 1997). Therefore, women come to discipline and survey their own bodies by engaging in practices which produce their own bodies according to the dictates of idealized normative construction of feminine embodiment. The power of surveillance enforces discipline through normalization procedures that constrain women by training them to desire such controls through individual self-discipline. Female bodies collude with their oppressors by voluntarily submitting to external regulation, transformation and improvement via exacting and normalizing disciplines of diet, makeup and dress. Women become active producers of their bodies through internalization and pursuit of continually shifting ideals of femininity propagated by cultural and media images advocating self-containment, self-monitoring and self-normalization. Women's bodies come to be tailored, by women, to conform to social ideals which are historically specific (Bartky 1992; Bordo 1995).

Disabled bodies are constructed and interpreted as inactive, passive unproductive and incapable of 'complete' or 'normal' lives. Culturally prescribed appearance norms portray defective bodies as inadequate, and reinforce the traditional conceptualization of the disabled body as deficient and in need of reconstruction or 'improvement' (Begum 1992; Garland-Thomson 1994, 2002). The disciplinary practices of physical normalcy, which are learnt early and unconsciously, create a standard of physical normality, as the disciplines of femininity create the ideal women (Wendell 1996). Feminine body ideals and standardization of female bodies tend towards the normate—the corporeal incarnation of culture's collective, unmarked, normative characteristics (Garland-Thomson 2002). Disabled women are deemed as 'incomplete' women, in terms of both physical appearance and productive and reproductive capacities.

Being 'Normal'

The twin ideologies of normalcy and beauty posit female and disabled bodies as pliable bodies to be shaped infinitely to conform to a set of standards called normal and beautiful. Socialized into such patriarchal ideologies, disabled girls grow up feeling uncomfortable with their own bodies for being deficient and thus not beautiful. The primary focus is on looking or seeming 'normal' while additional onus is to be capable of fulfilling one's productive and reproductive responsibilities within the home. Thus, the thrust for normalization is both gendered and ability-centred—to be able to walk, to look normal and present a feminine self that does not jar with the notion of a complete woman, along with being able to deal with the gendered work responsibilities. The authority assumed by the State and the patriarchal medical and social system are all aimed at normalizing the disabled female body (Meekosha 1998; Silvers 2000). As a result of such ideologies, disabled girls and their families seek 'normalization' through medical and rehabilitation strategies that are often experienced as painful and require long periods of time spent away from the family. Many disabled girls spent months in different rehabilitation centres or hospitals undergoing surgery to enable them to walk 'properly'—these surgical and physiotherapy procedures were sometimes extremely painful but were endured for the future benefit of the girls. Seema, a girl with arthrogryposis, says that she was in hospital for two long years for six surgeries and post-operative treatment to straighten her legs so that she could walk with special shoes and callipers. For girls with more severe impairments, mobility aids were experienced as painful and restrictive and girls, who could not use their callipers at home for daily life activities such as bathing and toileting or even household work, discontinued its use after adolescence when they realized that options for normalization were limited. At home, Sheela crawls to get her chores done faster as she can move with more ease than in her mobility aids.

Further efforts to normalize the body focused on attaining gaits that camouflage the impairment through mobility aids so that disabled girls walk straighter like 'normal' people. Malini says her wish to have a calliper became stronger when she realized that she could walk straight wearing it. Without the calliper she has to walk with a hand to her knee, but that used to emphasize her impairment and call attention to her in public spaces. The mobility aid helped Malini to present herself as 'normal' and like all other women. 'Without my callipers, I would have had to walk with a terribly lopsided gait'. Lekha uses her callipers when she goes out of the home, as she feels more dignified when she is able to project herself as a 'normal' woman. With the coming of modern technology, disabled girls now have a choice of attuning their mobility aids to their feminine self. Seema had been given metallic callipers with black leather boots and she felt 'extremely manly' in them. Lekha and Seema have requested for plastic callipers that can be worn with different shoes and under their clothes, which allows them to express their femininity. 'I am happy that I can wear my calliper inside my clothes when I go out such that the calliper is not visible to all. I bought fashionable sandals to go with the callipers. Now I can wear platform heels also if I want with my calliper'.

Disabled girls are socialized, like all other girls around them, into learning the ideals of physical appearance, appropriate feminine comportment, acceptable behavioural and other qualities and social expectations of their present and future roles. These ideological constructs are further concretized through the social interactions within families and communities. While families silently but subtly direct disabled girls towards more conservative modes of living, the larger community outside generally expresses its pity and disgust openly. Seema says that whenever she goes out of the home crawling, people tell her family members, 'Why do you bring her with so much trouble?' Similarly Sheela narrates, 'They look at my legs and say her life is wasted because she can't walk'. Disabled girls are made to recognize that although they are expected to conform to other 'feminine' norms, they are excluded from gendered notions of sexuality. This affects the ways in which disabled girls experience, adapt and deal with culturally valued notions of femininity, desirability and attractiveness.

For disabled girls, the performance of the gendered identity comes to be felt most acutely during adolescence. The onset of menstrual processes is viewed both in anticipation and trepidation—one to celebrate their womanhood and the other to fear for managing the period. Seema's menses started after all her younger sisters and she found it to be extremely embarrassing. 'Everyone used to ask me if my menses had started. Sometimes I used to worry that I would never become a woman'. On the other hand, Swati, who has severe cerebral palsy, was scared about negotiation of impairments with the periodic needs of her cycle. 'I could not move about during that time, my clothes would get soiled so easily and my mother had lots of extra washing to do'. For these girls with locomotor impairments, thicker pads that remain in place and are difficult to dislodge are the most convenient. Smita feels comfortable using thick cloth pads because of her weak legs and unstable hips. Malini recalls that she used to have more problems during her periods at home as she did not wear the calliper at home. 'Keeping the cloth pad in place was difficult as one of my legs is thin and the muscles don't have much power. Cloth pads are thicker and do not fall out easily or shift fast'.

Socialization into gendered impaired identities means internalizing that disabled women are 'incomplete' and hence do not require feminine adornments in terms of dress or ornamentation. Malini recalls in college, boys of her class used to taunt her, 'see how the disabled girl is dressed up'. She herself started feeling that she should not look feminine and abjured dress codes that signalled her growing femininity. Seema points out that people in her village do not prefer to see her dressed up. 'If I wear good clothes or jewellery they will say, "see the disabled girl, all dressed up". They say many things like, "see how she is and so much of desire to dress up."' Reflecting these attitudes, many disabled women, frustrated by their bodies and their expectations from it, adhere to conservative ways of dressing, choosing clothes that downplay their femininity. Sheela prefers to wear skirts and blouses because it does not hamper her movement by way of crawling. Seema wears nightgowns citing convenience of movement in such clothes. While they cite convenience for adopting adolescent dressing styles, disabled girls express clearly the negation or denial of their sexuality through their adherence to adolescent dress codes. This is one of the reasons why many disabled women shun the traditional saree, not just because it is difficult to manage so much cloth along with the needs of their impairments but also because that is a sign of burgeoning womanhood that is denied to many women with disabilities. Sheela says, 'It is very difficult to crawl around in a sari, as so much of cloth hampers one's movements'. Malini revealed, 'When I wear my calliper, the fold of the saree often gets stuck on the calliper and makes my balance precarious'. Yet for women with mild impairments the saree becomes the tool with which one can conceal the extent to impairment and assume the veneer of normalcy. Malini and Jahanara use the saree to conceal their impairment, and walk slowly to hide the difference in gait.

The female body is implicated in symbolic religio-cultural practices and as part of their socialization into their future roles as wives and mothers, all girls are trained in the socio-religious rituals and practices of families. For disabled girls while such participation is never compulsory, yet participation in such rituals is an assertion of their gender identity. In many families where Lakshmi puja is performed on a daily/weekly basis, disabled girls cite difficulties in performance of rituals as they cannot adhere to notions of cleanliness associated with offering prayers to gods. Girls who crawl or move on their hips find the performance of rituals difficult, as they are unable to adhere to the norms of cleanliness associated with puja. 'As I move by dragging my feet along the ground and holding on to them for keeping my balance, I cannot hold the utensils of the gods in the same hand and touch them to my feet'. Seema is forced to do the rituals when her family goes to visit relatives. 'How will I take the evening puja lamp from room to room?' Thus, for many of these disabled women, the experience of impairment influences their performance of religious rites. Malini rues the fact that she cannot enter most of the temples because of her impairment. Many of the temples can be reached only by climbing long flights of stairs and Malini finds it difficult to negotiate the steep steps in her bare feet (i.e., without her leather shoes and callipers) as temples ban use of leather.

The Labouring Body

Disabled bodies have been seen as incapable of engaging in labour, whether in domestic spaces or in productive work. For disabled women, this becomes a double bind as women are expected to shoulder the domestic responsibilities almost singlehandedly while also contributing to the family income, especially in low-income families both in urban and rural areas. The perceived inability of disabled women to deal with household work becomes a self-serving circle of denial, where disabled girls are denied training in household chores in childhood and adolescence, leading to aspersions on ability to engage with the same work in adulthood. In childhood, families almost always accommodate the impairment of the disabled girl, refusing to allow her to engage in domestic chores like their sisters. 'Mother always used to say "how can she do it?"' Yet in times of distress for the family, disabled girls have to take on more responsibility. When Malini's father lost his job, the whole family started working in piecework to ensure adequate income. Malini, being disabled, was considered unfit for income-generating work, but had to take over the responsibility of cooking for the entire family. She learnt all the household work at this age, from cooking, cleaning, washing to putting mud on walls, tending to their cow, cutting hay and so on. Similarly when Krishna's mother was hospitalized, she had to step into her mother's shoes. 'I was forced to take up all the responsibility for the home then, from cooking to cleaning, washing and supervising the work of the maid at home'.

There is an implicit difference created between the household chores and the labour required to maintain the family, and disabled women are seen as incapable of assuming sociocultural responsibility assigned to women for the entire family and household. Thus, the nature of responsibilities assigned varies depending on the composition of the household and the degree of disability, in case of single women with disabilities, while married women have to deal with all aspects of the domestic/household work, while being castigated as incapable by their natal and affinal families. While single women with disabilities also participate in and take responsibility for all aspects of the household work, their contributions are often negated and relegated to the realm of support rather than primary responsibility. Sheela says, 'I can do anything that can be done sitting down as I don't have any problems with my hands', and assists with the drying and de-husking of paddy, but her sister underscores the fact that she is dependent on others for many things. Similarly Seema, who washes the clothes and utensils for all members of the family at the nearby pond, finds her family highlighting her incapability to carry the dishes and the clothes to and back from the pond. From her childhood, Mita learnt all the household work from cooking, cleaning and washing to putting mud on walls, tending to their cow, cutting hay and so on 'My family always felt I would not be able to cope so I wanted to show them I could'.

Marriage plunges a woman into the realm of adulthood and full responsibility, and married disabled women also have to cope with cooking for the entire family and household work such as cleaning, washing clothes and utensils in their affinal family. Amita has to undertake all the housework from fortifying the house walls with a mixture of cow dung and mud, to cutting vegetables, cooking, cleaning the utensils, washing clothes, bringing water, gathering fuel from the gardens behind the house as well as making *biris* to support the family. Reconciling the performance of the household work with the needs of their impairment is a skill that married women with disabilities develop. When Amita has to fetch water for drinking and cooking from the tube well 500 metres away from their house or carry loads of gathered firewood from the garden, she uses buckets or other such containers to carry water and an improvised trolley cart for the firewood, in order to complete her responsibilities. Zainab uses buckets or other such containers to carry water to her home, especially if neither her husband nor her daughters are available to help her with the task. If husbands are at home and willing, married disabled women request them to fetch the water but mostly, they have to manage by balancing the water-filled containers carefully and walking slowly. Women expect and receive very little help and support from their husbands who, socialized into dominant gender culture ideologies, consider helping with 'womanly' household work demeaning.

For disabled women earning a living is often an imperative in order to survive, but many look for work in order to keep themselves engaged and prove their worth to the family and community around. Disabled women from economically poor families engage in different kinds of work that entail hard labour, despite the connotations of incapability associated with disability, and weakness associated with both gender and disability. Anita worked as a helper in a hotel cutting vegetables, cleaning and washing the utensils and the tables, where no concessions were made for her disability. Aparna used to assist her father in cultivating land that they took on rent, from readying the land by tilling it and breaking the mud into fine soil, to sowing the crop and checking for weeds, and finally to cutting the crop and binding them in bales and also beating them to de-husk the paddy. On his death, for many years she managed farming all by herself. Sulekha almost singlehandedly shoulders the responsibility of making puffed rice for their family business, working for 11 hours every day, frying the rice and packing it in the sacks. Engaging in productive work helps disabled women to challenge ideologies that negate their worth as productive members of the family. Barring the most severely disabled girls, others engage in different kinds of work, based on their capabilities and work that is available locally—from unskilled work like making puffed rice and *biris*, to semi-skilled work like embroidery and tailoring, to working in factories, schools and similar organizations.

The Desiring/Desired Body

Impaired bodies are constructed as incomplete, flawed and undesirable in terms of feminine qualities of beauty, grace and physical perfection. Disabled girls come to learn of their unacceptable, undesirable bodies through the process of socialization during adolescence and adulthood. The childhood and adolescence exhortations by family members towards the disabled girl not to engage in physical labour were as much for accommodating her impairment as for sending the message that her capacity to labour was limited and hence expectations to fulfil the roles and responsibilities that other women had was unavailable to her. Similarly, subtle yet speaking silences within the family convey the clear message that impaired female bodies are not deserving of the patriarchal male gaze or attention. 'I was always made to understand that I was different from my sisters, and could not have the same aspirations'. In Sheela's family, marriage alliances for all of her younger sisters were sought, but no one ever spoke of her marriage. Many of the disabled women with severe disabilities experience an insidious process of de-sexing, which compares the girl with the boys of the family, negating her femininity and sexuality. 'My mother says I am like her son as I will never leave home. I am their elder son and my brother, their younger son'.

The ideal type of the good girl, a woman who is physically unimpaired, beautiful and capable of physical labour, plays an important role in the representation of disabled women as un-marriageable (Ghosh 2016). Impaired female bodies, which are viewed as ugly and disgusting, are also doubted for the capacity to engage in labour to maintain the household. As Seema's mother pointed out, 'can she work like any of us? Who will take care of the household work?' The larger community in which the family and the disabled girl are located are sure that their impairments will interfere with the performance of the role of the lady of the family. Hence, functional capacity becomes one of the primary reasons for disabled girls not being considered fit for marriage. Sheela's sister feared that her sister would not be able to cope with the work at home. 'Which man will feed her for not doing the household chores?' Malini was afraid that she would be beaten up by family members for not being able to complete the household work in time. Amita's mother opined that, 'even good girls are beaten up by their husbands and in-laws, and deserted. My disabled daughter would be worse off if she got married'.

Disabled girls feel that, judged against the imaginary norm of femininity and the ideal *bhalo meye*,[1] they are found wanting in all relationships that allow women to express their sexuality. Ideologies of feminine attractiveness represent impaired bodies and disabled women as undesirable, unfit for attracting the attention of possible partners and incapable of entering relationships that require women to assume roles of wife and mother. For disabled girls also, the imperfection of the impaired bodies becomes the sole reason for their rejection in intimate relationships. Mita says that she never received any proposal from boys because she was disabled. Bred and socialized into patriarchal ideologies that emphasize the desirability of women, disabled girls feel that men experience shame and rejection for having an impaired partner. Sheela felt that her husband would be embarrassed to accompany her in public places. 'If we had to go to a relative's house or a social function, I would have to go with him. Does it look good that I will be crawling beside him? People would stare and pass comments. Will any man like to have a wife like me?' The patriarchal society in which girls are located also teaches them to doubt their capacity to bear and rear children. The body is experienced as restrictive in terms of the expectations from it and fears about its reproductive capacities. Lekha reiterates her mother's opinion, 'how can I perform all the responsibilities of a mother when I cannot even walk? How will I carry my child? How will I rock her to sleep? If she is ill how will I soothe her or take her to the doctor?'

The social negation of their femininity and sexuality is experienced both within families and in the wider public spaces through

---

[1] Here *bhalo meye* means 'good woman', who is both a morally upright woman as well as a woman with all functional capacities required for taking on familial and marital responsibilities.

representations, analogies and pejorative expressions of a disabled identity. The dominant ideologies of acceptable roles of women cast disabled women as dependent, incapable and weak and therefore to be restricted within private spaces. The venturing of disabled women into public spaces is seen as a transgression of norms of acceptability, which is both gendered and ability-centred. Whenever Sheela goes out in public transport, people make her feel as if there is nothing as worse as a disabled woman. 'People say, "oh what a sad thing to happen, if only god had not taken away both legs, if only she could walk, what a punishment for such a beautiful girl". It was as if all my beauty would now be wasted as I cannot walk'. When Lekha crawls along with her family, people often say to them, 'Can't you carry her? Why does she have to crawl?' When Sheela goes to board a vehicle, co-passengers wanting to help her grab her arms, not realizing that if they hold her hands, she will not be able to move at all. The gaze is experienced more sharply for disabled girls whose impairment is clearly visible and Lekha recalls being aware of being stared at all her life. 'But if I go out of the house crawling, instead of with the callipers, more people would stare at me'.

Norms of appropriate behaviour, however, are used to curb the freedom of disabled girls, with threats of loss of reputation as a 'good girl'. Disabled girls experiencing their bodies as restrictive in sexual relations, find their freedom further restrained in terms of protecting their reputation as a morally upright woman. Seema's mother told her, 'If some boy forces his attention on you, everyone will blame you that you cannot control yourself'. Lekha's mother urged her not to incite or excite the local boys, who used to heckle her. '*Ma* says ignore them as they are like dogs and will stop barking after some time. I know it is my fate to listen to such things'. Fear of being shamed and ostracized because of reputation as a 'loose' disabled woman prevented girls from interacting with boys in the public sphere. Seema revealed that she has consciously never allowed any man to get close to her. 'How can I? Just imagine, people would say, "she is like that and look, how she is flirting with boys"'. Sheela does not talk to men and boys, because rumours about her liaisons with them could ruin her reputation in the village. 'Mother says, what will happen if my disabled daughter's reputation is maligned?' The onus of maintaining their reputation as 'good girl' in the moral sense is doubly important for disabled women, as they feel that they already have lost status as a physically and functionally perfect woman. Despite the denial of their sexuality, disabled women fear repercussions, both physical and social, over any sexual attention that they might receive. The process of negation and denial of the sexuality of disabled women proceeds from suppression within the household to encounters in the public sphere, that serve to reinforce the ideologies and lead to withdrawal of disabled women, sometimes reluctantly, from the arena of sexuality (Ghosh 2016).

CONCLUSION

For girls and women with disabilities, the sociocultural ideologies around gendered disabled bodies influence the experiences of their bodies in different domains of everyday life and social contexts. Impaired bodies are experienced as both equal to and yet different from other female bodies—while women with bodies marked by impairment always interpret their bodies from the lens of gender, they also turn the internalized able-bodied gaze on themselves to interpret their everyday lived experiences as fraught by barriers to gendered performances. Disabled girls attempt to carve out a feminine self, according to the dictates of the socially acceptable representations, thereby modifying and justifying such performances as dependent on the exigencies of their bodily impairments. Thus, disabled femininity is constructed, nurtured and contested within the domains of the sociocultural valuation of bodies and the ideas around the activities and practices in which such bodies are to be implicated. While most disabled women accept their impaired bodies as something which is devalued and 'wanting' in day-to-day practice, the impaired female body engages in all of the activities and practices that govern daily lives of these women.

In the performance of a normative femininity within the demands of an impaired body, disabled women redefine the ideal of an acceptable body and performance in different aspects of their lives, according to the imperatives of their impairments. Such redefinitions are allowed by family and community, with the unspoken control over their expressions of sexuality and femininity. The ideal type of a 'good girl' looms large in lives of women with disabilities, and is interpreted as women who conform to and actualize the ideal notions that the gender culture attributes to women, even if they do not possess unimpaired 'normal' bodies. Thus, disability structures the lived experiences of disabled women, in terms of fulfilling the expectations from female bodies, in terms of beauty and appearance and in the expected roles of productive and reproductive responsibilities. The devaluation of impaired female bodies in every domain of life ensure that disabled women are pushed into the margins of society.

REFERENCES

Bagchi, Jasodhara, ed. 1995. *Indian Women: Myth and Reality*. Kolkata: Sangam Books.

Barnes, C. 1992. *Disabling Imagery and the Media: An Exploration of Media Representations of Disabled People*. Belper: The British Council of Organisations of Disabled People.

Bartky, Sandra Lee. 1992. 'Foucault, Femininity and the Modernisation of Patriarchal Power.' In *Feminist Philosophies*, edited by J. Kourany, J. P. Sterba and R. Tong. Upper Saddle River, NJ: Prentice Hall.

Begum, Nasa. 1992. 'Disabled Women and the Feminist Agenda.' *Feminist Review* 40 (Spring): 70–84.

Bordo, Susan. 1993. 'Feminism, Foucault and the Politics of the Body.' In *Up Against Foucault*, edited by C. Ramazanoglu. London: Routledge.

———. 1995. 'Reading the Slender Body.' In *Feminism and Philosophy*, edited by N. Tuana and R. Tong. Boulder, CO: West View Press.

———. 1996. 'Anorexia Nervosa.' In *Women, Knowledge and Reality: Explorations in Feminist Philosophy*, edited by A. Garry, and M. Pearsall. New York, NY: Routledge.

Castelnuovo, S., and S. R. Guthrie. 1998. *Feminism and the Female Body: Liberating the Amazon Within*. Boulder, CO: Lynne Rienner Publishers.

Davis, Kathy. 1996. 'From Objectified Body to Embodied Subject.' In *Feminist Social Psychologies*, edited by S. Wilkinson. Buckingham: Open University Press.

Dube, Leela. 1989. 'On the Construction of Gender: Hindu Girls in Patrilineal India.' In *Socialisation, Education and Women: Explorations in Gender Identity*, edited by Chanana Karuna. New Delhi: Orient Longman.

Foucault, M. 1979. *Discipline and Punish*. New York, NY: Pantheon Books.

Garland-Thomson, R. 1994. 'Redrawing the Boundaries of Feminist Disability Studies.' *Feminist Studies* 20 (3): 583–97.

———. 1997. *Extraordinary Bodies: Figuring Physical Disability in American Culture and Literature*. New York, NY: Columbia University Press.

Garland-Thomson, R. 2002. 'Integrating Disability, Transforming Feminist Theory.' *NWSA Journal* 14 (3): 1–32.

Ghosh, Nandini. 2016. *Impaired Bodies Gendered Lives: Everyday Realities of Disabled Women*. New Delhi: Primus Books.

Harraway, D. 1997. 'Gender for a Marxist Dictionary: The Sexual Politics of a Word.' In *Feminist Readings*, edited by L. McDowell and J. P. Sharpe. London: Arnold.

Meekosha, H. 1998. 'Body Battles: Bodies, Gender and Disability.' In *The Disability Studies Reader: Social Science Perspectives*, edited by T. Shakespeare. London: Cassell.

Sarkar, Tanika. 1995. 'Hindu Conjugality and Nationalism.' In *Indian Women: Myth and Reality*, edited by J. Bagchi. Kolkata: Sangam Books.

Shakespeare, T. 1994. 'Cultural Representation of Disabled People: Dustbins for Disavowal?' *Disability and Society* 9 (3): 283–99.

Silvers, Anita. 2000. 'Disability.' In *A Companion to Feminist Philosophy*, edited by A. Jaggar and I. M. Young. Oxford: Blackwell.

Thapan, Meenakshi. 1995. 'Gender, Body and Everyday Life.' *Social Scientist* 23 (7–9, July–September): 32–58.

——— ed. 1997. *Embodiment: Essays on Gender and Identity*. New Delhi: Oxford University Press.

Wendell, Susan. 1996. *The Rejected Body: Feminist Philosophical Reflections on Disability*. New York, NY: Routledge.

Chapter 7

Emergence of Epistemological Questions of Crip Queer across Shifting Geo/Bio-political Terrain

Janet Price and Niluka Gunawardena

Over the last decade, mainstream discourse around disability in South Asia and globally has had a broad political focus aligned to the material restrictions and prejudice faced by disabled people. Sexuality/disability was limited to a framing by special interest groups, and wherever questions were raised globally, there was little apparent geographic variance in the normatively structured conceptualizations of the non-sexual, non-reproductive disabled adult or, conversely, the perversely sexual individual with intellectual or psychosocial disabilities. The discourse oscillated between these two settings, overlain by a gendering which added the desire for but impossibility of motherhood for disabled women. Disabled people continued to be viewed, not universally and without exception but in most places and contexts, as heteronormative yet without desire, unmarriageable and unable as well as unsafe to bear and rear children (Addlakha et al. 2017).

Yet, such apparent uniformity of perception and conceptualization negates regional specificities of sex, sexuality, identity and expression, especially in the context of post-colonial subjectivities. It is misguided to speak of universal embodied norms and hence by virtue, universal abjections, when there is no absolute, hegemonic narrative discourse of an ideal embodied being.

Through this chapter, we hope to tell stories of people's experiences of sexuality and disability over time in South Asia,[1] building a disability–sexuality epistemological framework of embodiment and desire that, whilst structured by South Asian knowledge and positionalities, is informed by extant discursive analysis in the North. Avoiding the creation of a grand narrative, we investigate what insights a geo-specific focus can bring to understandings of non-normative subjectivities (national, corporeal and desirous) and offer new ways in which disability–sexuality can be used as a contextual and locational analytical lens to build new knowledge. This is not to discount the discursive influence of geodisability knowledge like international medical discourses and Hollywoodized notions of desirability and bodily cohesion, rather it is to investigate both regional narratives of disability and sexuality and explore localized manifestations of such global narratives in South Asia.

OVERLAPPING MOVEMENTS

Existing epistemologies of disability–sexuality are largely informed by critical disability studies, post-modern and post-colonial scholarship and queer studies, and the field is strongly interdisciplinary and malleable in its scope, historically located yet with resonances in the present. Although not widely recognized as a single field of enquiry, there is an emerging analytic field, focused not only upon the crucial figure of the 'queercrip' but rather drawing upon a growing body of work that aims to understand how disability–sexuality works across terrains and through time to make the world 'otherwise' (McRuer 2006).

---

[1] The plan for the chapter was to incorporate India, Pakistan, Bangladesh and Sri Lanka as the main foci of the chapter with acknowledgment of a wider geographical spread to Nepal and Myanmar. However, the limitations of writing from disabled embodiment have reduced our scope.

In *Disability Nationalism in Crip Times*, McRuer (2010) aims to build a tentative and speculative understanding of post-colonial and transnational theories by weaving together moments of importance to the development of queer and crip thought. We summarize them here to offer a background and then, in the following section(s), proceed to rework them around contextualized findings.

NORTHERN MO(VE)MENTS

The first moment is marked for McRuer by 'opposition' and 'binary modes', following the argument that the emergence of industrialization in Europe in the late 1700s led to the naturalization of heterosexuality and of gender, with women's role affirmed within the domestic space of the home against the public workspace. The solidification of the oppositional divide between labouring space and domestic provided for the emergence of homosexual acts between men and allowed for the drawing of a distinction between male industrial and social roles and those of the home-caring female, thus enabling the naturalization of heterosexually distinct roles and locations around home/work/leisure.

This industrial stimulus also marked, for disability studies, the time of the emergence of the social model, tying disability to oppositional expectations of an able and 'fit' labouring body, masculine, naturalized as heterosexual. The disabled body was effectively a broken male body, gendered female in its inadequacies, within the public gaze (Shildrick and Price 1996). The solidification of female domestic space provided a site for the care and nurture of young, old and disabled bodies, further naturalizing gender roles, aided by the displacement of rural structures of interdependency in home and work, both across gender and dis/ability.[2]

---

[2] The solidification of the oppositional divide between labouring space and domestic provided for the emergence of homosexual acts between men and allowed, as John D'Emilio (1983) proposed in what McRuer (2006: 166) refers to as the classic "Capitalism and Gay Identity", for the drawing of a distinction between male industrial and social roles and those of the home-caring female, thus enabling the naturalization of heterosexually distinct roles and locations around home/work/leisure.

The second movement of 'alterity' and 'difference' works to check the notion that sexual binaries and homo/heterosexual identities will be found in similar modes all across the world. Scholars and activists working across the Global South from Western scripts have produced counter-narratives of gendered identity and embodiment that set tradition against modernity, transforming and at times exoticizing postcolonial histories. McRuer holds, 'if homosexual identity emerges in the West, we should not automatically expect to find it in other places and times' (2010, 168). Processes of compulsory heterosexuality must, of necessity, be disrupted, gendered/disabled identities acknowledged as located and specific. Although expanding, disability politics globally does not produce the same (non)disabled identities everywhere in response to compulsory abled-bodiedness. The UN Convention for Rights of People with Disabilities advances its global advocacy, yet, despite refusing a fixed definition of disability, it aims at identical subjects rendered global, only for them to re-emerge non-identical, within different times and places.

McRuer's third moment is one of what he terms 'generative incoherence'. He argues we should neither 'expect to find "homosexual identity" in other times and places' nor particularly coherently in the West' (2010, 168). Gendered hetero/homosexual embodiment are established, if at all, as unstable situations, in shifting, adaptive moments, whilst different regions, other cities of the world share the delights and secrets of their unfolding, ever-changing 'cultures of desire', each offering novel encounters with the potentials of queer life (p. 168). Within the LGBTQ[3] clubs and cafes, a reliable, gay identity cannot be found, neither in the West nor in other times and places. As queer cultures flourish under economic globalization, these gay cultures may have more to share with each other—as Halberstam says, a 'metronormativity'—than with other non-heteronormative people within their state. And the groups found in rural areas/small towns may themselves share more at what Akhil Katyal terms a 'regional level', not geographic so much as 'a traffic of signs and forms of culture (2010, p. 24)'. Specific cultures/places/times meanwhile reveal transgender lives and 'other

---

[3] Lesbian, Gay, Bisexual, Trans, Queer (LGBTQ).

non-identical queer modes of being' at the centre of negotiating the emergence of gendered fluidity (p. 168).

With disability, McRuer suggests that although moments that establish new knowledge forms have less clarity, it is possible to identify the emergence of 'metropolitan' disabled identities that are located globally but with differing understandings such as the ever-strengthening but always shifting figure of the UN advocated 'person with disabilities' and the para-athletes whose performance highlights disabled exceptionalism.

The fourth moment marks the 'uneven bio-political incorporation' of both gay and disabled men and women against histories of colonization, independence and the creation of new nation-states. (McRuer 2010, 168). At moments of scarcity, terror or national/local disruption, Puar (2007) argues these bodies are marked by queer, bio-political and necropolitical processes, simultaneously targeting some for life and some for death. Globalization, fundamentalist ideologies and the spread of fear constitute bodies of colour, queer and anomalous bodies as anti-national, contagious and terrorist lookalikes, a tendency exacerbated by Trump's American presidency. And whilst homonational ideals feed the narrow dreams of queer conformism, increasingly incorporating right-wing anti-Muslim views (Sircar 2017), it is the 'able disabled', those readily integrated into nationalist fantasies of normalcy and neoliberal cultural imaginaries of productivity who escape the destructive tentacles of the web of globalization as it pulls in those deemed excessive, targeted by maldevelopment, for quarantine or elimination (Mitchell w Snyder 2015).

SOUTH ASIAN EPISTEMOLOGIES

Whilst McRuer has offered us a strong base to begin analysis of disability–sexuality epistemologies, we are wary of simply following his script and nor would he propose we do so. The complex history of sexuality in South Asia has received close attention from religious/spiritual, postcolonial and sexuality scholars but disability histories within South Asia have received comparatively limited attention. Miles (2001) argues,

> The emergence of Asian disability materials, embodying concepts and practices based far from the historical European roots in Semitic religion,

Greek philosophy and Roman law, underlines the dangers of constructing 'universal' theories on a Eurocentric experience base.

What he ignores, however, is the manner in which over time and with travel, from medieval times and even earlier, culture came to incorporate not only European but also Chinese and East Asian influence. Whilst drawing on historical material we mark rather a foray into analyses of how sexuality–disability in South Asia, the related discursive trends, embodied experience and social dynamics of this intersectional terrain may offer ways of interpreting and intervening in the world differently, of 'becoming', along other pathways.

First Move: Categorical Generation of Anomalous Embodiments

Foucault (1990) and other scholars asserted, although not without contention, that it was only into the late 19th century that distinct forms of sexual-emotional categories that divided individuals between 'heterosexual' and 'homosexual' spaces were identified. They suggest that in earlier periods, although people performed sexual acts with both same-sex and other-sex partners, they did not acquire separately labelled identities. Scholars of the history, sexuality and oral/textual traditions of the South Asian geographical region offer a divergent analysis of the history of same-sex love, desire and relationships. Within both male and female lives, same-sex relationships have been written about, exalted and presented in many contexts, across a wide geographic range, as companionate and sometimes sexual friendships, preferable to male–female marriage, which was primarily for the purpose of procreation (Charu 2010; Vanita 2012). Unlike the oft-repeated claim that it was the Muslims who brought homosexuality to India, scripts and oral poetry dating from the second-century BCE through the mediaeval and colonial era and into the present include stories of same-sex love (Vanita 2012). They speak of individuals within named categories—taxonomies of local and esoteric terminology for same sex relations—that identify not simply sexual acts but desire, ways of living, roles, creation of relationships, fluid gender status and sex changes, same-sex births and acceptance of all these shifts within a wider community.

Interwoven with these tales are indications of shifting forms of embodiment, particularly the emergence of the Hindu and Buddhist deities bearing many limbs, multiple heads or animal tails. Understood through the epics as godlike, these multiple, anomalously embodied 'monstrous' beings bear spiritual powers yet carry human resemblances, both not-I and I. They serve to shake the secure and proper boundaries of human being, opening individuals to vulnerability, unpredictability whilst occupying a liminal space, interweaving the magical and demonic. As Shildrick argues in *Embodying the Monster* (2002), a productive reading of such corporeality reveals not simple oppositions but rather the ambiguity of the monstrous other who haunts the self-same. Haraway writes of 'queering what counts as nature' (1992, 300), the interweaving of human/deity that can be perceived through a disability framework, something that interestingly has been little developed by Asian academics except Ghai (2002). Widely recognized by current-day worshippers who identify newborn children, normatively diagnosed disabled, as reincarnations of deities, such as Lakshmi, born with multiple limbs, who became Vishnu in the eyes of those queuing long hours to worship her (*Evening Standard* 2007).

The generation of shape-shifting and fluid deities often occurs in a queering of heterosexual reproduction, sometimes generated by paternal shape shifting and play as and when Vishnu assumes his beautiful Mohini form to which Shiva is attracted and, in a Dravidian/Puranic legend, they have intercourse, Vishnu bears a child (Vanita 2000a). The power of the symbolic doubling of 'maternal imagination' and the eros generated by two queens creates Bhagirath, born without bones as a 'blob' of matter, of skin, flesh and mucus, an embodiment without the necessity for male intervention (Vanita 2000b). His morphology signals the co-tangibility of his generation from the eros of the meeting of two 'yonis' which, when rendered into his fleshy corporeality, represents 'the memory of the intimacy of mucus' (Irigaray 1993, 170).

Shildrick notes that from the 16th century, texts in Europe cite sources back to Hippocrates and Aristotle as highlighting maternal imagination or maternal impression as the cause of infant anomaly. Whilst mild variations such as birthmarks were put down to a desire for strawberries, for example, the birth of infants with 'grossly disordered morphology' was 'taken as evidence of far more dangerous and disruptive passions' (Shildrick 2002, 33). In addition, in Western eyes, the joining of two women in desire was deeply disruptive. However, South Asian histories suggest that this queering of desire as two women come together was not such a fearful site of disorder but perhaps more a field marked by the power of the doubling of eros. Familiar with the fluidity of symbolic manifestations of the deities and living through era where sexuality itself was accepted as fluid multiplicity, the generation of figures replicating rare and thus magical forces offered—and continues to provide—ongoing symbolic protection against the many vulnerabilities experienced in day-to-day life.

In researching specific examples of disabled sexuality, scholars such as Ghai (2002, 2015, 65–66) early identified figures within religious history and myth that linked disabled figures with sexuality whilst postcolonial scholars of sexuality such as Thadani (1996, 116) highlighted ancient sculptural figures of corporeal excess within temple architecture, engaged in sexual activities. Such anomalously embodied presentations have rarely been identified as figures of disability, escaping from any binary of non/disabled or cripped identification and rather existing in non-identical moments of cripqueering. This enables indigenous epistemologies and cosmologies across South Asia, folk and animist systems of belief and major regional religions—Hinduism, Buddhism and Islam—with their attendant rituals, relations and practices, to develop localized spatio-temporal hierarchies of these liminal anomalous bodies and fluid sexualities. Found within temple and shrine architecture, a space of sexual performance is created in which any attempt to distinguish between hetero- and homosexual acts dissolves. Non-normative embodiments are imbued with exceptionality and assigned desirability or undesirability through cultural narratives. Perceivably transgressive desires for excessive bodies are found widely in folklore and religious narratives, often in the form of myths surrounding exceptional characters such as small people, multi-limbed demigods and other 'others' with extraordinary corporeal forms or skills deemed fantastical outside the context of such narratives. Yet this discursive ordering of subjectivities is significantly shaped and conditioned by a regionally specific form of ontological dissonance. Ideologies of contagion, virtue, contamination and (im)purity, including karmic narratives of embodied immor(t) ality, exceptionalize corporealities by virtue of their non-normative attributes, often 'read' in symbolic terms.

The ongoing repetition of familiar religio-symbolic devices is based on a narrative framework that is not individualistic in its nature and orientation. Rather, it is a discursive framework that regulates and manages bodies and desires in a collective manner. Transgressive desires and the desire for transgressive bodies are given meaning through interwoven values—exemplary, holy, deviant and immoral—produced/productive through ethno-religious narratives. These require an understanding of the wider cosmologies of embodied normativity and desire in South Asia which, understood through the lens of disability–sexuality, raise questions that, despite the growing strength of disability discourse in the region, have rarely been addressed.

Second Move: Colonial Eugenics and Discursive Nationalisms

These cosmological narratives unwind and travel through to the present day, inflecting disability/sexuality. However, back in the 18th and 19th centuries, the geopolitics of European colonialism within South Asia was propagated through exploration and trade, a process that mirrored the relationships established by China and countries of the East. Unlike them, European intentions expanded to the establishment of trading centres, economic control via the East India Company and, ultimately, military invasion and the establishment of imperial rule. These 'eugenic colonial' processes worked through rules of hierarchical differentiation, marking indigenous populations by a racial ableism, which excluded them from privileges of citizenship. Cast as subjects not citizens, their labour generated imperial profit, their reproduction a supply of workers and consumers to help build trade, and of fighters to protect European possessions, such that individuals were subsumed within disciplinary regimes managed by a burgeoning bureaucracy.

The bio-politics of South Asia incorporated notions of Oriental sexuality, a source of fascination to the West for 'its sensuality, its tendency to despotism, its aberrant mentality, its habits of inaccuracy, its backwardness' (Said 1978, 205). Through the continual reproduction of historical and geographical codes of thought, discourses and images, the Orient, as Said argued, solidified its epistemological coherence as strange and foreign whilst reflecting an image that enabled the West to see itself as superior, democratic and justified in its rule. Yet, Westerners looked to precisely this distinction of Orient from Occident for a less rule-bound, more erotic and guiltless experience of sexuality in the early 20th century.

In 1857, the Indian war of independence shifted the power balance and led to attacks on indigenous cultures. Prior to this, cities such as Lucknow, Delhi and Lahore had a flourishing Indo-Persian culture and were the sites of a hybrid network of shifting sexual and emotional relationships involving courtesans, nawabs, poet-scholars, householders and servants. These were cities where women and men indulged in 'pleasure, play and fun', publicly sharing their love and desire through songs and the ghazals. And, in more private spaces, 'rekhti', poetic conversations, served, as Vanita (2012) argues, as a route to the ambiguous, more private, female–female relationships that proliferated between the beloved and her lover.

Simultaneously, the enforcement of race norms and regulation of proximity between Indians and Britons meant that planters, settlers and other colonial officials who had previously established long-term affairs, even marriage with their Indian 'bibis' were widely discouraged. They deserted Indian wives and abandoned their Anglo-Indian children (Ghosh 2006). Mixed-gender and race encounters were viewed as amoral, illegitimate and obscene by the migrating Christian missionaries. With the British colonial takeover, alterity and fluidity were replaced by a more oppositional and fixed social make-up of bourgeois, predetermined gender and sexual roles, with a strong disapproval of homosexuality. Mirroring other European powers, the missionaries extended their proselytizing Puritan zeal and imposed a new order of moral hygiene across local societies. Heterosexual same-race/class marital relationships were established as the disciplinary norm, with oppositional gendered roles for men and women very firmly distinguished, similar to, but never the same as, those they mirrored in the West.

The 1850s saw a strengthening of the colonial desire to regulate and discipline the sexual, moral and hygienic practices of the lower ranks of the army, British and Indian, including of the sex workers they used, both in the UK and across the Empire. Prescriptive hygiene practices for troops were accompanied by Contagious Disease legislation (1864 to: UK Repeal 1886; India Repeal 1915) that instituted medico-legal forces establishing new norms of able-bodies fit for an imperial future against malnourished, infection-prone, morally inadequate and sexually contagious working-class men and women (Mort 1987). By this period, Said argued, '"Oriental sex" was as standard a commodity as any other available in the mass culture', increasingly uniform, managed as a utility, tied by a web of demands and expectations, much as with sexual relationships in the West (1978, 190). Resistance emerged through major campaigns against the legislation on moral and scientific grounds, led by maternal imperialists such as Josephine Butler, not only freeing individuals but serving to resist the mapping of neighbourhood and community terrain through bio-political means (Burton 1990; Mort 1987).

The late 19th and first half of the 20th centuries in South Asia, up to and following independence of the nation-states from colonial power, were marked by major geo-spatial, ideological and corporeal shifts. Borders of terrain and community, desires fulfilled or denied and millions of individual bodies were all incorporated into efforts to maintain a hegemonic order of able heteronormative bodies. With the growing pressures of communal violence, the struggle for order served to simultaneously create and obliterate disability. Intervening in these discursive trends, the ideological and disciplinary practices of eugenics revealed the hegemonic desire for perfectible bodies in intersection with colonial discourses of race and with localized narratives of nationalist and religious corporeal ideals and typologies. The early 20th-century growth in eugenic groups across India, notably in Madras, Mysore, Shimla and Lahore, discursively built notions of morality and racial purity, initiating campaigns for improvement in heritable quality and for birth control (Ahluwalia 2010). In both categories of sexuality and disability, this pre-independence period saw caste, race and religious distinctions increase in power within the wider India. An emphasis on oppositional strains between self/other, gender norms surrounding the figure of the ideal protector of wife and community, an increased divisiveness between religions, and able-bodied norms that emphasized the position of the racially, physically and socially fit as opposed to the eugenically unfit and ill-bred individual together brought about a major push towards a remapping of the Indian population and of the land.

These norms structured colonial bureaucratic expectations of indigenous deviations from the ideal. Hindu and Muslim civilizations were seen as degenerate, the women as abject and many men as effeminate, in comparison to the valorized masculine ideals of colonial powers (Chakravarti 1989). Much preferred by colonial leaders, martial races such as the Sikhs were constituted as fit, strong and capable, given positions within the army, and held as standing ready to defend their land. In comparison, the Bengali babu or clerk occupied a position about which a feeling of effeminacy—*chakri*—was fostered. Small and weak, near-sighted from office work and unable/unprepared to offer protection, they were viewed as a perverted, 'artificial and unnatural class of persons' (Sinha 1995, 5). Colonial approaches to social reform of the status of women into the 20th century led by Hindu caste reformers and middle classes looked to the regulation of female sexuality and the upholding community honour. Whilst the British focused on child marriage and sati as examples of necessary reform, within Hindu caste groups women were seen as 'guardians' of the 'race' and upholders of caste status. As the 'idealised *pativrata*', she herself entered into gender and sexual reform with zeal (Gupta 2001, 8, 24). However, women took on a greater moral load within all communities, Hindu, Muslim and Sikh, and any threat to their sexual purity came to be seen as a threat to and dilution of the race and to the idea of nation, as the struggle for independence across pre-independence South Asia grew.

This was followed, in turn, by the violence against nation, community and self that scarred the periods of India/Pakistan partition and independence. This ontological violence of ableist heteronormativity was addressed through the interstices of the post/colonial partitioning and fracturing of the nation-state, utilizing discourses of embodied statehood and nationalist cohesion. On the one hand, the notion of Bharat Mata, Mother India, strengthened as a rallying cry as independence struggles grew. The anthropomorphized maternal nation, representing female purity, self-sacrificing nurture and fertility, was a high caste maternal figure, deemed post-desire, desexualized (Naaz 2017).

She was never 'a Dalit Bahujan or Adivasi or Muslim or tribal woman or that of any other minority community. She must belong to not only the upper caste but upper class too' (Singh 2016). This ideological female form served as a route for some Hindu men, via the expression of a hyper-masculinized identity, to wreak violence and shed blood in the name of shoring up India's metaphorical and actual boundaries. This contributed to the fighting around independence and the horrors of partition, whilst the symbolic link between the fertile mother and the prosperous nation tied Indian men to a filial role whose duty was to revere, protect and help build the state.

Divisions between the religious communities, fostered by the British, climaxed at partition, when many millions found themselves religiously on what was regarded as the wrong side of the new state borders and, as people moved state, hundreds of thousands were killed and injured on all sides—women, men and children, Hindus, Muslims and Sikhs. The widespread rape of women during partition, within the boundaries of the new nations of India and Pakistan, was likewise seen as an attack by the Muslim and Hindu/Sikh races respectively upon the integrity of the new nations themselves, bringing shame to communities and undermining notions of national and individual autonomy. The newly independent nations were constituted of the productive and resistant terrain and boundaries drawn upon the broken and sexually violated bodies of women, marked by the loss of the land necessary to the country's full embodied identity, much as a disabled body may be understood as marked by loss. Tied to concepts of honour and purity was a demand for silence about the violation of women that still affects all three of these countries (Menon and Bhasin 1998). The Bangladesh Liberation War against West Pakistan, leading to independence in 1971, also saw mass atrocities, major loss of life and injury, and genocidal rape of women. Eugenically focused massacres of students, intelligentsia, religious minorities and armed personnel extended imperial necropolitical targeting (Wikipedia 2017). The internal struggles in Sri Lanka between Tamil and Sinhalese grew in part from colonially instituted and eugenically inspired divisions linked to nation building that set the different ethnic groups against each other, again fighting through the figures of women and the ideals of purity, fertility, respectability and authenticity (De Mel 1996; Sabaratnam 2010). And the broken figure of

'Bharat Mata', of woman-as-nation, continues as a symbol of disability affecting the nations of Pakistan and India, with Kashmir continuing to the present day as the unhealed wound within the conjoined body.

Third: Metropolitan Moves and Local Expressions

Ongoing challenges against the continuing encroachment of remnants of colonial laws such as those against gay men's relationships and against disability regulations developed into a 'period of intensification in the early 1990s that advanced strategies for the recuperability of previously abjected forms of bodily difference' (Puar 2014). Many countries in South Asia follow histories and quotidian specificities of embodied existence that serve to influence emerging distinctions and alterities in sexual and disabled representations, structuring epistemologies that influence issues such as identity politics, citizenship and justice.

As McRuer (2010) points out, post-colonial scholars seek to ensure that a Western homo/hetero-sexual binary is not automatically replicated in states of the South Asia. 'Moments of alterity' arise through non-normative figures such as the hijra, *kothi*, gay and lesbian, *shamopremee nari* and *du-gana*[4] across different historical contexts, different countries with Muslim, Buddhist, Christian and Hindu citizens. A 'generative incoherence' of moments of becoming reveals fluid and unstable positionalities across sexuality and disability in response to glocalized changing economic and social pressures and as those in the present reach back and reclaim namings from the past. Looking back 40 years, Thadani points out sexuality in India was understood through individualized and personal sexual activities. Women from small towns referred to the pleasures of 'lesbo-sex' (Thadani 1997), a privatized practice taking place in local beauty salons, whilst men had

---

[4] Hijra (assigned male at birth, having a feminine gender expression and able to avail of a 'third gender' legal status), *Kothi* (assigned male at birth, 'receptive' partner, having a feminine gender expression), gay and lesbian (male or generic homosexual and female homosexual roles), *shamopremee nari* (woman loving woman Bangla), *du-gana* (two women who splice and eat a doubled nut or fruit, with the 'masculine' and 'feminine' roles being arbitrarily assigned to each depending on the part each happens to get). S. P. Shah, 2015; Hena, 2012; Vanita, 2012, 139.

more established terminology to draw upon—*Kothi, Panthi*[5]—describing the roles each partner played during sex. Expression of a 'gay/lesbian' identity was questioned as a Western imposition,[6] even as it began to become established in cities, in part linked to the economic liberalization moving across South Asia (Karimjee 1987). Sexuality was simultaneously viewed by right-wing groups as a degenerative and amoral influence on religious values, by doctors as an illness requiring psychiatric intervention, by left-leaning feminists as an irrelevance (Ghosh 2011), and by indigenous radical feminists as a struggle against the compulsory heterosexuality of South Asia that demanded local terminologies appropriate to Indian cultural homo/sociality. Meanwhile, in 1993 the self-identified lesbian organization Sakhi noted the rapid loss and physical destruction of 'gynefocal, matrilineal and lesbian histories' and mythology, traditions of the peripheries, of rural areas (Thadani 1996, 120). This knowledge was often specific to small areas and mutable over time rather than permanently fixed. Shortly after this report, the release of the film *Fire* by Deepa Mehta about a lesbian couple stirred anger and fear amongst the right-wing BJP about moral contagion and the potential wildfire spread of lesbianism, yet the protest was countered by supportive rallies, not only women identifying in public as lesbian, perhaps for the first time visible in India) but also protests in favour of free speech (Ghosh 2011). The gradual re/emergence of sexual identities, both historical and new, rather than the labelling of sexual behaviour was parried by attacks on and the loss of images and stories of same-sex identity and activities from past to present, of individuals committing suicide, as the societal elimination both spread and was fed by fear of the contagion.

In the previous decade as HIV spread within South Asia in the context of broadly negative public opinion, small liberal elites of 'out' LGBT individuals were identified within an unevenly constituted

---

[5] *Panthi* (male 'non-receptive' partner, often identified in relation to kothis); Shah (2015, 649).

[6] Karimjee's work, 'The Eastern Disease?/The Western Disease?' shows culture specific images of herself together with text describing sex between women through both orientalist and lesbian feminist frames. She was the first woman living in the UK from a Muslim background to publish an 'Out' piece of lesbian work (Gupta 1996: 173–74).

population of 'MSM', many impoverished, and enumerated and regulated by HIV discourse, a language of sex, illness, disability and death. The increasingly governmental HIV/AIDS development discourse affected not only identifying 'MSM' but also sex workers, injecting drug users, migrant workers, members of the trans-population and married 'MSM', bringing together wide-ranging non-identical queercrip individuals negotiating their positionalities in relation to the ambivalence of sexual and disability rights identities. Later, in India, the campaign for repeal of Section 377, the 'sodomy' clause which led to heavy criminalization and police harassment served to help many focus in this disparate community, providing legitimate causes for campaign and serving to build confidence, alliances and identities in their demands for rights, care and decriminalization (Misra 2009).

In the late 1980s, across most of South Asia, disability was structured as a welfare or medical concern, underlain by belief in locally informed religion and superstition. Disability organizations, largely led by non-disabled people, met the needs of single impairment groups such as blind or deaf people. Charitable by nature, such groups ran residential institutions and educational and development programmes, practices tied into colonial investments in the region. Institutionalization was and continues to be, on the one hand, a profoundly desexualizing experience, particularly for disabled women, supported by the stories of mass sterilization of inmates (Paryay 1994) and of women in a mental institution being left naked in the ward (Women with Disabilities India Network 2012). However, as Foucault argued, sexuality is rather the focus of close attention, monitoring, management and regulation at every level (Foucault 1990). Those institutionalized are punished for any evidence of contact with the other sex, taught to perceive themselves as non-sexual, to manage into invisibility signs of wet dreams or of menstruation. Young women with learning/psychosocial disabilities face the threat of sterilization, with their mothers, in particular, deeply concerned to prevent the potential of visible and shaming pregnancy whilst resigned to the possibility of rape against which they feel less capable of protecting their children (Khanna R. 2004). Young adults are directed towards socially sanctioned same-impairment marriages, negotiated through a small number of web and social groups. Yet, the options are so limited that some women will chose to become sex workers rather than live at home facing the disapproval and shame of their families or marry and face the violence of husbands' anger (Price and Goyal 2016). However, the challenge by outsiders to what they perceive as local disability prejudice and discrimination frequently misconstrues the interdependence in communities, the care, adaptations to and support for vulnerability. Other histories also circulate, as the tales of shared desire expressed in same-sex relationships, sanctioned within disability residences, highlight (Vanita 2017).

What also gets lost in thinking disability within the near past is the impact of intersectional aspects of self and the multiple social forces that form disabled women's lives. Metropolitan writers, disabled and not, are often disengaged from and cannot conceive of the local phenomenologies and interdependencies facing disabled women living under conditions such as those in the parts of India and Pakistan where patriarchy is an overwhelming force, infusing every aspect of men's and women's existence (Addlakha et al. 2017). For young women planning their futures, these gendered and sexual constraints marking family honour and shame dominate in the policing of their everyday lives, serving to discipline their clothing, comportment, movements and aspirations, and to mediate the ubiquitous violence they face (Goyal 2017).

Whilst no large-scale public movement for disability rights grew within South Asia until the late 1980s and 1990s (Mehrotra 2011), in 1995, a new Indian Disability Act was established but with limitations on independence and rights and almost no recognition of reproductive or sexual rights (TARSHI 2017). It incorporated minimal provision of state welfare support, although for a tightly defined group of people with difficult to come by medical certificates of disability. It is, however, interesting to trace earlier and specific moments within the metropolitan discourse around disability/sexuality, particularly as it unfolds in relation to the UN Convention. Disability protest movements arose in the post-Vietnam period in the USA, the UK, Scandinavia and Latin America in the second half of the 20th century. The formation of modernist, welfare, liberal and left conceptions of disability, developing differentially across regions, saw an incoherence amongst disability ideas as the call for rights for disability grew internationally. Underlain for some by liberal fantasies of the sovereign body with its capacity for freedom, autonomy and choice, a body drawn upon in the name of the 'free society' beloved of Western liberals and those enamoured of the independent state, these calls discounted the nature of disabled embodiment amid demands for equal treatment. For disabled people, particularly many disabled women from the Global South, the struggle for disability rights grew throughout the 1990s, incorporating amongst many other claims, those for sexual rights. In pursuit of their claims, there existed a necessity to frame disability as a globally recognizable condition, standardized by uniform rules and regulations, structured by the claim to a common humanity.

It is notable that whilst the range of disability models was stimulated by preceding left politics, liberation struggles and anti-imperialist ideals, the disability claims ultimately were reframed in line with feminists' and LGBT's battle for identity rights. Codifying a legalistic standing for the UN convention, much of the argument and theory come from the Global North, those very places which had sought to maintain imperial domination. As Shaaf notes, 'Voices from the South are rarely in evidence, particularly in the context of sexuality' (2011, 114). Through the UNCRPD (2006) signed in 2006, naturalized and conservative sex and gender roles are reiterated and reinforced by the social model of disability, itself taken as the basis for the constitution of disability on a global level,[7] propagating concepts of 'people with disability' that sideline differences between majority and minority world in embodiment, interdependency and how neoliberalism has played out. Previously, Standard Rule 9 on Equalization of Opportunities for persons with disabilities on 'family life and personal integrity' had emerged as a model in 1993 after the Decade of Disabled Persons, offering potential sexual rights and freedoms, recognizing those moments of alterity within their sexuality. Ultimately, the disciplinary processes of UN Convention-building reiterated a more narrowly framed and less diverse understanding of a performative disability role that focused on the reduction of the concepts of sexual rights and the imposition of heteronormative family-oriented sexuality. The more conservative forces such as the Holy See and some Islamic and Catholic countries

---

[7] UNCRPD website Introduction.

were fearful of opening both a road inimical to marriage and the family and a pathway to morally contagious 'rampant sex' (Shaaf 2011, 124). A similar group also challenged the incorporation of sexual and reproductive health into the convention on the basis that it might open a road to abortion and, with an uncomfortable mix of bedfellows, even to euthanasia of disabled adults and babies. The ultimate framing of sexuality for disabled people was thus constrained, with mention of sexual rights limited whilst protective measures and policing of sexual boundaries were established. As Ruiz (2017) argues, the social construction of disabled sexuality was pared back within the convention, returning it towards a medical framing of sex/uality. And following Foucault, it is important to recognize that within the UN system and its ideal of universal rights, power/knowledge is exercised through norms constituted around and against the multiple embodied expressions of sexuality, at their most productive when operating through the hegemonic norms of post-colonial institutions, whose ideal figure is the abled, white, straight male.

Overall, the metropolitan spread of universalized notions of disability rights has inflicted a wave of epistemic violence against the localized cultures and knowledge of South Asia, who viewed disability and sexuality through multiple differential localized lenses, many of which are now lost. Some were longstanding with strong historical roots, as discussed in the first move above, linked to local myths, environments, deities, to differing phenomenologies of embodiment and to a recognition of the fear, anxiety, vulnerability and awe of contact with another (Shildrick 2009). Some knowledge was newer, tied into the struggles for independence and the aura around those with liberation wounds, whether identifying with the pride of the new, independent national body or with shame and the loss of integrity, as discussed in the second move. And, most recently, modernist knowledge of disability, benefits and rehabilitation planned in legal and government offices, as expressed in Disability Rights Bills, have clashed with neoliberal practices and thought focused only on austerity measures, incorporation and utility of a disabled being.

With the onset of neoliberal demands, some disabled people are neglected, starved, excluded and die, maybe in increasing numbers.

However, over the years, many have been incorporated into the rhythms and interstices of community life, of rural ways where they have found a niche. As globalization and urbanization lead to changes in the rural constituency with land being expropriated for mining, forest and other industries, and as villages drain of young men and women and are shorn of those who will make them co-productive, who will help them grow both in population and in wealth, only old people, children and those with disabilities remain, while the struggle for survival harshens with rural production outsourced to industry. With the loss of roles and interdependence, shifts in phenomenological experience and alteration in marriage prospects, disabled people are seen increasingly as discarded prospects of capitalist success.

This latter metropolitan/neoliberal tension highlights how the 'uneven bio-political incorporation of disability/sexuality' that manifests fails to take account of the different ways of being/becoming of disabled people. This emerges particularly strongly in a 2017 journal on disability and sexuality with a focus on the Global South. Many of the articles which speak the language of 'metropolitan' disability fail to get to grips with the daily lived experience of disabled women in the majority world, who face not only conditions of environmental access that limit independence but also cultural norms of sexual control, sexual violence and low-level but continuous familial harassment, unthought of as framings of disability and sexuality, but which mark some for inclusion in families, others for quarantine, deemed unmarriageable and/or used as foci for sexual violence (Addlakha et al. 2017).

Meanwhile, the work of disability and of gender/civil rights groups in India, Sri Lanka, Bangladesh and beyond makes visible the concurrent challenges and possibilities of the non-identical moments and of disabled people growing into a world that offers potential, hope and, for some, the emergence of localized cultures of desire, in contrast to the marginalizing forces previously outlined. Through blogs and stories, both indigenous to South Asia and drawing on knowledge from across the world, they provide a window to the ways in which people draw together resources for survival under duress.

1. A disabled, female-to-male disabled, transperson works in a tribal village in India and offers benefits and family/sexuality advice (enabled.in 2011).
2. A metropolitan group of non/disabled people runs a course addressing disability and sexuality in a Muslim area, compelled to advertise under cover to protect those involved.
3. A woman forcibly committed to a mental asylum by her husband, who then absconded with her children (Beckenridge 2017), shares creative writing and poetry on blogs.
4. A group of disabled activists from Sri Lanka and India plans a disability arts festival, developing local talent and cripqueer work.

These examples instantiate an understanding of the creative differences that emerge whilst living and working as a disability activist within the region, rather than repeating the more generalized knowledge that emerges through a Metropolitan epistemology.

FOURTH: BODIES—DISPOSING AND PRODUCING

So what of disability–sexuality knowledge as neoliberalism spread its tentacles around the globe in the 21st century? The ratification of UNCRPD and production of new disability laws in the countries of South Asia are aspects of how metropolitan, intersectional approaches are expanding. Despite rights promised through the UN and the mantra of 'Nothing About Us Without Us', the distances and differences of global time–space and the contexts of cripqueer are too great, at odds with each other, to result in reliably meaningful achievement of universal rights.

Erevelles (2010) cautions that the very institutions that are designed to protect, nurture and empower those at the intersectional margins may invisibilize them and erase them as argued earlier in the third section. Such erasure happens through the institutional framings of normativity and deviance and the regulation of the boundaries between them. Rhetoric surrounding the gendered health of a nation (mother nation) and anxieties surrounding contagion underpin such frameworks, which in turn naturalize and justify institutionalized forms of differential treatment and inequity. In South Asia, such frameworks help constitute ideas of disability–sexuality whilst resistance serves to restructure critically ontological marginality, especially in relation to institutionality and governmentality. Disabled women's health and fertility is one clear area of intervention here. The uneven incorporation of cripqueer subjectivities into the landscape of post-colonial nation states and global economies further identifies how non-normative bodies are designated and categorized locally. International/national disability and gender rights charities encroach, structurally and discursively, into ever more marginal spaces arguing for intersectionality, but their standardized programmes and research narratives prove impossible for many to engage with. The fluid social constitution of much disability, derived from context, environment, economy and alliance results in many of those in need falling outside of disability definitions of both state and charity and, thus, being erased from the script.

The rural/urban/metropolitan differential is strongly marked in South Asia across the strong power and familial relationships lived day to day. Educated young disabled people learn the languages of the UN, academy and institutions that advance globalized rights concepts and cultures to escape their limited local potentials. However, they become isolated from regional cultures and localized expressions that emerge as non-identical cripqueer modes of being, resistant to uniform disability speech and acts. Development and globalization progress in distinct ways where the majority world serves not as a producer of goods but as a provider of raw materials, bodies and ideas, leading post-colonial scholars to think disability differently. The result is that disabled people and those living with debility contend with the ontological and phenomenological experience of what Grech terms 'neocolonized bodies' (2015, 12).

Increasing numbers are deemed to be an excess, 'disposable bodies', affected by major disaster such as the Bhopal chemical explosion, the collapse of Rana Plaza, terror regimes and environmental disaster. They campaign for recompense, their problematic bodies persisting under partial erasure. Hope is a trace that floats through their memories as others attempt to manage them into absence. Puar argues, they 'confound attempts to fold easily into and out of the distinctions between living and dying, and to reflect shifting, capacious, porous and contradictory parameters of bio and necro politics' (2012, 163).

Large populations of poor in South Asia face the depletion of reserves available for living. There are growing numbers of debilitated bodies, surviving on maldistributed resources. One-third of India's children face hunger despite the country's huge wealth. Managed by neoliberal demands on trans-global bio-political bodies—economic, military, political, environmental and pharma—the benefits of prosperity and consequences of austerity are the focus of disciplinary norms that serve to regulate individual bodies as they gradually lose capacity. 'Slow death', Berlant says, is a state of prolonged exploitation of an individual's resources of survival, 'the physical wearing out of the population... very nearly a defining condition of their experience and historical existence' (2010, 754). To those who work in the informal sector, bonded labourers and slaves, subsistence farmers, tribal and indigenous peoples, and the women who not only work in these spheres but who are simultaneously expected to manage households, the notion of a free society, with the exercise of autonomy and choice, is a fantastical mirage. They face the everyday experience of exhaustion and debility, a condition neither unusual nor appearing to require specific attention. Not part of a defined disability community, cripped and queered by their resistance to the governmentality of state law and bureaucracy and the corrosion of daily wages, large numbers of neo-colonized bodies lack recourse to material assistance despite bureaucratic recording and face the inevitability of a necropolitical slide into absence and death.

Neoliberalism also demands 'productive bodies' yielding ever-increased profits from available resources. The female body is a container to be filled with a surrogate child, each surrogate pregnancy part of an ever-expanding assemblage in India's cities. Managed by discursive regimes of reproductive health and eugenic normativity, monitored by Big Pharma with health data conveyed electronically to potential parents overseas, all is well until the foetus/child proves aberrant. At which point their value falls and all contracts are void. There are myriad productive bodies, predominantly amongst the socioeconomically marginalized, including those made available through the HIV/AIDS industry: those willing to sell body parts to others, their suitability checked against DNA and antigens; those who sign up for drug, vaccines and cosmetic tests, compelled to sell themselves to aid the health and perfectibility of others, to enable them to gain in status within consumerism's hierarchies of beauty and desirability; those deemed 'the able disabled', apparently fit and capable of productive work, entitled to symbolic support and recognition though not necessarily financial resources in exchange for their inspirational value to the politicians and bureaucrats seeking to impose austerity (Titchcovsky 2003). As Khanna says, these processes have 'simultaneously engendered social mobility for Queer (*and I would add, Crip*) folk, otherwise excluded from masculinist political economies' (2010, 45).

CONCLUSION: FINDING BALANCE WITHOUT CONSTANCY

In tracing the movements around disability–sexuality epistemologies in South Asia, we have followed patterns of the past as they e/merge in our current relationships to disability, of the epistemology and ontology of disabled desires, the engagement with and resistance to state, body and self, economies, cultures and environments. In addition, through these we have traced the generative flow of ever-renewing cripqueer affiliations in South Asia.

This chapter has not been about providing answers but rather about offering provocations to think, see, feel and hear the world differently. Cripqueer epistemologies challenge established ways of being and accepted approaches to doing disability politics from a South Asian context. We aim to stimulate the opening of doors to the development of further new knowledge both locally and from other regions and contexts across the globe, in the process creating a demand for the current universalized knowledge to be specifically situated and as appropriate restricted to within the Northern context from which the majority currently emerge.

REFERENCES

Addlakha, Renu, Janet Price, and Shirin Heidari. 2017. 'Disability and Sexuality: Claiming Sexual and Reproductive Rights.' *Reproductive Health Matters* 27 (50): 4–9.

Ahluwalia, S. 2010. *Reproductive Restraints: Birth Control in India, 1877–1947*. Champaign, IL: University of Illinois Press.

Berlant, Lauren. 2011. 'Austerity, Precarity, Awkwardness.' Available at: https://supervalentthought.files.wordpress.com/2011/12/berlant-aaa-2011final.pdf (accessed May 2, 2018).

Burton, A. M. 1990, January. 'The White Woman's Burden: British Feminists and the Indian Woman, 1865–1915.' *Women's Studies International Forum* 13 (4): 295–308.

Chakravarti, Uma. 1989. 'Whatever Happened to the Vedic Dasi? Orientalism, Nationalism and a Script for the Past.' In *Recasting Women: Essays in Colonial History*, edited by Kumkum Sangari and Sudesh Vaid. New Delhi: Kali for Women.

De Mel, Neloufer. 1996 'Static Signifiers: Metaphors of Women in Sri Lankan War Poetry.' In *Embodied Violence: Communalising Women's Sexuality in South Asia*, edited by Kumari Jayawardena and Malathi de Alwis, 168–89. New Delhi: Kali for Women.

D'Emilio, J. 1983. 'Capitalism and Gay Identity.' In *Powers of Desire: The Politics of Sexuality*, edited by A. Snitow, C. Stansell and S. Thompson, pp. 100–116. New York: Monthly Review Press.

enabled.in. 2011. 'New Life for Disabled Transgender–Kiran.' Available at: http://enabled.in/wp/new-life-for-disabled-transgender-kiran/ (accessed July 22, 2018).

Erevelles, N., and A. Minear. 2010. 'Unspeakable Offenses: Untangling Race and Disability in Discourses of Intersectionality.' *Journal of Literary and Cultural Disability Studies* 4 (2): 127–45.

Evening Standard. 2007. 'Toddler With Eight Limbs Branded "Reincarnation of Hindu God" to Undergo Life-saving Operation 05/11/2007. Available at: https://www.standard.co.uk/news/toddler-with-eight-limbs-branded-reincarnation-of-hindu-god-to-undergo-life-saving-operation-7261460.html (accessed May 2, 2018).

Foucault, M. 1990. *The History of Sexuality: An Introduction*. Vol. 1. Translated by Robert Hurley. New York: Vintage.

Ghai, A. 2002. 'Disabled Women: An Excluded Agenda of Indian Feminism.' *Hypatia* 17 (3): 49–66.

———. 2015. *Rethinking Disability in India*. New Delhi and Abingdon: Routledge.

Ghosh, D. 2006. *Sex and the Family in Colonial India: The Making of Empire*. Vol. 13. Cambridge: Cambridge University Press.

Ghosh, Shohini. 2011. *Fire*. New Delhi: Orient Publishing.

Grech S. 2015. 'Decolonising Eurocentric Disability Studies: Why Colonialism Matters in the Disability and Global South Debate.' *Social Identities: Journal for the Study of Race, Nation and Culture*. doi:10.1080/13504630.2014.995347.

Gupta, Charu. 2001. *Sexuality, Obscenity, Community*. New Delhi: Permanent Black.

Gupta, Sunil. 1996. 'Culture Wars: Race and Queer Art.' In *Outlooks: Lesbian and Gay Sexualities and Visual Cultures*, edited by Horne Peter and Reina Lewis. London/New York, NY: Routledge.

Haraway, Donna. 1992. 'The Promises of Monsters: A Regenerative Politics for Inappropriated Others. In *Cultural Studies*, edited by Lawrence Gossberg, Cary Nelson, Paula A. Treichler, 295–337. London: Routledge.

Hena, Hasna. 2012. 'Women-Loving-Women: Issues and Concerns in Bangladesh Perspective 400–427. In *Women-Loving-Women in Africa and Asia*, edited by Saskia Wieringa. ILGA. Available at: http://ilga.org/women-loving-women-in-africa-and-asia/ (accessed May 2, 2018).

Irigaray, Luce. 1993. *An Ethics of Sexual Difference.* Translated by Catherine Porter and Gillian Gill (p. 170). New York: Cornell University Press.

Jaramillo Ruiz, F. 2017. 'The Committee on the Rights of Persons with Disabilities and Its Take on Sexuality'. *Reproductive Health Matters* 25 (50): 92–103. https://doi.org/10.1080/09688080.2017.1332449.

Karimjee, Mumtaz. 1987. 'The Eastern Disease?/The Western Disease?' In *My Mothers, My Sisters, Myself (Series)*. *Spectrum Women's Photography Festival Exhibition Catalogue*: A Collaboration with *Ten_8 International Photography Magazine Issue 30*, by Elaine Kramer, Liz Heron, and Pratibha Parmar. London: Ten 8.

Katyal, Akhil. 2010. 'No "Sexuality" for All: Some Notes from India.' *Polyvocia— The SOAS Journal of Graduate Research* 2: 21–19. Available at: https://www.soas.ac.uk/research/rsa/journalofgraduateresearch/edition-2/file58285.pdf (accessed August 2018).

Khanna, Akshay. 2010. 'A Refracted Subject: Sexualness in the Realms of Law and Epidemiology'. PhD Dissertation, University of Edinburgh. Draft shared on email, in Katyal, Akhil. 2011. *Playing a Double Game: Idioms of Same Sex Desire in India*. PhD Thesis, SOAS (School of Oriental and African Studies). https://eprints.soas.ac.uk/13103/ (accessed May 1, 2018).

Khanna Renu et al. 2004. *Consultative Meet to Design a Perspective Building Workshop on Gender and Disability: Report on the Proceedings.* Women's Health Training Research and Advocacy Cell, M. S. University, Vadodara.

McRuer, R. 2006. *Crip Theory: Cultural Signs of Queerness and Disability.* New York, NY: New York University Press.

———. 2010. 'Disability Nationalism in Crip Times.' *Journal of Literary and Cultural Disability Studies* 4 (2): 163–78.

Mehrotra, N. 2011. 'Disability Rights Movements in India: Politics and Practice'. *Economic & Political Weekly* 46 (6): 65–72.

Menon, Ritu, and Kamla Bhasin. 1998. *Border and Boundaries: Women in India's Partition.* New Delhi: Kali for Women.

Miles, M. 2001. 'Studying Responses to Disability in South Asian Histories: Approaches Personal, Prakrital and Pragmatical.' *Disability and Society* 16 (1): 143–60.

Misra, G. 2009. 'Decriminalising Homosexuality in India.' *Reproductive Health Matters* 17 (34): 20–28.

Mitchell, David, with Sharon Snyder. 2015. *The Biopolitics of Disability.* Michigan: University of Michigan Press.

Mort, Frank. 1987. *Dangerous Sexualities*. London and New York: RKP. (Naz Petition).
Naaz, Hira. 2017. 'Women's Sexuality in the Indian Nationalist Discourse.' In *Feminism in India*. Available at: https://feminisminindia.com/2017/08/14/womens-sexuality-indian-nationalist-discourse/ (accessed May 1, 2018).
Nidhi, Goyal. 2017. 'Denial of Sexual Rights: Insights from Lives of Women with Visual Impairment in India.' *Reproductive Health Matters* 27 (50): 138–46.
Paryay. 1994. 'Hysterectomy in the Mentally Handicapped'. *Issues in Medical Ethics* 2 (1): 6–7.
Price, Janet, and Nidhi Goyal. 2016. 'The Fluid Connections and Uncertain Spaces of Women with Disabilities: Making Links Across and Beyond the Global South.' In *Disability in the Global South: The Critical Handbook*, edited by Shaun Grech and Karen Soldatic. Switzerland: Springer.
Beckenridge, Jhilmil (2017) My Family Colluded to Have me Put in Mental Health Facility in *Sexuality and Disability* http://blog.sexualityanddisability.org/2017/01/family-colluded-put-mental-health-facility-story-survived/ (accessed September 19, 2017).
Puar, J. K. 2007. *Terrorist Assemblages: Homonationalism in Queer Times*. Durham, NC: Duke University Press.
———. 2012. 'Precarity Talk: A Virtual Roundtable with Lauren Berlant, Judith Butler, Bojana Cvejic, Isabell Lorey, Jasbir Puar, and Ana Vujanovic'. *TDR: The Drama Review* 56 (4): 163–77.
———. 2014. 'Disability.' *TSQ: Transgender Studies Quarterly* 1 (1–2): 77–81.
Sabaratnam, T. 2010, December 18. Chapter 18: 'The First Sinhalese—Tamil Rift.' *Sri Lankan Tamil Struggle*. USA: Ilankai Tamil Sangam. Available at: http://www.sangam.org/2010/12/Tamil_Struggle_18.php (accessed May 2, 2018).
Said, Edward. 1978. *Orientalism*. London: RKP (1991, Penguin).
Shaaf M. 2011. 'Negotiating Sexuality in the Convention on the Rights of Persons with Disabilities.' *Sur International Journal on Human Rights* 8 (14): 113.
Shah, S. P. 2015. 'Queering Critiques of Neoliberalism in India: Urbanism and Inequality in the Era of Transnational "LGBTQ" Rights.' *Antipode* 47 (3): 635–51.
Shildrick, Margrit. 2002. *Embodying the Monster*. London: SAGE.
———. 2009. *Dangerous Discourses of Disability, Subjectivity and Sexuality*. London: Palgrave Macmillan.
Shildrick, Margrit, and Janet Price. 1996. 'Breaking the Boundaries of the Broken Body.' *Body and Society* 2 (4): 93–113.
Singh, Poonam. 2016. 'Bharat Mata and the Ideal Indian Woman.' *Feminism India*. Available at: https://feminisminindia.com/2016/04/29/bharat-mata-indian-womanhood-2/ (accessed May 2, 2018).
Sinha, Mrinalini. 1995. *Colonial Masculinity: The 'Manly Englishman' and the 'Effeminate Bengali' in the Late Nineteenth Century* (Studies in Imperialism). Manchester: Manchester University Press.

Sircar, O. J. 2017. 'New Queer Politics in the New India: Notes on Failure and Stuckness in a Negative Moment.' *Harvard Journal of the Legal Left* 11: 1–36. Available at: http://dspace.jgu.edu.in:8080/xmlui/handle/10739/588 (accessed May 2, 2018).

TARSHI. 2017. *Sexuality and Disability in the Indian Context*. Working Paper, 2nd ed. New Delhi: TARSHI.

Thadani, Giti. 1996. *Sakhiyani: Lesbian Desire in Ancient and Modern India*. London and New York: Cassell.

Titchcovsky, Tanya. 2003. *Disability, Self, and Society*. Toronto: University of Toronto Press.

UNCRPD. 2006. 'Convention on the Rights of Persons with Disabilities and its Optional Protocol (A/RES/61/106), specifically Article 23 – Respect for Home and the Family'. Available at: https://www.un.org/development/desa/disabilities/convention-on-the-rights-of-persons-with-disabilities.html (accessed May 2, 2018).

Vanita, Ruth. 2000a. 'Ayyappa and Vavar: Celibate Friends.' In *Same Sex Love in India*, edited by R. Vanita and S. Kidwai. New Delhi: MacMillan India.

———. 2000b. 'Krittivasa Ramayan: The Birth of Bhagiratha' (Bengali). In *Same Sex Love in India*, edited by Ruth Vanita and Saleem Kidwai. Translated by Kumkum Roy. New Delhi: MacMillan India.

———. 2012. *Gender, Sex and the City: Urdu Rekhti Poetry, 1780–1870*. New Delhi: Orient Blackswan.

———. 2017. *Gay and Lesbian Love Stories*, edited by Ashok Row Kavi. Delhi: Juggernaut Books. Available at: https://www.facebook.com/permalink.php?story_fbid=1880231955594514&id=100008231828251&comment_id=188027646559063 (May 2, 2018).

Wikipedia. *Bangladesh Liberation War*. Available at: https://en.wikipedia.org/wiki/Bangladesh_Liberation_War (May 2, 2018).

Women with Disabilities India Network. 2012. *Women with Disabilities in India*. Available at: https://womenenabled.org/pdfs/mapping/Women%20with%20Disabilities%20in%20India.pdf.

Chapter 8

Ethics and Practice of Care
A Focus on Disability

Upali Chakravarti

INTRODUCTION

Care is a fundamental requirement of human existence because at different points of time in our lives we need care arising from our physical and biological vulnerabilities. Care is also something we may not be able to do for ourselves, and may have to rely on others. Care is understood essentially as a private or individual concern, a one-way relationship between the carer and the recipient. Care is also regarded as the prime responsibility of the family, with the tasks routinely falling on women for whom it is seen as a natural and almost instinctive behaviour.

This narrow and self-limiting thinking has also dominated care advocacy and policy makers. However, when the issue of care and carers became a subject of study for social researchers and emerged into the public domain, care moved from a private concern to a public issue. In the process, it also became an area of debate for competing ethical values and opened up to popular, academic and political scrutiny. This is reflected in the changing patterns of formally organized care and support for informal care. According to Michael Fine (2004), the changing patterns of care have become the cause of long and heated debates, often expressed in controversies and open conflicts between protagonists. These changes are evident in almost every sphere, from disputes over the 'work–life' or work and family balance and the development of formal childcare services, to the deinstitutionalization of care for people with disabilities and mental health problems, and the expansion and reorganization of community care programmes to help older people remain in their homes.

CARING AND CAREGIVING: COMMUNITY, FAMILY AND GENDER

Dalley (1998) has focused on dependent people and the women who usually care for them, drawing attention to the ideology—the pattern of beliefs and attitudes—which underlie action. Competing ideologies outline alternative social policies for the provision of care for dependent people, namely familism and collectivism. At the affective level, a distinction can be made between 'caring for' and 'caring about'. The first includes the tasks of tending another person; the second deals with the feelings for another person (Parker and Graham, cited in Dalley 1998, 8).

Caring for and caring about are deemed to form a unitary, integral part of a woman's nature (which cannot be offloaded in the 'normal' state of affairs). In the 'extra-normal' situation of a child being chronically dependent beyond the constraints of dependency dictated by its age—through sickness and disability—the mother automatically extends and is expected to extend her 'caring for' function. Just as the affective links which form at birth are tied into the mechanical links of servicing and maintenance in the case of healthy children, the same affective links in the case of disabled and chronically dependent family members get tied to the servicing and maintenance functions. In the public sphere, the same forces are at work; women go into the caring occupations because their natures and their intertwined capacities for caring for and caring about are thought to suit them well for those types of jobs.

The mixing of the caring functions (for and about) has implications for both parties in the caring relationship. Love, in this context, often becomes fractured or distorted by feelings of obligation, burden and frustration. But the prevailing ethos of family-based care suggests that 'normal' tasks are being performed and roles enacted are straightforward, expected and unproblematic. According to Dalley, evidence suggests that the boundaries of obligation and willingness are indeed carefully delimited, and the willingness to care is highly relationship and context specific. As long as a daughter or son with disability is a child, caring falls within the normal parameters (even though it may be arduous). Once the child becomes an adult, tensions in the caring relationship may develop and love, obligation, guilt, dislike and may all be intermingled.

The ambivalence frequently felt by those involved in the process of caring is made more problematic because public discourse insists that there can be no separation between caring for and caring about. Official and lay commentaries on community care policies all assert the conjunction of the two.

For men, the entanglement of caring for and caring about does not, broadly speaking, exist. Men, it is recognized, can care about, without being expected to care for. The man is expected to provide the setting within which the provision of care may take place, and the finances for it, if he has no wife.

Thus, in a society where standards of success are measured in terms of the public sphere of male achievement, and where female work, both at home and outside, tends to be dominated by routine, often physically onerous and often unrewarding activity, the cost women pay is high. Why do women accept this cost? The common view is that it is located in women's special relationship to the function of caring, their capacities for self-sacrifice and sense of altruism. Both men and women hold this view. This raises the issue of ideology and internalizing of values. A view that holds women to be caring to the point of self-sacrifice is propagated at all levels of thought and action; it figures in art and literature; it is present in social welfare policies, and it is the currency in which the social exchanges within the domestic sphere are transacted. Once this central tenet—of women's natural propensity to care (in contradistinction to men's nature)—is accepted, the locus for that caring then becomes determined. With woman as carer, man becomes provider; the foundation of the nuclear family is laid. It becomes the ideal model to which all should approximate.

For most women, especially the working-class women, the model results in a triple burden—child rearing, housework and wage labour. The nuclear family and the roles associated with it may not always exist in concrete form; but as an ideological construct, it is of crucial significance. Land and Rose have discussed how fundamental to the ways of seeing women in modern society is the notion of altruism (H. Land and H. Rose, cited in Dalley 1998, 17). They call the personal servicing that women do—caring for and caring about—as compulsory altruism. Land and Rose show how social policies have been built on the same assumptions—to such an extent that the altruism which women come to see as naturally part of their character becomes compulsory. The policies could not be implemented and the structure would not function if women declined to be altruistic. They cite both the Beveridge proposals and current community care policies as examples, suggesting that they reinforce the traditional pattern of enforced dependency and compulsory altruism. This is not to be against the

> [e]xpression of free altruism which potentially lies within community care—and self help strategies… the feminist hostility to community care turns partly on the needs and interests of women which are to be masked once more in altruistic services to others and partly on the needs and interests of the cared for. In considering the needs and interests of both, feminists accept a central insight from The Gift Relationship. Titmuss demonstrated that for the gift to be safe, that is non-injurious to the recipient, it had to be freely given. (p. 14)

This, according to Dalley, is the nub of the problem. To be critical of community care policies is not to be critical of the importance of caring for and caring about, or of the necessity of enabling disabled and chronically dependent people to live 'normalized' and 'ordinary' lives. Nor is it to deny that people want to be cared for in familiar surroundings, and to be cared about by people about whom they themselves also care. But because there is consensus at the level of public discourse (both official and lay) that community care is the right policy on both ethical and pragmatic grounds, feminists run the risk of being severely criticized as self-interested and uncaring. It is important that they contest these judgements: to fight for women's rights is to fight for justice just as it is to fight for the rights of any disenfranchised, subordinated or devalued group; to question the nature of community care is to seek solutions which are equitable, comfortable and acceptable for chronically dependent people as well as for women as (potential) carers.

For the moment there is widespread acceptance of the way things are. Women have internalized the altruistic ideal; society has capitalized on it. Scathingly, Dalley argues that with women being prepared to remain or return to the home to care, society is provided with a readymade 'reserve army' of nurses—an army which does not need hospitals to be built for it to work in and does not need wages to be paid it, because, it is assumed, its members are already provided for by being dependent on and supported by, wage-earning men. It is this 'reserve army' which is increasingly being activated to provide the community care that policies and politicians have been calling for over recent years—a form of care that is largely uncosted and unmeasured, which can be invoked by planners and politicians without its costs being borne by official resources. Women are offered little option as to whether they participate as carers or not. Indeed, a choice is not available to those in need of care.

In a review article published in the *New York Times*, Nussbaum (2001) develops further the arguments on disability and society on the basis of three books on the issue of caring for dependent persons. She argues that the need for care suggests both major criticisms of the dominant theories of social justice as well as major changes that should be made in the political arrangements. To begin with, she poses the question: Who does all the work that extreme dependency requires? In most cases, according to Kittay (1999) and Williams (2001), this work is done by women, since women are far more likely than men to accept part-time work and the career detours it requires. Fathers who agree to help care for a child, who will soon go off to school, moreover, are much less likely to shoulder the taxing long-term burden of care for an extremely disabled child or parent. Citing the example of the USA, most women who do such work cannot count on much by way of support from an extended family or community network.

Much of the work of caring for a dependent is unpaid; nor is it recognized by the market as work. And yet it has a large effect on the rest of such a worker's life. For persons who can afford hired help—most of it is from women who are themselves even though paid, neither paid highly nor as generally respected by society as they should be for performing a vital social service. Kittay and Williams posit that a just society may be the one that would also look at the other side of the problem: the burdens on people who provide care for dependants. These people may need many things: recognition that what they are doing is work; assistance, both human and financial; a chance at a rewarding career for themselves; and participation in social and political life. Williams shows that it used to be assumed that women, who were not full citizens anyway and did not need to work outside the home, would do all this work. Women weren't asked whether they would do this work: it was just theirs to do.

One now thinks of women as equal citizens who are entitled to pursue the full range of occupations. Also, we now generally think that they are entitled to a real choice about whether they will assume the burden of caring for the extremely dependent. But the realities of life in a society that still assumes that this work will be done for free, 'out of love', still put enormous burdens on women across the entire economic spectrum, diminishing their productivity and their contribution to civic and political life. Theories of justice have virtually nothing about these problems. Instead, Kittay believes that these theories have done real harm, shaping one's practical political ideas through their subtle effect on the ways one speaks and thinks. For example, she suggests plausibly that attacks on providing welfare for non-working mothers are influenced by images of the citizen as an independent worker that come to us from centuries of social-contract thinking. Thus, Kittay holds that more perceptive philosophical theorizing is important to address these issues in practical political life. Even if not immediately, theoretical conceptions shape public arguments, giving people the concepts they use and shaping the alternatives they consider.

This takes one to the issue of the caregivers. Both Williams and Kittay see the work of caring for dependants at home as a crucial issue affecting the social equality of women. Holding that women are often subtly coerced by social norms into shouldering the burden of caring for a dependent, Williams argues that any solution to the problem has different parts—one is the reallocation of domestic responsibilities between men and women in the home. The second is the role of the State. The State may lighten the burden of people who care for the dependants through a wide range of policies. Citing Berube (1998), Nussbaum suggests that the key to social justice for both the disabled and those who care for them lies in enlarging the imagination. If fellow citizens are not seen as parties to a mutually advantageous bargain, then one will never see value in the permanently handicapped. Value in the disabled elderly is seen only in terms of them as formerly productive people who deserve some recompense for that earlier productivity; this is surely not all that their dignity requires. Another point is that if little value or dignity is seen in dependent people, it is unlikely that we would see dignity in the work done by dressing or washing them, and we will be unlikely to accord this work the social recognition it should have.

According to Nussbaum, although in both theory and practice American society has moved beyond earlier versions of the social contract tradition, by insisting on human dignity as a central social value, it is nevertheless far from having shaken off the dark implications of the idea of a social bargain for mutual advantage, because disabled dependents are still not regarded as full participants in it. Therefore, the adherence to human dignity as a basic social value remains partial in America. Thus, as pointed out by Gauthier (as cited by Nussbaum 2001), while the elderly have paid for the care they receive by earlier periods of productivity, the handicapped have not. Nussbaum states, quoting Berube's phrase that 'a more capacious and supple sense of what it is to be human' is crucial if we are to think more clearly about problems of justice.

STATE, SOCIETY AND DISABILITY

Most of the recent literature on caregiving indicates that research in the area of caregiving or care work in India is concentrated in the area of ageing. The focus is on both formal and informal caregivers in the locations of the home, institutions and other alternative facilities for the aged. The research highlights the growing need for formal care in the present scenario where the joint family system is breaking down, kinship ties are weakening, and children who are supposedly the carers of aged parents are seeking alternate solutions. Non-institutional care is very dependent on the caregivers within the home who are primarily women (wife, daughter, daughter-in-law, sister, etc.); even in the formal or semi-formal set-ups (ashrams etc.), it is the women who are not necessarily professional nurses who provide the care required by the elderly.

The international trend of increasing aged population, especially in developed countries, has also led to an increase in the role definition of the professional nurse as the formal caregiver. Although the nurse as a caregiver is professionally trained, she is also supposed to be caring and gentle, be like a family member and yet keep her emotions under control unlike women within the family. The underlying philosophy for the nursing profession is to do caring work 'for the love of it' apart from it being a paid job so that it remains a lower paid profession in relation to other types of skilled work. The expansion of nursing as a profession within the expansion of the medical system has led to research in the area of remuneration and benefits for nurses, ways and methods to deal with caregiver stress in nurses and, also, its regional and social basis of recruitment, especially in India.

Concern about disability has a long history, which has reflected the economy, the level of technology, class interests and ideology of the times. Hence, in this context, it is important to understand the development of the welfare state and the various social welfare policies regarding disability and rehabilitation the world over. The term welfare is popularly associated with some form of economic or non-economic benefits to persons who need support, which they are not able to otherwise secure for themselves. The provider of such support can be a governmental body, religious body, occupational guild, and non-governmental or voluntary organization. However, in the context of a welfare policy, it is the role of the government that comes into prominence. Many theorists and social analysts have attempted to formulate the kind of welfare policy that should be adopted by the state. Thus, variations in social welfare policies are seen as guided by variations in the values and ideologies of given societies, variations in the techno-economic bases and market fluctuations within and around given societies, and also that social welfare policies are a camouflage for inherent class and interest group conflicts in society. Thus, there are different social and economic models of welfare.

The public policies of the liberal countries, including those that have never been governed by social democratic parties, for example, Canada and the United States, and those governed by such parties for a long period, for example, Great Britain, are residual and assistential. Such welfare state policies provide services and benefits based on proven financial need (means tested) rather than as a matter of citizen or worker's rights. There are exceptions, such as the universal health services in Canada and Britain. The liberal model assigns welfare responsibilities to the private sector, once the minimums are guaranteed by the state. But towards the end of the 1970s, the boom of post-war economic growth came to a halt and caused global recession. The growth in the welfare state globally came to an abrupt end in many countries. Simultaneously, the collapse of the Soviet Union and the nations of the socialist block in the late 1980s led to the reshaping of the capitalist world and a possibility to pressurize for a return to the laissez-faire liberalism by reducing state interference to a minimum. The theoretical perspective of the neo-liberals gained prominence and advocated the rejection of the welfare state principle. Thus, by the 1980s the welfare model was being countered globally. Public expenditure was cut back, affecting social expenditure that suffered the most.

The case for the market providing services is being ably presented by economists who argue that services collectively organized by the State are seen as a temporary economic phenomenon peculiar to a specific historical phase in the development of large-scale industrial societies. They were needed as social supports when the masses were poor, in times of war, and when the future of capitalism was uncertain. These conditions, it is argued, are no longer prevalent, and the 'welfare state' should wither away and people should resort to a self-regulating market. Private responsibility should replace public paternalism.

INDIAN SCENARIO

A significant part of Harriss-White's indictment of the Indian State is that there is little in the way of constitutional provision to safeguard the special rights of the people with disability, emanating from their special needs. The Indian Constitution established that people with disabilities are entitled to the same social, economic and political rights and privileges as other citizens of India in the Fundamental Rights and Directive Principles of State Policy. Article 41 of the Constitution is the only article that explicitly mentions people with disability, but it appears under Part IV of the Constitution, for example, under the Directive Principles.

A fuller understanding of why the people with disability never came under the purview of the Indian welfare state model can be obtained from Nirja Jayal's analysis of the Indian welfare state. In re-examining whether India is, or ever was, a welfare state in the sense in which Western political theory and practice define it, Jayal argues that indeed it is true that India does not fulfil many of the definitional criteria associated with the welfare states of the West. In the world of its origins, the institution of the welfare state was historically inspired by the intention to provide a corrective mechanism, compensating for market-generated inequalities. In India, according to Jayal, the assumption by the state of welfare tasks—however narrowly defined—paralleled the embarkation on a state-directed and essentially capitalist path of development. Thus, the Indian State can be characterized as an interventionist and developmentalist state, with only a limited welfarist orientation.

It is suggested that the Indian State may be more appropriately characterized as an interventionist rather than a welfare state. Interventionism can subsume a welfarist orientation. The primary purpose of interventionism and its inspiring and guiding force was developmentalist. This was not a state that self-consciously and deliberately took on the responsibility of providing for its citizens in clearly defined areas which bore some relationship to the idea of needs, especially basic needs. Instead, the paramount concern of the post-colonial Indian State was the project of modernization. The developmental initiatives of the state were largely directed to the industrial sector. In the strategy of development planning, the economic component of development was privileged over its social and political aspects. This approach necessitated the acceptance of structural inequalities.

Thus, according to Harriss-White (1999), 'in setting its current welfare priorities, the state has ducked responsibility for people with disability and is currently unwilling, rather than unable, to substitute for the market or the various charitable institutions proxying for the "community"'. Given the wider framework of the political economy in which the state is retreating from its earlier welfarist obligations, which may not have ever been put into practice but were recognized at least at the conceptual level, the debate on disability is tending to be confined to a state versus NGO, and an institutional versus community based rehabilitation (CBR) paradigm. However, the issue being missed out is that from the point of view of the people with disability, the State and the NGOs, or institutions and CBR, are not contradictory but complementary to each other. The stability of state resources, the framework of rights and the capacity to reach widely into the countryside, which only the state has, are a necessary component of any disability programme even when the NGOs are a part of the service delivery system, and CBR facilitates the incorporation of the disabled into their communities.

This survey of the different approaches to welfare indicates that, in sum, welfare is not an adjunct to the economy but a part of the economy and impacts the experience of health and disability. The only alternative to state failure is the state itself because it is only the state which can provide continuity of services.

THE CONTEXTS OF CAREGIVING

Since caring is the fundamental and integral part of any looking after, whether it is a child, an aged person or a child with disability, it is important to understand the contexts of caregiving. The organization of caring in a given society is closely linked to the way in which the society organizes different aspects of social relations. According to Dalley (1998), within the context of the family under normal circumstances, responsibility for fulfilling the caring, nurturing function in relation to the rearing of children and the servicing of adult family members falls upon women. Women are also expected in 'extra-normal' circumstances to care for the chronically dependent (the disabled and elderly) persons. In traditional societies, because there is relatively little specialized division of labour, caring becomes absorbed into a larger collectivity if none of the functions is demarcated by a public–private dichotomy.

According to Dalley, what has been termed as the social construction of dependency is of a different order in such societies as compared to its capitalist construction. In the latter, those who cannot work (for wages) due to physical or mental impairment, or those who have passed beyond the age limit imposed by society on the end of working life, automatically become dependent either on the state or on the family. She also argues that their dependency is not intrinsic to their physical or chronological condition; instead, they have been 'socially constructed' as dependent because they are arbitrarily ruled out from being party to the bargain or contract which non-dependent individuals are able, or obliged to enter into with society. Hence, systems of support and care may vary according to the degree to which the confinements of the disabled are compounded by the social constraints of marginalization and stigmatization, or mitigated by the social supports of integration. In societies, which do not have formal segregated care systems, the principal structure of kinship provides the basis for caring. She further states that in situations where society takes on responsibility for providing care, the form of care adopted has tended to be modelled closely on the familial model.

The above argument probably explains why most national and international research on caregiving is increasingly focused on the aged. The aged are viewed as people who had contributed to the nation's economy, and hence have a right to have state policies to support them in their old age. While a person with a disability is viewed as a non-contributing entity, in fact a 'burden' on the State's resources as the person will never contribute economically to society, and hence hardly deserves any support. The family of such a person is also consigned to the realms of a 'non-entity', almost as a punishment for having produced such a non-productive child. This larger view is internalized by the parents to such an extent that they too have no expectations from the State to provide them any support.

ETHICS OF CARE

Joan Tronto in her book *Moral Boundaries* (1993) explains that ethics of care is:

> a set of moral sensibilities, issues and practices that arise from taking seriously the fact that care is a central aspect of human existence… a species of activity that includes everything that we do to maintain, continue and repair our 'world' so that we can live in it as well as possible. That world includes our bodies, ourselves and our environment, all of which we seek to interweave in a complex, life-sustaining web.

Under ethics of care, the practice of caring would be highly valued within society. A central role for society is to meet the essential needs of citizens. In many cases, this must be by care. Far from being hidden, caregivers would come to represent a norm, fulfilling an essential societal obligation. Social structures and attitudes would need to be set up to encourage and enable caring relationships. A broad range of social policies promoting care would be required.

Ethics of care would challenge the way legal rights and responsibilities are commonly understood. Much of the law is based on the assumption that we are competent, detached and independent people who are entitled to have our rights of self-determination and autonomy fiercely protected. Legal rights and rules operate to draw boundaries around ourselves and protect us from interference from others. However, the reality is that we are ignorant, vulnerable, interdependent individuals, whose strength and reality is not in our autonomy, but our relationships with others (Meyer 2004).

The law should start with a norm of interlocking mutually dependent relationships, rather than an individualized vision of rights (West 1997, 356).

DISABILITY CRITIQUE OF CARE

The main critique is that many writers on care have presented the issue from the carer's perspective, such as the calls for 'carers' rights'. Care has been presented as a unidirectional activity. Attempts to define care, the central aspect of an ethic of care, have tended to reinforce the notion that we are looking at an activity which one person does to another.

The traditional division between the carer and the person receiving care fails to capture the dynamic in caring relationships. It tends to emphasize the vulnerability of some, rather than recognizing the vulnerability of all. It paints the 'cared for' as passive. By talking of caring relationships, we can recognize that we are all givers and receivers of care.

Care, it is said by many care ethicists, is a good thing because it meets the needs of others. Put that way, it is easy to see how it plays into the individualized model of care. This way of understanding care may be said to reinforce the individualized model of disability because it locates the 'problem' in the body of the person with disability, which is met by the care. In particular, it assumes a norm for bodies, and disabled bodies are those departing from this norm, and so requiring care which can bring them back to the norm.

According to Herring, one particular way that care ethics is in danger of doing this is by emphasizing the burdens of care. A common tactic (understandably) of organizations promoting the interests of carers is to emphasize the burdens and disadvantages that carers suffer because of their work. This supposedly paints the disabled person as the cause of disadvantage. Unintentionally, it can imply that disability is 'a problem', which carers pay as the cost for solving (Herring 2014).

CARE AND POWER

Ethics of care assumes that care is good and something to be prioritized. This overlooks the 'dark side of care'. In particular, it ignores the paternalistic edge that can accompany care.

Woods contends that disabled people have never demanded or asked for care! He says, 'We have sought independent living, which means being able to achieve maximum independence and control over our own lives. The concept of care seems to many disabled people a tool through which others are able to dominate and manage our lives' (Shakespeare 2000, 63).

What is captured in these quotations, but often lost in the ethics of care literature, is the way that caring for another can amount to an exercise of power. The image is of one person, strong and able, stands above and over another who is frail and physically vulnerable, forced to rely on the former's strength and goodwill. People with disability are already marginalized by society and can be further disempowered by the nature of care. At its worst, care can objectify the person with disability. This, it should be emphasized, is often the result of 'carers' trying to be kind.

According to Kelly (2011, 562–65), in the context of disability,

> [C]are is haunted by the spectres of institutionalization, medicalization and paternalistic charities which, in varying degrees past and present, systematically marginalize people with disabilities… In the name of 'caring for' individuals or society at large, disabled people have been subjected to multiple forms of oppression, including forced sterilization, painful and ineffective physical 'therapies', physical and emotional abuse, and of course, institutionalization.

Fink argues that the failure to include evidence of the lives of disabled people has had several effects: First, it has perpetuated the continuing tendency of discourses of care to constitute disabled people as an inevitable burden on their families, thereby setting up a dichotomy between 'normal' families and families with disabled members. This suggests that one set of relationships is benign and 'the other is problematic and pathological'. Second, it has elided the ways in which care relationships can be understood as being built around elements of reciprocity and interdependence—failing, thereby, to acknowledge that in some places and at some times, we have all experienced giving and receiving care (Fink 2004, 14).

CARE ETHICS AS PUBLIC

That the distribution of public resources can be a matter of care counters the notion that a care ethics is suited only for the private sphere of intimate relations and not for public policy. Many have already addressed the different ways the scope of care extends beyond intimate relations. Joan Tronto (1993), Sarah Ruddick (1989), Michael Slote

(2001), Virginia Held (2006), and Nel Noddings (2002), among others, invite us to imagine what a society that governed by a social policy on a care paradigm might actually look like. The virtues that guide care in intimate spheres can introduce new values into the public domain. We can argue for a public ethic of care based on the idea that we are all embedded in nested dependencies. It is the obligation and responsibility of the larger society to enable and support relations of dependency work that takes place in the more intimate settings, for that is the point and purpose of social organization—or at least a major one.

Rather than see the emphasis on dependence and connection as limitations, I have suggested that we see the emphasis of these in a care ethics as resources. Acknowledging the inevitable dependency of certain forms of disability, setting them in the context of inevitable dependencies of all sorts, is another way to reintegrate disability into the species norm. According to Kittay, it is part of our species typicality to be vulnerable to disability, to have periods of dependency and to be responsible to care for dependent individuals. We as a species are unique (or nearly so) in the extent to which we attend to dependency, most likely because we experience the long dependency of youth. When we recognize that dependency is an aspect of what it is to be the sorts of beings we are, we, as a society, can begin to confront our fear and loathing of dependency and, with it, of disability. To sum up, Kittay says that when we acknowledge how dependence on another saves us from isolation and provides the connections to another that makes life worthwhile, we can start the process of embracing needed dependencies (Kittay 2011).

REFERENCES

Berube, M. 1998. *Life as We Know It: A Father, a Family and an Exceptional Child*. California: Vintage.
Dalley, G. 1998. *Ideologies of Caring: Rethinking Community and Collectivism*. London: Macmillan.
Fine, Michael. 2004. 'Renewing the Social Vision of Care', *Australian Journal of Social Issues* 39(3): 217–32.
Fink, Janet. 2004. *Care: Personal Lives and Social Policy*. University of Bristol, UK: Policy Press.

Harriss-White. 1999. 'On to a Loser: Disability in India'. In *Illfare in India: Essays on India's Social Sector in Honour of S. Guhan*, edited by B. Harriss-White and S. Subramanian, pp. 152–53. New Delhi: SAGE.

Held, Virginia. 2006. *The Ethics of Care: Personal, Political, and Global*. Oxford: Oxford University Press.

Herring, Jonathan. 2014. 'The Disability Critique of Care.' *Elder Law Review* 8, Article 2. Available at: www.uws.edu.au/__data/assets/pdf_file/0003/733764/Herring_02.pdf.

Jayal, N.G. 1994. 'The Gentle Leviathan: Welfare and the Indian State', *Social Scientist* 22 (9–12): 18–26.

Kelly, Christine. 2011. 'Making Care Accessible: Personal Assistance for Disabled People and the Politics of Language.' *Critical Social Policy* 31 (4): 562–65.

Kittay, E. F. 1999. *Love's Labour: Essays on Women, Equality and Dependency*. Abingdon: Routledge.

———. 2011. 'The Ethics of Care, Dependence, and Disability.' *Ratio Juris* 24 (1): 49–58.

Meyer, Christopher. 2004. 'Cruel Choices: Autonomy and Critical Care Decision-Making.' *Bioethics* 18: 104.

Noddings, Nel. 2002. *Starting at Home: Caring and Social Policy*. Berkeley, CA: University of California Press.

Nussbaum, Martha. 2001. 'Disabled Lives: Who Cares?' *New York Review of Books* xlviii (1): 34–37.

Ruddick, Sara. 1989. *Maternal Thinking*. New York, NY: Beacon.

Shakespeare, Tom. 2001. *Help*. Venture. Available at: https://disability-studies.leeds.ac.uk/wp-content/uploads/sites/.../Shakespeare-help4.pdf.

Slote, Michael. 2001. *Morals from Motives*. Oxford: Oxford University Press.

Tronto, J. C. 1993. *Moral Boundaries: A Political Argument for an Ethic of Care*. New York, NY: Routledge.

West, Robin. 1997. *Caring for Justice*. New York, NY: New York University Press.

Williams, J. 2001. *Unbending Gender: Why Family and Work Conflict and What to Do About It*. Oxford: Oxford University Press.

PART 3

Knowing the Self and Writing Life

Chapter 9

Privilege or Marginalization
Narrative of a Disability Rights Activist

Nidhi Goyal

INTRODUCTION TO MY JOURNEY

I began my journey of being an activist not as someone who stood within the frameworks of any movement, not as someone who knew the theory of what being a feminist meant, or what it meant to be working for disability rights and gender justice. I began my journey from being a woman and then acquiring a disability as a teenager, almost half way through my current life. However unknowingly, I was in my own way working as a self-advocate, adapting to inaccessibilities, responding and altering my ethos and challenging norms and power structures. All through this I just knew one thing that I had a very supportive family—a privilege not very common for women or women with disabilities in India.

I think there are four instances of my life that were clear indicators of what I will be and what I would have to face in the future.

1. When I was wrestling with my male cousins at a gathering, only 10 at that time, a lady from the community pointed to my mum, watch your daughter, if she behaves like this how will she grow up and cope with her mother-in-law? And before my progressive strong

mother could respond, I remember turning around and replying, I will deal with it myself. But I knew since then that as a woman, social norms would try their best to leave few choices for me. I was expected to behave a certain way, engage with only 'girl like activities' and definitely had to shape myself to fit the future in-laws that I was assumed to have, and I had the clarity not to bow down to any of those.

2. When I was 13, we were playing a musical game in the garden of my apartment building. I remember digging my heels and refusing to continue the game until the adults took necessary action on the kid who was cheating and just getting away by being charming and funny—thus taking away the chance from and right of a less outgoing kid of the building to play. I didn't realize that dismissing 'slow', 'imperfect' bodies and minds was done in multiple ways. I only knew that if someone was too scared to or not in a position to raise their voice, I would stand up for them, with them, and support them.

3. When I acquired my blindness, my father's friend suggested to him that my disability be hidden for 3 years, so that I could be married off as soon as I was legal. This would be necessary if my father ever wanted to see me married else I would be a burden on him all his life and never be accepted by anyone for marriage. And my very tough and honest father said he would never hide the disability; he would never think I was a burden, and marriage was not the only thing that I was born for. I realized then that the ultimate role of the woman was still in 2001 considered to be marriage. That disability was assumed to be a shame and a burden and that people lived with a certainty that a disabled woman was not fit for marriage and would never find a partner.

4. When I wanted to apply for a postgraduate programme, I was specially called by the head of the programme to say that in her opinion—which by the way was based on very little knowledge and awareness and more on ignorance and prejudice—that she could not legally deny my right to apply to the programme, but for all intents and purposes I could not pursue the programme. The reasons given were: (a) I wouldn't be able to cope or perform because of my blindness and (b) Nobody would want my baggage (assumed by her since I was disabled) in the course. A meeting designed to

refuse admissions to a disabled student was not only discriminatory, it also told me that there was no awareness of how persons with visual impairment functioned or studied. Instead of educating herself, which would have been a far productive meeting, the concept was to create a disabling and disempowering environment. I defied her and made it into the course, where I realized that there was no understanding of reasonable accommodation, where the onus of altering the environment was on me. When I started performing well and ultimately topped the program, the attitude from negative stigma and the label of 'incapable' transformed to 'super normal' both extreme and problematic polarities which are designed to keep persons with disabilities away from the assumed 'normal'.

I did not know until then that I was already an activist in my own space, a self-advocate who was constantly battling situations, but I somewhere knew that I had allies, support, in the form of a family and some friends, which not many women with disabilities had. And perhaps the recognition of my privilege in having a support while many others didn't, was the most important thought that led to dissatisfaction in a journalistic, writing career. This had a combined effect of pushing me into a goal of working with and for women with disabilities with a commitment to creating a support and changing our/their lives for better.

Calling myself a woman with a disability, I brought two of my identities to the front and centre—being a woman and being disabled.

But a comment forced me to become more conscious of what further complexities were to follow within these intersecting identities and the various positions that we hold. I remember, a batch mate during one of my postgraduations in a discussion about persons with visual impairment said to me, you don't have any issues in life the only challenge is that you cannot see. She dismissed my experience of visual impairment because according to her I was not poor and disabled who for her are the 'real marginalized group'.

The absence of empathy was telling, but it also spoke that not being economically marginalized somehow reduces the experience of visual impairment—and does not make it different—from someone standing on other marginalized intersections. I started noticing that the outlook towards marginalizations was to rank them and compare one against the other, a completely meaningless exercise since that exhibits a flawed understanding in two ways. First of all that the check boxes of identities are not isolated, they exist in a context and climate which check boxes cannot factor in and secondly we are assuming that identity and positions that people occupy are rigid and never changing whereas they are fluid and are constantly evolving and transforming. The idea that marginalization can be double—woman and disabled—or triple—woman, disabled and poor—seemed to be problematic because they view marginalization as building blocks, which means you could work on remedying one marginalizing factor at a time, as if parts of someone's identity could be stripped in layers. But the truth remains that marginalizations and identities are like a web, complex and linked.

BEGINNING OF MY ACTIVISM

I began my official activist work in 2011 as a researcher and writer at a Mumbai-based non-profit, which suited my goals perfectly. Yes I wanted to work for and with girls and women with disabilities and I was always the one ready to take up edgy issues, issues that people found it difficult to speak about or were hesitant to raise. Again, I embraced my work on sexual rights of girls and women with disabilities, perhaps just the way I stepped into a life with blindness, with confidence, with a focus and without thinking of any larger consequences beyond my commitment.

In the women's rights space and the sexual rights space, talking on a large scale about sexual rights of girls and women with disabilities was a ground-breaking step forward. With Mumbai-based women's rights organization Point of View, I moved ahead in co-researching and co-authoring a pioneering online resource www.sexualityanddisability.org. It was exciting that conversations were finally starting but also a little unnerving to realize that disabled women before then were largely invisibilized and left out with regard to sexual rights and their issues.

As a young activist, I was aware that issues of girls and women with disabilities were being raised by a handful of disabled women, really the forerunners and leaders in what we could call the women with disability movement. They had laid down the foundation of the discourses at the intersection of gender and disability first in the 1990s, but they were the only and almost the same small group struggling and moving on till the end of the first decade of the 21st century when I joined the space. So where were the women with disabilities? How were their existential realities more compounded because of their multiple identities? Why were they invisible in the disability rights movement? How deep was the ungendering of persons with disabilities rampant in the country? And lastly but perhaps the most important—who defined the women in the women rights movement? Were women with disabilities not considered women enough to be included by other women?

My journey from 2011 has been a focus on advancing rights of girls and women with disabilities by working with a range of women's rights and human rights organizations nationally, regionally and internationally. Looking at the gaps that need to be filled, I have dived into research, writing, advocacy, training, campaigns and art for creating change. It has also resulted in me founding 'Rising Flame' to focus on gendered lives of persons with disabilities and rights of women and youth with disabilities. My journey for me has been a learning curve, a quest to understand the struggles of standing at the intersections of multiple movements, navigating the mindsets, and challenging power structures and hegemonic functioning at every stage possible. Here I humbly share some of my observations and experiences that I have had in this very short journey, conscious of the fact that I have a very long route to learn and grow.

ENGAGING WITH THE WOMEN'S RIGHTS MOVEMENT

In India, 1994 was the year when women with disabilities came to the radar of the women's rights movement because the State of Maharashtra gave orders to perform hysterectomy on the resident women of a mental hospital in Pune. The violations of bodily autonomy and consent were so grave that the alliance with the women's rights movement was formed, but unfortunately, this alliance was temporary and sporadic. What this helped in was the rise of voices of women with disabilities, the leaders in the women with disability movement. But when I joined activism at the end of the first decade of the 21st century, almost the same handful of names existed and were struggling to be heard and taken seriously. My conversation with one such senior activist told me that the complaint of the women's rights movement or probably some actors in the movement was that it was difficult to engage with the women with disabilities or their issues when these women didn't step out at all and were not visible or fighting for their rights. These women's rights actors had forgotten that sometimes social and infrastructural suppression could completely invisibilize someone and if the condition for inclusion was visibility then women with disabilities were naturally trapped in a vicious circle. But I didn't form my understanding of women's rights and women's rights activists based on the history or through conversations with senior women with disability activists alone.

I was at a women's rights conference in 2012. This was my first brush with a large conference of feminists, speaking about body and sexual rights for girls and women with disabilities when the question of prenatal testing as a technology linked with sexual and reproductive rights of women was being discussed. Some of the women clearly spoke that sex-selective abortion was not okay and that thought was pushed to form a law in India but it was okay for disability selective abortion. In reply, my co-panellist and I, both women with disabilities, started expanding the conversation and breaking down the thought behind disability selective abortion as follows:

- Nothing is black or white. We need to think through what it means to have a screening and then be aborted because of disability. It is the fear of 'deviance' that majority of people carry. Coupled with the ignorance of how persons with disabilities live a life with a disability. The invisibility of successful examples adds to the difficulty.
- It is the internalizing and perpetuating of the social stigma where disabled individuals are considered only as burdens to families and society.
- It is dominated by the medical model and influenced by doctors and medical practitioners who create a pressure to terminate a pregnancy in cases where the foetus is disabled or, in their terms, abnormal.
- Last but perhaps that which plays the most important part was that it is the lack of infrastructure and social security/governmental support in the country, which results on the family having to shoulder the entire burden of care. But this was true of disability as of so many other

conditions, including ageing, illnesses, accidents etc. What we were doing through bringing a medical solution, which was often forced, was simplifying this need for social security. It meant that governments were not forced to take further action and were left to go squat free.

Our primary arguments were that we are not advocating for changes in mindsets, changes in state provisions etc.; we are not creating an environment where women can make these choices without external pressures. Instead we are finding an easy solution of disability-selective abortion and saying that it is completely all right. On hearing this, one renowned non-disabled women's rights activist slapped our voices down and instead of presenting counter arguments to some of our arguments, she went on to say that we both on the panel—one with a visual disability and one with a locomotor disability—were in no place to present these arguments. As per her, most of the pre-natal testing was done for developmental disabilities and that we were very privileged in our position in society but also within the kinds of disabilities that existed to make such a statement. The other disabilities are far more difficult and we won't be able to understand the lived realities of such persons with disabilities and their families. It made me think of how categorizing others' privilege is easier than self-reflection of the privilege. Because weren't the forerunners of the women's movement women in the position of privilege? Aren't the women with privilege and power having the most access in the movement even now? I don't think privilege can be assumed necessarily a bad thing or something that makes an intent or an argument invalid. For me, privilege is something to be recognized, be humbled with and something that you can use to expand the sensitivity and empathy to experiences that the privilege has masked. Privilege is to recognize that some people are invisible and so consciously looking out for them, speaking with them is important. For me, if my privilege took me to that women's rights conference, while I continued to work with women across disabilities, it would be exclusion to not bring out voices of those who were not present there. Again, inclusion and change happen step by step and visiblising issues is perhaps the first step to visiblising the persons who live with it. For me, building movements and amplifying voices works collaboratively until a movement or persons are okay to stand on their feet. Women with disabilities needed the support and engagement of non-disabled women to visibilize their issues and the same applies to women with different disabilities—we may need each other to even enter spaces, voice our thoughts and rivet attention to our issues.

INCLUSION AND INTERSECTIONALITY

I see a few tricky and problematic areas in inclusion of women with disabilities in the women's rights movement and other movements. Although the disability movement globally has moved from the medical to the charity to the social model and beyond, in India with the diversity of cultures and geographies and progress we have a country/society that floats between these various models of disability. As the women's rights movement and other movements are a part of the society, we do somewhere internalize some pieces of beliefs that float in the society, and sometimes they are the prejudices and beliefs that make women with disabilities and their issues invisible.

I remember in 2011 when I was researching for the website that I mentioned above, I reached out to women's rights groups and some queer rights groups and asked if they would help me identify women with disabilities with a different gender identity and sexual orientation, one organization head told me that there were no disabled women who were lesbians. There were mental health issues and not disabilities amongst lesbians because of their suppression in society. The absolute refusal and the subtext of condescension for mixing the disabled identity with lesbians exhibited a hierarchy that actors belonging to one marginalized community have towards the other.

Even today the idea of visibility and approach to intersectionality is a complex one. Many actors in the women's rights movement tokenistically agree to include voices from marginalized constituencies. This is very reflective when often I am invited to women's rights convenings/conferences on the 'marginalized voices panel' where along with me is a Muslim woman and a Dalit woman. Now bringing some spotlight on voices that are invisible and working towards lifting ignorance is great, but what often happens is that these voices are only allowed space on exclusive panels and not in other areas of discussions. This ends up perpetuating the exclusion while the actors in the women's movement tick the political idea of inclusion and not the real inclusion.

What has stopped surprising me further is that when marginalized groups are brought together, they somehow are so grateful for the space, or are so focused on pushing for their issues to be included with the supposed mainstream that they forget the other women even on the 'marginalized panels'. It was hilarious when in a 2016 national convening, on a panel of Dalit women, Muslim women and disabled women, the Dalit women at the end concluded that our voices should be heard and we—all Dalit women and Muslim women—should be given space and we should not be marginalized. On hearing this, I smiled and calmly pointed out that may be she also wanted to add us—disabled women—and she casually replied 'Oh yes, I forgot'. When other marginalized groups are addressed and asked about disabled women in their community or region or religion, they often shrug and say 'we don't know', 'we haven't thought about them' or that 'they are in a bad shape they cannot get out of homes' and the conversations terminate there with an uncaring or pitying tone.

This attitude is not exclusive to non-disabled women either from the mainstream or the marginalized movement. The not caring for multiple identities or intersectionality as it is called is even present in the women with disability movement. At a global conference for women's rights in 2016 there was a vibrant mix of women and all groups were welcomed and encouraged. At the closing meeting of the women with disabilities, I suggested that may be our final representation should be done by the only transperson with a disability who was present at the conference, in order to lend visibility to this intersectionality as well, along with one woman with a disability. Others just shrugged away (with huge dislike) my suggestion of giving the important space of representation to someone who wasn't like majority of them.

All these encounters force me to sit and contemplate the human nature and behaviour of the actors embodying the movements, and many strands of conclusion come to me. We are not speaking enough to each other and that somehow in spite of our talks, our struggles and our openness, we are not able to look at people as a whole but within one identity or issue that marginalizes them the most. But I think that it is the human feeling of finally being heard, getting a space to present your issues, grabbing the opportunity to sync up with other mainstream movements and not being ready to share the piece of the pie that has been acquired finally and with immense struggles. But when we start with this attitude, somewhere the attitude and habit perpetuates and when the piece of the pie in terms of resources, visibility and space, becomes bigger and more frequent, even then we refuse to see the complexities and possibilities of intersectional existences.

ACCOMMODATIONS AND NORMALCY

I often have had the conversations of 'accessibility is expensive' with women's rights groups, because we see somethings as accommodations and some as not. So if you need electricity at night that is considered as 'normal' and not as an accommodation for people who are sight-dependent, only because they are a majority. If electronic copies of agendas of a meeting are requested, or braille feedback forms are needed, people consider it as an extra effort.

The other cost factor that is discussed even more is the need for a personal assistant for women with disabilities wherever needed on travels, in conferences and other spaces. We very largely talk about in our women's rights movement about co-habitation, community living, supporting each other and creating a healthy interdependent environment but these concepts fall by the wayside when it comes to girls and women with disabilities. They are left out from participation because having an extra person would add extra cost. Here is where expanding the understanding of accommodations is imperative. Women with disabilities may need assistance that is in their personal space; they may need transfers from wheelchairs to beds; they may need assistance in bathing or eating; they may need to hold hands to find their way, but they will bring equal intellectual, experiential and informational richness to conversations and dialogues or participation in activities and issues. If at all they are accepted with support person or an assistant, disabled women are often judged or marked lower on capability with an assistant as compared to them performing or travelling without one.

Thus leaving them with the two options—either to feel judged, or to not be able to maximize their capabilities with a support.

This scenario often results in the women's movement or actors in the women's movement engaging with women with either mild disabilities, or invisible disabilities, or those having a disability but high functioning, in short as close to perceived 'normal'. It is still the huge discomfort with diversity or with bodies and minds that don't function or react within the redefined 'acceptable'.

The push at the beginning of the women's rights movement globally was of defying the tags that the male world had planted on women of being weak, needing support and protection. But in this quest for being strong and fighting for our rights we somehow cancelled out the experiences of women who had very weak or failing bodies and minds yet very much women deserving equal dignity and respect. So for decades, stood the women with disabilities outside of the women's rights movement with bodies that may have been weak, minds that may have needed support in making decisions, existences which may have needed care. The movement today is evolving and changing particularly in India, but we still are somewhere unconsciously stuck in a zone of comfort and normativity. Most of the women with disabilities who are encouraged and included in opportunities are women who are high functioning—they resemble and perform the way non-disabled women would. This in itself is problematic because it sticks us in the old school of categorizing behaviour of fight like a man and cry like a woman. There is very little patience or support for bodies that are slower or not so forceful, for minds that take longer to process or may have inconstant ideas. This is evident in workspaces and systems, conferences, meetings, convenings, gatherings, celebration marches and parties and even in evolving areas of concerns like digital rights. We basically don't naturally think that the space also belongs to women with disabilities and that is the problem. I don't know if ignorance can be sighted as an excuse beyond a point. Learning and engaging is the key. But often we wait for women with disabilities to remind and speak for themselves. This sets a fatigue in the disabled women and they are forced to represent disability and make that ask of inclusion in some places and not in others, very much like prioritising their rights.

VOICES AND LEADERSHIP

How are movements built and voices amplified? How is leadership created? These are some of the key questions that women with disabilities are juggling with in India. I was recently speaking to a funder and they said that they would not fund the women with disability work of an organization based in a marginalized region of India because the leader of the organization was a man with a disability. 'What do we understand with leadership and building capacities to lead?' was the question that I was faced with in that discussion.

When there is someone with a disability, the lived reality of having a disability, facing access and other challenges is familiar. In wanting to advance issues of women with disabilities, nondisabled women/groups should not disregard the fact that men with disabilities also have some common lived realities. The question is not just if the current leadership is male, the question should extend to whether the current male leadership has the empathy towards nuancing the work for women with disabilities. The question should further be if the intent is to develop and support the growth and sustenance of separate women with disability leadership going forward. And the last question should be whether equal spaces, opportunities and dignity are awarded to women with disabilities? These are tough questions to ask and to answer.

To explain the criticality and the complexity of the question let me give you an example of another South Asian country here. (I refuse to specify which because of confidentiality issues for the disabled women there and their professional safety). There was a main network of persons with disabilities with a male leadership, which supported the institution of another country-wide network for women with disabilities. The women with disabilities leading the network of women with disabilities in that country seem to be doing good work. They bring up cases of violence against women with disabilities, talk about education and access, penetrate the government and UN bodies. However when they tried to take up specific issues on girls and women with disabilities and their sexual and reproductive health and rights independent of the main network and in collaboration with other women with disabilities in the country, they faced a huge resistance from the male leadership and they had to terminate the research and reporting process. The main points of resistance that stood out for us were that the women with disabilities network was autonomous so long as they took approvals from the main network; they kept the main network well informed of their activities; and the activities/engagements never challenged or superseded the main network's work. In short, it was limited autonomy and leadership. I remember when I tried to convince the women's network leader to continue the work and negotiate with the main network or even try and take a stand on the report we were writing, she said to me, I refuse to work against them, my career and professional growth will be destroyed. And those words stayed with me. It is a common occurrence where the disability rights movement needs to break down power and leadership and raise deeper questions about tokenism. If we are together battling the ablest power that does not mean that we carry the power circle of patriarchy or privilege amongst us (disability network and movements). Women with disabilities in this South Asian country working within these power structures were not only oppressed but had started the faulty style of leadership with the idea of rigid hierarchy based on power and access. These form cycles where control and empowerment go hand-in-hand. The main network encouraged the building of the women with disability network and enhanced the opportunities that women with disabilities would have otherwise received of exposure, of space, of visibility and of travel. But does this justify the penultimate control that rests with the male led main network? What would be the correct way to alter the situation-some say that such a pseudo network instituted by men should be disbanded, some suggest that they should completely divorce from the main network led by men but I don't think answers are black and white. The reach and the access to spaces, authorities and to funds may still be with the main network and pulling out of over all issues that impact persons with disabilities is not the way forward for women with disabilities because the overall issues are also our issues in addition to the specific gendered issues. A strategic capacity building of key actors in the movement but really of the women with disability networks would be an important step. The courage and the step forward will have to come from the women with disabilities movement. As for the main networks/movements dominated by men with disabilities they need to remember—just like women's rights movement—that they are not creating spaces for women with disabilities, the space also belongs to the disabled women.

CROSS DISABILITY WORK: WHAT DOES THAT MEAN?

I was collecting data for a research report to be launched in the end of 2017 where I was documenting cases of sexual violence against girls and women with disabilities and their access to the justice system in India. During this phase a case of sexual abuse of hearing impaired children at a 'special school' was brought to me through the other trainings and work that I do with the sexuality disability programme at Point of View and we decided to support them with facilitating connections with appropriate legal help. When our role as Point of View was over, I approached them for permissions to document the case and interview the hearing impaired alumnae of the school that were supporting the case. What followed was an unanticipated backlash. The woman (hearing impaired alumnus) was very annoyed that I was writing about hearing impaired persons when I wasn't hearing impaired and that I was eating into work opportunities for persons with hearing impairment. This disturbing confrontation again raised many questions and forced me to analyse the landscape.

What is the understanding of work across disabilities. Disability is not a homogenous group, but also each disability cannot live in silos. We need to talk to each other, raise issues of other disabilities alongside ours. What is the point if a cinema hall plays audio described films accessible to persons with visual impairment yet the access to such a hall is only through multiple and winding stairs obviously inaccessible for persons with a locomotor disability? The assumption here, in providing one accessibility feature and not the other, would be that a certain group would need access more than others. It also exhibits a limited understanding of accessible cinema, which would certainly include the hall as well as the film. The next assumption and that worries me the most is that we assume that a person can live only one disability at a time and refuses to consider the concept of bodies that have multiple disabilities, are fluid and ever-changing or deteriorating. It absolutely would refuse to fathom the concept of temporarily abled bodies and the concept of aging and disability—both of which might need multiple accessibilities in place. But how many persons with disabilities or actors in the movement would actually care and say that x is accessible for me but not for all persons with disabilities? May be not many.

Even within the movement some people with disabilities have a louder voice and push because of their position to speak or move. There is a marginalization and invisibility even within the movement, which is consciously being eroded by concerted efforts towards inclusion. These marginalizations are felt most by persons with invisible disabilities and those who were denied the label/recognition of disability and those who were denied independent voice as a result of lack of legal capacity. But the rift grows wider because of two main points:

1. People with disabilities have, to a certain extent, internalized the ableist lens that the society has. Being comfortable with one's own disability, the limitations and challenges cease to be a 'not normal' part of life very much like for the non-disabled persons. As a result, the attitude among many persons with disabilities towards disabilities other than theirs is that of unfamiliarity, charity or demeaning. Many actors in the movement end up creating a hierarchy within different disabilities but also then subconsciously bumping the non-disabled persons above all—the peak of the pyramid which is normal—and work towards it to feel accepted and included.
2. Acknowledgement and visibility by other non-disabled persons or officials (that matter) causes a crack between different disabilities and give rise to resentment and competition for rights and resources. At a conference in 2016, I clearly remember my co-panellist, also a woman with a disability, say that persons with visual impairment had a disability concession while reserving train tickets but persons with psychosocial disabilities did not get any such concessions. This in turn has been leading to persons with psychosocial disability resenting the provisions that persons with visual impairment had benefitted from.

For me, this raised very important questions of whose voices are amplified. Are we as a movement silencing some voices or not consciously including them? Or is it a combination with whose voice gets heard finally by authorities? Probably the non-disabled world including authorities is able to deal with certain disabilities more than others, again with the misconception that some disabilities closely resemble the normative realities that non-disabled persons have or simply with the thought that some people 'looked disabled' whatever that means.

Sometimes the feeling is not just of standing at the intersections of many movements, that is, women's rights, disability rights, sexual rights, but it is even about standing within a subsection of the movement while questioning and reflecting on the privileges and marginalizations that exist there.

CONCLUSION

In societies where the birth of a girl child is yet not celebrated—and it is not an exaggeration or a phenomenon reserved for rural India—the birth of a woman with a disability is not considered to be a happy moment. To disguise the apparent failure of the mother—since any 'abnormality' in child is often blamed on the mother—and preserve the prestige of the family, women with disabilities are frequently forced to hide their disabilities. It is a common story where deaf girls are stopped from using a sign on the road since their parents don't want others to know that the girls are deaf, or the parents to hide medical records of a daughter with a neurological, psychological or intellectual condition.

Social outing of a disability is another step of acceptance that families have to battle since the word disabled (or any others used instead in India) for that matter carry a lot of baggage of stigma and prejudices and misconceptions.

I was talking to mothers of children with cerebral palsy and or developmental disabilities and the first reaction that they hear from the health professionals is that they have given birth to almost a vegetable. It is luck and one must accept the condition as is and be fine till the child lives. A friend also shared that her mother was asked very seriously by a doctor when her sister was born with multiple disabilities whether the mother would like the doctors to 'take care' (end the life of) of the child. it would be very easy for them to end the existence with a simple needle and some medicines.

Women with disabilities and their families face multiple discriminations because of their various life contexts. It is never easy to be a woman who is constantly being judged for her worth or capability; it is not easy to be less valued than non-disabled women and certainly disabled and non-disabled men; and it is not easy when no numbers are present to validate the existence of a group. We as a country raise a voice on one gang rape when it is of a middle class young woman but stay silent on a similar brutal rape of a woman with an intellectual disability just months from the first incident.

We are still battling these difficulties today, but we also have support, and a thrust from expected and unexpected quarters. The challenge only arises when inclusion of women and girls with disabilities is seen as the 'in thing' or is as a result of the pressure created by funders. There is a huge tokenistic inclusion in disability rights discourses and the check boxes being checked in the women's rights dialogues. It is an exercise to maintain an image, or to have a 'feel good' factor of working with diversity. But the dilemma is should these tokenistic spaces and discussions be boycotted or grabbed as opportunities to create a bigger space for girls and women with disabilities.

Swimming in these murky spaces, I as a young activist, entered many organizations and movements directly where the intent was honest and sincere and peripherally where the opportunities, however slim, existed to push for issues of girls and women with disabilities.

But for me the real inclusion in minds and spaces will be when feminists challenge the dominant understanding of feminism and accept that there are multiple ways of being a feminist; that failing bodies or minds are not a sight of shame or weakness; when women's rights actors perform access audits of their places, systems or even communications, and are at least aware and making efforts to become more accessible and inclusive. Inclusion does not only mean clinically and politically providing reasonable accommodations (defined by UNCRPD), it means inclusion in discussions and inclusion in building a movement; it would mean engaging with girls and women with disabilities and treating their issues as ours. Inclusion for me would also mean that disability rights organizations become gender sensitive and treat women with disabilities, their issues and voices with equal dignity and importance.

Continuing to stand at the cusp of many movements, always believing I cannot be boxed into one identity and the same with the women who I am working for and with, I realize that intersectional and cross movement work is never easy. But there is a hope and a joy that women with disabilities are getting stronger and the veil of silence shrouding our issues is being lifted inch by inch in the last couple of years. In India, we have a criminal law amendment for women that have made provisions for girls and women with disabilities, there is a progressive disability law which considers in the multiple discriminations and challenges that women with disabilities face. All with the efforts of women with disabilities themselves but also due to allies in the women's rights and disability rights movements. We are today a group, however small, no longer invisible or silenced and will continue to come out and grow!

Chapter 10

Journey So Far
My Life with an Impairment

Sameer Chaturvedi

MY BIRTH AND AFTERWARDS

I was born in Gorakhpur Civil Hospital, where there was no facility for providing oxygen to a newborn. My mother was told by a gynaecologist that there were probably two babies inside the womb. The doctor gave a tentative date of delivery, which was around Christmas time, but my mother felt some unease in the first week of December itself. My father was not there to look after my mother as he was posted in Banaras and went back to resume his official work even as the doctor anticipated a delivery in a few weeks. When I was born, the medical attendants there were not sure whether I would survive. Six hours passed before I uttered my first cry. My twin brother was born healthy. My parents observed a developmental delay in me as compared to my brother. I raised my head when I was about six months old, something that usually happens in first 4 months of a child's life. My parents took me to Banaras Hindu University Medical College where doctors diagnosed me with cerebral palsy.[1]

---

[1] https://www.theweek.in/content/archival/news/india/gorakhpur-hospital-tragedy-children-death-oxygen.html

I believe, it is social reaction which makes a person realize the value society at large attaches to his or her body. In my case, the queries were polite as people often asked my mother:

'*Is bacche ko ye kese hua, Bhagwan ne diya hai toh vahi rasta dikhaenge*'. (How did this happen to the child? Since this condition has been given to him by God, he only will show you the way forward.) So, I became conscious of my body through the world (Merleau-Ponty 1996). There were times when playing with my siblings or cousins, the other kids reminded me of my bodily limitation (Hughes and Paterson 1997).

Kids enjoy playing games like *Pakran Pakrai, Lagripala* (both variations of the game Tag) *Chupan–Chupai* (hide and seek), *Khokho and Uuch–Nich*; these would be games requiring a certain amount of 'physical fitness' and normality for participation. However, I was included in playing most of them. More than my participation, I enjoyed seeing my co-participants, who could run faster than me. Such incidents led to some guilt regarding my body and made me to question my mother as to why they chose a hospital where there was no oxygen box. My mom blamed it on *Bhagya* (fate) because people who took her there were misinformed about the facilities in relation to childbirth.

Although seldom, but why did I ask such things to my mom, in the first place? As I see today, it was not only celebrated values like ability and functionality, which I was internalizing, but also ideals to which I was comparing my existence.

However, there is another side also to my life-story. I was a fun-loving person who loved to be part of every happy moment at home or in the neighbourhood. My experience of impairment did not always dominate my existence as I have other shades to my personality. This is not to, however, say that I was not affected by my impairment.

During our stay at Gorakhpur there was a lane near our home through which many marriage processions would pass. I would watch those processions from the terrace and try to match my steps to the tune of the accompanying music. I loved to dance, even as my siblings were a bit shy.

I started walking at the age of two and a half years. My impairment impacted my body balance. I used to fall down frequently. But it was never a big deal for me to get hurt. A cut on the body would make me feel good. I took it as a marker of being a fighter or a hero. I am not sure but I might have been embodying these ideas from the famous cartoon series 'He-Man'. But once I hurt myself badly. I lost my balance and banged the back of my head on the door, and it started bleeding. My sister and my brother, who themselves were kids then, managed to climb the big gate of our Saharanpur residence to inform our mother, who was out visiting a neighbour.

My mother believed I was unconscious for a little while. I remember one thing though. On our way to the nursing home, my mother panicked, and there was constant effort from her to not let me close my eyes, which irritated me as I was conscious. Stitches never bothered me and who would complain when suddenly you become the centre of your parents' attention. The next morning, my mother gave me *haldi vala dudh* (turmeric milk) that I hated the most, but the best part about getting hurt was that I was subjected to care that made my mother allow me to watch cartoons of my choice. I was free from getting scolded by her over watching it at a stretch for more than a couple of hours. Also, I enjoyed my look in the mirror. The white bandage over my head gave me a sense of excitement, maybe because it reinforced the idea of being warrior who cooperated with the doctor stitching the wounds.

As I grew, my parents became concerned about my education. When we were at Saharanpur, they started sending me to a playway school in our locality along with my brother. They took me to some institution for spastic people where medical practitioners reaffirmed after seeing me that I am intellectually fine and physical rehabilitation would be beneficial for me. Actually, at the time of my birth doctors predicted that I would not be impaired intellectually. Some even said that I will be 80% fine physically too. So, from the very beginning, the expectation was to attain maximum normalcy[2] (Foucault 1976[1973]).

This belief was further strengthened when the physiotherapist, who used to visit me, told my mother that I could attain complete normalcy. Physiotherapy became a daily routine. I used to find it pretty boring. Also, stretching exercises were painful. My parents knew that I had a

---

[2] For Foucault, the very consciousness that an individual is in pathological state and in need of medical gaze is discursively constructed.

craze for cricket. They used to motivate me by saying: 'If you want to play for India focus on the exercises to realize your dreams'.

I come from a Brahmin family of believers. It is something which I inherited through the socialization process. I was told not to be superstitious, but to believe in God. In their own terms, my parents always pushed me to do well. I remember the day when my father made me read an interview given by Sudha Chandran, an orthopaedic impaired dancer/actor who sees Idea of God as the source of positivity. She believes that God has sent each of us, whether impaired or non-impaired, with a purpose. Her interpretation, however, only represents one side of the story. The negative tendency to associate impairment with punishment given by God is widespread (Miles 1995). Here, the role of television is immense.

As we know, television is the medium that tries not only to reproduce but sustain the sanctity of Hindu cultural ideals (Mankekar 1999). Television plays a vital role not only in perpetuating the idea of normality but in spreading it across every section of the society. For example, I was fond of Ramanand Sagar's *Krishna*. There was an episode in which Lord Krishna through his magical powers made a hunchback walk straight again.[3] It made me believe that God can heal my pain by blessing me with a healthy body and the desire to become a normal person was further consolidated.

I have learned that both the Ramayana and the Mahabharata discredited disabled characters by putting them in bad light, but as a kid I was not aware of these nuances, before obtaining a degree in disability studies that highlighted ableism in Hindu culture (Ghai 2002, 88–100; Mehrotra 2013; Miles 1995). The very act of Lakshman deforming Surpanakha for me was the symbolic of victory of good over evil. I used to feel that I was normal but when I wasn't able to do something or if people around me or within my family pointed towards my impairment and blamed me for not being serious enough about my physical therapy to improve my condition or left me out of social gatherings, I used to feel bad. Like when one of my cousins remarked that he only wanted to take my brother out for a movie: 'It is not that easy to take Sameer along for a movie. There are some pragmatic issues'. Outside of my family, my life was not only about how I experienced my body or the normalizing

---

[3] https://www.youtube.com/watch?v=9KTq6wc8wyw

process but also how a person with an impairment and his/her family pushed to struggle because society is not barrier-free (Oliver 1996).

SCHOOL LIFE AND BEYOND

Accessibility and acceptability were the major issues I faced during my school life. Authorities in most of the schools showed their scepticism in giving me admission. I remember there was a missionary school where the principal said that they didn't have adequate infrastructure to give me admission. Also, if I hurt myself who would take responsibility? This was the kind of attitude shown to my parents. Almost every school was willing to take my brother but not me on the grounds of my impairment. Those days we were in Lucknow when one day my mother took both of us to a school for admission. They allowed my brother admission but not me and cited the reason that I hadn't cleared the entrance test. My mother was about to take me home when somebody from behind said:

'*Ye kaha padhta hai?*' (Where does he study?)

My mother said: '*Inko bhi admission ke liye laye the, par office me jo sir baithe hai unhone mana kar diya*'. (I had brought him for admission, but the person who was sitting in the office refused.)

She was the principal of the school. She enquired about my intellectual ability from my mother, and said: 'If he is intellectually normal, then there is absolutely no problem and we can admit him and also since his brother is going to be around he should not face any problem'.

My mother was ecstatic that I got admission in school. Overall, both relief and joy marked my entry into schooling.

I cannot recollect the reason but I used to go outside the classroom very rarely. It was because of my fear of hurting myself by falling down. Also, teachers were bit protective about me especially after I fell down in a school corridor and lost half a tooth. This made some people in the school administration say that this place was not suitable for me and that was the reason my parents kept reminding me to be cautious while moving outside of class.

All students were nice to me but nobody really ever asked me whether I wanted to play with them. At times, when any of my classmates stayed back in class for their own personal reason, I was the one who initiated the dialogue. I love to interact with people around, but I don't really remember any long conversations I had with any of my classmates. It was just casual chitchat. I am not sure that my classmates ignored me because of my impairment as suggested in some of the literature related to disability studies (Murphy 1995).[4] I tried showcasing my skills in stand-up comedy. I still remember one of my jokes about *Motu Ram*, an imaginary character that I used to embody. The whole class would burst into laughter. I took it as a success at that time, which shows how I had internalized the ablest attitude of mocking a body that appears different.

There was a teacher who also happened to be the son of the principal. His favourite pastime was to beat me. Once I fell down while I was about to sit. He saw it from outside and came inside the classroom and started hitting me. Once I heard him discussing with his colleague '*Parents samajte nahi hai isko special school me bhejna chahiye*'. (Parents do not understand; they should send him to a special school.) His statement was not challenged by the other colleague as they were not used to seeing an impaired at regular schools.[5]

In the annual fest of school, I participated in the racing competition, which I wanted to win. But in comparison to other participants I found myself moving quite slowly. The race was finished in two minutes. I was disappointed to the core for not having won. A teacher gave me a consolation prize that I reluctantly took. I do not understand why society wants to construct an inspirational picture of an impaired person, even when he hasn't achieved a milestone. It is this kind of attitude that needs to be challenged, as it is dehumanizing.

Also, I fail to understand why society views impaired persons as asexual, who do not have any idea regarding heterosexual intimacy. There was one Plonza Khushwaha; I met her when I was in kindergarten. I confided to my brother about her, who shared my feelings

---

[4] Murphy argued that the very sight of disabled create anxiousness among non-disabled which make them avoiding disabled that in turn renders invisible status to disabled.

[5] https://cafedissensus.com/2017/09/16/dear-mom-now-its-my-turn-a-personal-account/

with my family. My parents did not encourage it, as I was too small to be in love with someone. But, I had a cousin who was ten to eleven years older than me who took interest in my love life so I told him that like any romantic hero of Bollywood, I managed to tell her:

'*Plonza mujhe tumhari aankhon ka kajal accha lagta hai*' (Plonza, I like the kohl that you put in your eyes.)

He laughed and said but the girl does not seem to be from an upper caste. He jokingly further said if at all I'm thinking of a future with her, there is a need to build a suitable career. For that to happen, I would have to start studying really hard and top the class. Also, he advised me to concentrate on my physiotherapy sessions. So, unknowingly, I was internalizing societal ideals about what it takes to be a suitable match, such as a good profession and a healthy body.

During those times, I used to play *Ghar–Ghar* at my locality, where I always wanted to play the role of an understanding husband who cares for the well-being of his wife. My understanding of man and his role and duty was not that different from Lord Rama in *Ramayana*.

After some time, my father was transferred to Banaras again, and this time we shifted along with him. My sister and brother got admission in St Joseph's Convent School but the principal politely said no to me. As I anticipated, my parents decided to get me admitted in a nearby public school. First, I did not enjoy it. For the first time, my brother was not there at the same school where I was going to study. Second, my siblings got admission in a convent school. I used to think that those who study in such schools not only have good language skills but also have a high social status.

I joined the public school. Initially, somebody from my family dropped me to the school, but later it was decided that I would take the rickshaw service provided by the school at a monthly charge. Initially I had some scepticism regarding the school but gradually I started enjoying the atmosphere. I used to pick up things quite quickly. Probably, I benefited from studying in a school that had very low class strength. I was doing well in my studies, and that kept my confidence level high.

School authorities were concerned about my safety and I was asked not to leave class during the lunch breaks. I did comply with the administrative demand but used to feel a bit odd as nobody at my home ever stopped me from taking part in outdoor activities. Slowly but surely I did challenge the commandment of the school administration of not letting me go outside the class. I also told my mother to have a word with the principal regarding this, as I wanted to enjoy my school life like any other kid.

I started going outside the classroom to play with the students of my class as well as from other classes. One day, while playing with other students, I lost my balance and fell down. There were bruises on my head. Somebody came with the first-aid box. A discussion ensued between some teachers and the principal. They looked very concerned about my well-being.

The principal said, 'We have to take precautionary measures. *Aaj Sameer ko ghar bhej dete hai*' (let us send Sameer back home). But this incident forced me back into the classroom during lunch breaks. Thinking about the incident, I was kicking myself for falling down. I did well in my studies, as the school atmosphere was more relaxing than other schools and provided much needed empathy which every student needs.

After a few years I qualified the entrance test of St Mary Convent School. My name was among the merit holders. For the first time I saw my father expressing his joy as he picked me up in his arms to embrace me.

I joined the school in the hope of doing good but only suffered. It was the first time in my life I was studying in a school where class strength on average was 60. It was a full-fledged English medium school, and their mode of instruction was completely in English. This was unlike my previous experiences, where teachers preferred talking in Hindi while delivering a lecture. Every day I used to feel a bit anxious entering the class because I was not able to follow the lectures. For the first time I was studying in a school where classes were at the first floor; it was a cause of concern for my parents as well. The school administration was quite positive while giving me admission saying that 'it would be managed'. It was decided that I would not be part of the assembly. So, it felt like a repetition of my experience of the school in Lucknow where I was denied an opportunity to establish a bond with my classmate. It was the first time I felt lonely.

There were some nice students around who used to encourage me to participate more in the class as there was constant effort from my side to hide myself. Some students accompanied me to the washroom on the teacher's instructions. But there was a kind of divide between me and my fellow classmates. I don't know how much that was influenced by the ideas of normality and abnormality (Hughes 2007), but it was a gap that never appeared to get bridged. On the contrary, I wanted that kind of school life where I was party to all the activity that is happening around me, whether it is bullying a fellow student or having a fight with a girl student over the sitting arrangement. My class teacher's decision to make me sit beside her did not help my case either. Maybe I never belonged in that place. I did not go for the picnic. I was not part of the group photograph at the school because I was late. All these things partly contributed in my not doing well in class.

On the suggestion of the teacher, I was shifted to the Hindi medium school, which was situated opposite our place at Banaras. I did really well at that school. In one of the classes, I was among the top three students. It was a school where students were from the economically and socially weaker sections of the society. From relatives of vegetable sellers to relatives of temple priests, the students came from many diverse backgrounds. I bonded well with most of my classmates. I'm not sure if it had something to do with my class status or culture of Banaras, which seems to privilege collectivism over individualism. Most of my friends did come to see me off after we finished school, and I could tell that they were not patronizing me. Yes, there were times when people did mention my impairment, but it was never a basis for my exclusion. I was one of them.[6]

Keeping my best interest in mind, my father took a transfer to Noida. The shift was thought better from the perspective of my education as well as health. He thought it was a better place where all the facilities (including medical facilities) could be easily accessed. My parents admitted me to the nearest school in our neighbourhood so that I could walk down to the school. So, early in the morning I used to cross a road, pass by a colony to reach to my school. Often I was punished for coming late to the school. It was never a problem for me. The only thing that bothered me was the behaviour of my classmates. It was, in a way, reminiscent of my experience at St Mary's School, where from the morning assembly to the last class of games I

---

[6] https://cafedissensus.com/2016/08/14/reflecting-on-my-memory-my-life-with-disability/

used to be stationed inside the class. I decided to break this chain by hinting to my classmates that I too am interested in playing football. I participated in a couple of games and I really enjoyed myself. I was, however, also experiencing other changes in my life. I was in my teens then and went through some biological changes that impacted my personal as well as academic life. I was not able to share with anyone what exactly I was going through. It made me not only change schools but cities as well. It shaped me into what I am today. It was after this phase I started advocating for sex education for persons with impairment. I used to motivate myself by thinking about the best thing that had happened to me so far.

The school from where I did my 11th and 12th was not a big and famous one and classmates' behaviour was not that great either. But, by then, I stopped bothering about these issues. I remember that school for one teacher. I do not know what he exactly saw in me. Motivation from his side pushed me to work harder. I could perform to the best of my ability, and this teacher also helped me in finding a dedicated scribe.

For the first time in my life I used a scribe in classes 11th and 12th. In the school where I studied earlier, I only used to take extra time in which many schools never gave me full one hour to finish the paper. I remember the principal of one of the schools directing the teachers: 'Provide Sameer with question paper before the assembly'.

I was only given 25 to 30 minutes extra by the school. No teacher really motivated me to use a scribe as this teacher did in classes 11th and 12th. I was one of the toppers in class 12th.

LIFE POST SCHOOL

I managed to secure admission in the Department of Sociology at Hindu College, University of Delhi. I decided not to be dependent on anybody and to concentrate only on my studies. I was anticipating similar kinds of attitude from students that I experienced in my school days. But it turned out to be quite good.

Faculty members associated with the Department as well as my classmates treated me on equal terms. After a long time, there were people in my life whom I could call friends. People with diverse kind of interests who cared for each other. At home, my siblings as well as my cousins knew about my likes and dislikes, desires and infatuations. I did not want to pass through as somebody who has no feelings, asexual (Kim 2011). So I opened up with my friends about what kind of girl I would love to date and build a life with.

Things were fine between me and all the friends until they decided to leave me alone to make me learn how to lead a self-dependent life. It was something I did not enjoy. They stopped waiting for me and were running away from me. I used to feel a bit sad about the whole scenario and fear that what if somebody asked me: Where are your friends? Why are you alone?

I wondered how carrying my bag had become a burdensome task for my friends. I was told that they were doing this for making me self-dependent and we were still friends. I made it clear to them that I think there is no one who is self-dependent. Still, I am not sure whether they were right or I was wrong.

While at Hindu College, I tried my hands at dramatics as well. I did all the things which I desired.

People really appreciated my acting skills. But I was never really asked to accompany my colleagues when they went outside Delhi to perform. Even I did not push for it, as I needed some assistance in getting ready. Maybe, I was doing things I always wanted to do but not able to liberate myself from the 'personal tragedy' (Oliver 1996, 15). The same thing happened when the department was planning to go for a field trip to Mumbai. I withdrew from it because I did not want my classmates to see me as vulnerable.

The major issue I faced during my graduation was the hazard of commuting to the University of Delhi. I missed classes almost for a month. I availed a carpool service at a high price but it was worth paying ₹1,500. I enjoyed every bit of my cab ride with the students who were studying in different colleges of the North campus of the University of Delhi.

It was very difficult to get quality scribes to write the college exams. There were no preparations from the university's side to make the whole process disabled-friendly. Every year during my graduation, I remember going to the University Health Centre two days before the commencement of exam to get the no objection certificate to avail services of the scribe. As we only used to get 15 days to prepare for exams, these administrative procedures never helped the case of a student like me who was not good at mugging assignments. I learned a lot from classroom engagement, and pursuing both an undergraduate as well as postgraduate degree in a discipline like sociology made me evaluate inequality in a social context. For example, the main reason behind women inequality is not their bodies but the patriarchal social structure which not only renders women's bodies vulnerable but also does not provide enough opportunities to them to avail all the opportunities of their professional lives.

Writing my MPhil dissertation on 'Disability Studies' was the best thing that happened to me in Jawaharlal Nehru University. It enhanced my critical perspective. One of its strands, social model of disability sees marginalization of persons with impairment in the way society has been structured. Like staircases and printed texts perpetuate existing negative attitude that excludes impaired persons from attaining quality education and a desirable job.

It made me realize that why only one kind of body is privileged over the other and one kind of intellectual activity over the other. Actually, it is the non-impaired who have made social rules that label life of impaired persons as unworthy. It made me understand the necessity of challenging such ablest values and that's how my own perspective towards my body changed from a personal tragedy to the celebration of the impairment. It also made me understand the diversity within the disability discourses.

CONCLUSION

From my childhood up to now, there is a marked shift in my experience of being an impaired person. Viewing the society from the lessons learnt from disability studies not only makes accessibility and acceptability a core issue, but it makes us construe a person with impairment as diversity. At a personal level, it has made me assert for self-determination.

For me, there is a need to propagate the kind of reflective exercise in the society that can create oneness among members of the society, on the one hand, and respect for individual differences, on the other. Also, if impairment causes physical discomfort, which it does, non-impaired ones are not beyond physical suffering.

As I believe, persons with impairments must be competing in the job market with their non-impaired colleagues. We can be good husbands, wives, caregivers and lovers.

Let's imagine a world beyond stigma.[7]

REFERENCES

Foucault, M. 1976[1973]. *The Birth of the Clinic*. London: Routledge, Tavistock Publications (first published in English in 1973).

Ghai, Anita. 2002. 'Disability in the Indian Context: Post-colonial Perspectives.' *Disability/Postmodernity: Embodying Disability Theory*. London, New York: Continuum.

Hughes, Bill. 2007. 'Being Disabled: Towards a Critical Social Ontology for Disability Studies.' *Disability & Society* 22 (7): 673–84.

Hughes, Bill, and Kevin Paterson. 1997. 'The Social Model of Disability and the Disappearing Body: Towards a Sociology of Impairment.' *Disability & Society* 12 (3): 325–40.

Kim, Eunjung. 2011. 'Asexuality in Disability Narratives.' *Sexualities* 14 (4): 479–93.

Mankekar, Purnima. 1999. *Screening Culture, Viewing Politics: An Ethnography of Television, Womanhood, and Nation in Postcolonial India*. Durham, N.C.: Duke University Press.

Mehrotra, Nilika. 2013. 'Cultural Conception of Disability in Haryana.' In *Disability, Gender and State Policy: Exploring Margins*. Rawat Publications.

Merleau-Ponty, M. 1996[1962]. *Phenomenology of Perception*. Delhi: Motilal Banarsidass (first Indian edition, first published in English in 1962).

Miles, Michael. 'Disability in an Eastern Religious Context: Historical Perspectives.' *Disability & Society* 10 (1): 49–70.

Murphy, R. 1995. 'Encounters.' *The Body Silent: The Different World of the Disabled* (pp. 140–58). London, Los Angeles, Berkeley: University of California Press.

Oliver, Michael. 1996. 'The Social Model in Context.' *Understanding Disability*, 30–42. London: Macmillan Education.

---

[7] https://www.patientsengage.com/conditions/living-with-cerebral-palsy-parents-encouraged-independence

Chapter 11

Narratives of Growing with A-typicality

Asha Singh

INTRODUCTION

Sometimes small events in different parts of the globe are momentous as they deal with poignant issues; however, they influence the big picture with slow strokes. The wheelchair user April Coughlin created one such moment by introducing disability as a disadvantaged porous state, conveying that most individuals go in and out of marginalization in a world characterized by uniformity (Simon 2013). Simon reported Coughlin leading a march with banners of Temporarily Able Bodies (TAB) in *The New York Times*. TAB participants were drawing dismissive public gaze on the rights of people with disability just like circumstantial barriers faced by each individual. TAB captured parallels in exclusion that could be language disability for Hindi speaker in Karnataka. Inability of urban youth in drawing water from a well or ageing individuals unable to read fine print may as well find temporary disabling contexts. Besides specific impairments, long life, uneven resources or being members of minority groups will pose challenging barriers, creating disabling moments for people.

Being wheelchair-bound reduces access, opportunity and choice, in addition the inflexible social attitudes disallows discussions on everyday concerns of people with disability. There is an urgency for paradigm shift in societal orientation towards 'disability'. Society seems ignorant of the confluence of factors that limit opportunities for a large growing group of people with specific 'typicality' or needs. Disability as a discipline needed to organize itself and examine the physical features, attitudes and values, enlarging the social ground of typical and atypical continuum.

THE CHAPTER FORMAT

I share some ways in which we as a family shaped social encounters for my daughter who defied typical norms with some handholding to wade through a world geared towards uniformity. She forced us to review her skills by forceful declarations. 'It is hard to put what is in my mind on paper' or silences or just stoic inaction to indicate inability. Guided by her needs, we alternated use of special school for learning difficulties and a public school to build her skills. Reframing typical norms became primary to de-restrict opportunities and enhance participation for her. Routines and rhythms even in many art courses are designed for people who are more typical. Children with contemplative or slow to respond disposition often fall in the cracks unless pushed. What follows are personal narrative stories of ways to enable the atypical to walk along creating a space for their pace.

Similar to the emergence of women studies or Dalit studies, disability studies evolved to centre stage, facts that need normalizing in society to promote equality and equity of opportunity and choices. The lived experiences of people with atypicality need constructive facilitation to enhance quality of life for all. Coming to terms with limitations cannot be diffused by jolts and distasteful experiences often putting parents in a cycle of 'chronic sorrow' (Cameron et al. 1992, 96–112). Motivation has to be fuelled by stories of trials and triumphs.

Traces of addressing diversity are rewarding and provide recognition to individuals. The founder of Centre for Cellular and Molecular Biology in Hyderabad in the early 1990s described academic as well as the details of the state-of-the-art facilities for research, participation and engagement that included notice boards in Braille, conference chairs with writing fixtures on the right allowing ease of note taking for left-handed people. Sharing rare disability infrastructural details in formal seminars evoked squeals of delight from lone or couple of left-handed persons. Recognition of difference became assertion of identity and privileging liberation in right-handed majority. Providing facilities to meet special needs is significant to circumvent the danger of negativity in atypical children (Barbour 1996, 12–15; Gorman 1999, 72–77).

Anecdotes of joy in being part of social physical world is significant for what schools with lifts, accessible toilets and other barrier-free fixtures would do for the social and emotional well-being of children with limitations. Addressing individual challenges are acts of empathy, besides being steps in coexistence of many competencies and statement of inclusive attitudes in society. Infrastructural support is visible support of different competencies; however, the invisible challenges continue to rest in small intended acts of commission and unintended omission as raised by the protesters. Exclusion and neglect can be cognitively repressive and emotionally damaging. This chapter examines disabling encounters and experiences contingent on individual-specific atypical wiring of the intellectual system. The attempt is to address systemic barriers such as dominance of print-based learning, assessment based on reproduction of facts on paper or strong forces of competition that dis-privilege children who may be 'learning disabled'. Socialization, schooling or occasions for or absence of social interaction can be contexts or experiences creating isolation, rejection or exclusion. 'Stereotypical normative behaviours' not only in educational settings including a range of social situations can be daunting for individuals. There is often no attempt or time to explore the difference.

Research is testimony to the possibility of achievements beyond the 'fixed-ability' learning (Swann et al. 2012), and evidence from research affirms that '… human potential is not predictable, that children's futures are unknowable, that education or exposure has the power to enhance the lives of all' (p. 1).

Teacher education programmes in India lay emphasis on standardization, competition or setting target for predictable outcomes.

The majority of society supports uniformity in classroom teaching—learning, methods of assessment and evaluation of knowledge. The proponents of inclusive education need to challenge and change this 'deep-rooted orthodoxy' review processes of learning and the role of the teacher (Slee 2012, 895–907). The assumptions of how learning is conceived and presence of specific practices support one kind of ability, oppressing the individual who displays differences in comprehension and expression. Identifying barriers to inclusive thinking, values and practices will animate discourses on disability and seriously encourage appreciation of diversity in learners.

THEORETICAL CONCEPTUALIZATION

The contents in this chapter present evidence of influencing social acceptance of variation by alternating intervention and collaboration to nurture 'potential' and 'presence', thereby shaping social construction of ability–disability. The individual negotiations are parental involvements modifying social expectations and perceptions of disability in a wide range of educational–social settings. The argument is guided by a constructivist theoretical framework to explain experiences of disability as observed, perceived and interpreted by parents (Parry and Dan 1994; White and Epston 1990). The leanings in the discussions are resonant with the social model of disability adopted by the World Health Organization (Finkelstein 1993, 9–16; Smith 1999, 117–44). Disability is largely viewed as the interaction between societal expectations and abilities of the individual. It is often stated that disability becomes a problem due to non-conformity to social expectations, rendering social spaces as disabling.

The text essays examples from the journey of a mother and child negotiating norms in socializing a person with an atypical disposition. It would be worthwhile to state that irrespective of ability or disability, children thrive if a dyadic relationship is premised on implicit trust and belief in the individual. A positive, consistent and caring relation with a significant other is necessary for individuals to thrive and more so in instances of atypicality.

THE STORY OF A JOURNEY

Encounters with time lag in emergence of competence beyond typical range began early with delay in head control. I slowly adjusted to unsolicited concern 'no head control, how many months?' The unfolding of developmental variance was conveyed as a palpable challenge to me, 'the mother', by continued commentaries. I soon learnt to convert distress reaction to warning signals and forces to be 'coped with'. I could not influence friends and relatives to refrain but I heeded by doubling my inputs. Their words seemed to bare facts and unclothe reality that I was evading or did not wish to address. The comments also left me helpless. Experiencing agony was never ending.

A young friend on seeing Maya at nine months after a gap of four weeks exclaimed 'she is just the same'. My expression spelt recoiling within, still she furthered my agony adding her expectations to see Maya sitting and pulling herself to standing position. She articulated thoughts I was procrastinating. 'Developmental delay' put the fear of tsunami. Such remarks induced anxiety, generated helplessness, but after some setback we doubled our efforts in reaching the expected goals. Social understanding of ability and disability need not always revolve around empathy and emotional sensitivity or medical deficit model. These are moments to shape caregivers for rising to intervene for the sake of the child.

Challenges of socializing children

In such instances of despondency, my route was to seek similarities in the socializing of my first child. I consoled myself by noting that socialization of the young necessitates facing childhood problems in magnitudes that varied. Socialization of the older sibling had also raised conflicts such as playground bullying. The response to which was 'no violence in return', just ignore and follow your game. I was helpless in both, however; the inference I drew seemed to indicate empowering individuals according to the context. Intervention either in the physical domain or in the social domain would emerge from experiential inputs or interactions. As parents, the epistemic principle was empowerment for Maya to craft a social space; however, it is easier said in hindsight. To realize that past is history, future is mystery and that the present is a gift of 'now' is tremendously difficult.

Seeking comfort in the ways the older sibling had matured was both redeeming to the self of the mother and functioned to lift spirits in destabilizing moments in the socialization of daughter Maya.

Seeking and reaching out to certain experts served to be reassuring 'Put her in a school, she will catch up on speech being with children', suggesting to widen her social network as small families sometimes did not provide enough stimulation. Some professionals demoted any vision of a bright future 'your child will not be a lawyer or teacher', referring to our professions. The words seemed sharp verbal attacks mocking our existence, 'Not hiding the reality' seemed brutal almost sadistic. Frequency of such encounters slowly made us strong, enabling of not harbouring parental injury and rise from the ashes to challenge professional certainty of diagnosis. We sang, read books and took the children to parks, book fairs, providing all experiences children enjoy.

SUPPORTIVE ENVIRONMENTS: ENABLING FAMILIES

At two years and two months after a new year's eve party, Maya walked independently and the news brought honest relief, joy and laughter from a few friends. Often attitudinal change begins with small circles of intimacy. Positive forces can be sourced from few friends. Their trust and faith brought tidings from their circles of intimacy. Small supportive groups generated belief and positivity and unflinching support and trust for nurturing the optimal. We stuck to a small circle of friends spending evenings together playing, spreading objects for Maya to feel, touch and create in the midst of adult chatter. Few friends are enough to create ripples of positive gratification in comparison to many.

Maya's father explained quite early to her that she was 'Maya', meaning 'illusion'. Maya as a little child would often repeat, *Main hoon bhi mein nahi bhi hoon, idhar bhi hoon udhar bhi hoon* (I am there, I am not there, I am here and I am there). This playful philosophical orientation has inadvertently guided Maya in her life's journey encountering social challenges, adapting, adjusting and creating spaces in social contexts. Quite unconsciously, she built a shield to diffuse rejection that she identified quickly, 'I am the oldest in the class', 'no one comes to my birthday party', 'I was left in the class, everyone went for Annual Day

Practice'. Collateral advantage of using philosophical analogy has been absence of self-labelling in fact enabling. Strategies for empowerment had to be modified; in later years, there was an active attempt to train Maya to ignore infantile interactions that became very significant as the years progressed.

THE EARLY YEARS

Bringing up a child is joyous as well as demanding of meeting the needs of another 'self'. Each young child responds as guided by individual disposition that initiates and shapes the nature of interactions with the caregivers in the environment. However, in situations of difference, the adult may have to train for specific inputs as also learn to deal with weak social support. The process of socializing a child with a difference requires responsiveness as guided by atypicality. Some new learning may be negotiating isolation and social systemic resistances.

The dyadic relation encountered small triumphs and many trials as social contexts are arrangements for neurotypical individuals. With delayed speech, the child needed to be in environments with continuous linguistic inputs, despite doctor's recommendation the entry to preschool needed to clear many procedures.

Of course, reaching out to experts for remedial inputs with the knowledge that early detection early intervention benefits children was a task that needed new forms of courage. Self-propelling motivation and belief is the only force to nurture and reckon with and diffuse social barriers.

> As a three-year-old preschooler in an 'inclusive' set up, Maya was admitted with her own helper. This had become necessary as she was also younger than other peers and needed to be in a linguistically rich environment. The family ensured that the helper's presence was there for her safety and to tell us what was happening in school. Such a conversation helped Maya understand the idea of going with a helper unlike other children to be a conscious decision in her favour. (At a preschool, Rajkumari Amrit Kaur Child Study Centre, 1986)

The Child Study Centre, despite university affiliations and guided by child development professionals, created this modification only after recommendation from an All India Institute of Medical Sciences-certified speech therapist. Often, one family pursues and treads the path not travelled to open routes for further such requirements. Disability needs social representation within public spaces, and then hesitation to discuss atypical features opens dialogue and in turn routes for others to seek developmental inputs. Families need to be counselled and encouraged to deal with differences in public domains and seek opportunities for their children.

As advocates of disability studies, it is necessary to imbibe value of certain norms and structures and not dismiss all boundaries. For instance, the biological pattern or the species-specific behaviour boosts adult compliance for the care and well-being for the survival of the baby. The anxiety or distress from tactless comments has to be sublimated. The spirit to help children to bring out the optimal rests in a positive belief. A transformed force of faith in the child's individual potential can bring miracles. Human infancy embedded in the longest period of dependency compels holding and nurturing environments to be a necessary condition for human development. In the light of the developmental demands supported by neuroscience research, the significance of the early years is undisputed. If the baby displays any variations to a neurotypical pattern, the dyadic relation is obliged to modify and refigure the dynamics. The journey of parents and daughter in the various stages of the lifespan presented a range of negotiations, resistances and silences peppered with rebellion. With initial lack of confidence, the family pushed the child in different ways, assisting Maya evolve from a baby who reacted to the second dose of the DPT immunization to becoming a teacher who assists teachers in a leading private school.

THE FORMAL SCHOOL

Maya and the family did face humiliation in not complying with the pace of other children. The teacher shamed both mother and child for inability to move ahead and not being ashamed. It did not occur to the teacher that perhaps Maya needed promptings and push to engage in the classroom dynamics. Not all children swim out from deep emersion, without floating assistance and cajoling. The utter dismay at the child being ridiculed in front of the classmates left me heart broken. An angry-faced child stomping out of class saying, 'I don't know how to do', brought relief. An open confession of inability that the teacher was unable to identify. This experience forced the mother to seek a special school for the dyslexics. It was a delayed decision, but sometimes a new path emerges with time. Maya thrived under the individualized tutelage and developed immense confidence and pride in academic work. Specially devised language teaching enhanced comprehension across the curriculum. The school worked on building academic potential. Maya developed good language skills and writing proficiency. Total absence of non-academic social contexts and interactions became a concern for the family. The mother felt a wider exposure would enrich Maya's life chances.

The family started a search for an inclusive school, which in the late 1990s was difficult to find. Educational settings and social frames were still ruled by norm-based deficit model. Quirk of circumstances brought admission for Maya in a leading school. There is immense gratitude for easy inclusion; however, that was only a start, sustaining a meaningful relation was a rather bumpy ride. The school and the classroom were set for children habituated to work in groups, give weekly class tests and adeptly following group instructions. Even if some children were not competent, they silently followed; the numbers in class did not permit possibility of individual attention; however, they managed with low performance.

Maya clearly resisted lack of attention and would not want to do anything without reassuring nod or validation, specially tasks based on cognitive processing. No essay could be written without some approval of initial work. The teachers had been apprised but could only intervene once in a while. Moments of attention heightened the concentration to allow for a general understanding of curricular transaction. Maya was also very sharp to exclusions such as 'not been given the class test' on the assumption that she would not be able to perform. Frank and forthright reproduction of classroom interactions alerted the mother, who then provided innovative solutions such as creating a question paper for the child. This practice was permitted, and we kept the paper formal. Besides collaborative acts, the mother also made interventions in assessment processes, requesting leniency for flawless grammar or overlooking accurate spelling in non-language subjects.

Reduced syllabus and focused content were permitted to assess comprehension. However, the school was unprepared for assessing the learning process not reproduction of facts. In their opinion, the focused content and objective-type assessment in academic structure disadvantaged other non-learning disabled children. The mother persisted that, for Maya, competition was not the aim but being enabled to be a part of the existing social contexts of which schooling is a significant component. The social contexts have to assist individual capacities rather than disabling the differently abled. With persuasion, a space for assistive assessment was created. Flexibility in assessment was a small step in impacting academic norms in the school system. Maya and family had stirred a micro-social system to adapt to the differences in needs of individuals. As cautioned by disability scholars, disabling environments have to be dealt with to create facilitative systems (Lenny 1993, 233–40).

There is huge indebtedness to the public school, for willingly admitting Maya providing experience of mainstream education. It helped her grow in real social contexts of competition, forging an individualized space beyond contest. However, crossing hurdles is not a one-time feat or 'happily ever after'. Consistency and continuity in negotiating mountain loads of curricular content was an all-time challenge. Parenting in general and parenting of child with varying abilities is a full-time task centred on alertness to test routine, agility in setting the paper and social finesse in getting child-led assessment. Social stereotyping or astounding assumptions never failed to throw bewildering surprises 'you are quite intelligent what happens to your academics?'

Insensitivity was often brought to my notice by my daughter's frank reproductions of everyday school encounters. Maya also became aware that her mother's visits enhanced the quality of school experience and in later years would often remark 'come to school, its action time'.

Involving parents is useful as they have instinctive insights that can energize pedagogical action, a fact that Maya internalized more than the school. We made sure that Maya had a variety of inputs choosing teachers with care (Jeynes 2012, 710).

Self-Regulation of Parental Diffidence

Maya was enrolled for music lessons and the teacher chose small goals. She rejoiced at successes provided by individual attention within group teaching. Such small gestures impacted both the mother and daughter. Maya performed as part of the choir gaining pride in stage performances. Rewards from the gamut of experiences propelled a renewed vigour in the aggressive socializing of atypicality within deeply norm-ridden social structures. Classroom dynamics posed different kinds of encounters everyday increasing my belief that schools may profess 'inclusion' but the groundwork to deal with real issues is incomplete. Schools often viewed the mother as overambitious, constantly monitoring or having unrealistic dreams (Goddard et al. 2000, 279–83).

Emotional balance was often rocked by friends raising anger towards lack of initiative of inclusive actions by school. Despite much debate and critical views about the inefficiency of the school, the mother with mixed energy of confidence and diffidence continued to keep a consistent vigil. Science teachers would insist on spelling accuracy despite knowing the dyslexic diagnosis, English teachers would go wild with red marks, disgusted at Maya's inability to crack the phonetic idiosyncrasy of the English language. Maya had been trained to work through sight words, magic 'e' and other mnemonic devices; however, sequential memory did not always stand in good stead. Her frustration was in exclusion from co-curricular activities.

'I sat all day in class as all children were practicing'. The mother went to intervene and shift focus from cultural excellence to team performance including children who may be different. Convincing the school of possibility of teamwork and its social benefits for individual children needed persuasion as the 'annual day' is a big event showcasing institutional achievements and, in the words of the school authorities, 'is attended by invited guests, dignitaries and parents'. Waving aside the feeling of exclusion from the parent category, the mother relentlessly urged, 'Don't school performances need trees, or people to make crowds? As children, we took turns to do such passive roles'. The principal smiled and the mother felt reassured of her daughter's presence on stage not anticipating the irony that followed. 'Give me old torn clothes for the show, I am a beggar in the school annual ballet'. The role allocation was hilarious and the comic element evoked immense laughter. It became a family legend enhancing conspiratorial camaraderie in reconfiguring societal norms. Such instances are ubiquitous and reported by other parents. The deep structures in prejudice and assumptions have often resulted in humour.

Many years later, when Maya visited a leading institute for disability certification, the guard at the door stopped them to be informed 'we have an appointment'. The mother said they had an appointment with the doctor. Without missing a beat, he questioningly pointed towards Maya, '*yeh maand buddhi hain?*' (Is she retarded?). Maya's hard stare seemed to make no dent in his fixed frame of reference and firm belief that disability fractures are skill of interpretation. Maya has often regaled family, 'the guard called me "*maand buddhi*"'. In an institutional setting for the differently abled, the presence of such dismissive labelling seemed ominous. There is a growing concern for disability sensitivity not getting enough international attention and action.

Social Initiative: Involving and Engaging

In the regular public schools, a range of activities are offered to build among students awareness of social inequities and contentious issues. Maya had come to the grade where she needed to be part of such an initiative. In a chance encounter, one of the teachers had observed Maya telling a story to a small child. She proposed that as part of Socially Useful Productive work, Maya should do storytelling sessions in the kindergarten classes. Maya used puppets and simple props to engage the children. She was received well until the mother was summoned by a teacher in the KG section to be informed that Maya was eating children's lunch. A panic-stricken mother rushed to the school to find that after one storytelling session, some children wanted to 'share what they had' contingent on the theme of the story 'share what you have'.

The teacher walked in only to see Maya biting off a bit from many lunch boxes. The episode was a big setback, as vulnerability of individuals for social isolation and labelling was quite fragile. The humiliation, the violence on individual dignity and the possibility of being judged seemed so easy without sufficient evidence or any chance for individuals to defend themselves. Despite the oppressive forces of majoritarian beliefs, differently abled groups have asserted their visibility through special abilities, through specific inputs and imagination of motivated individuals. The affirmation of rewards is energizing and serves to be a catalyst in surviving and reviving from situations of severe seclusion and rejection.

STORIES ABOUT SOCIAL IDENTITY, INCLUSION AND DISADVANTAGE

Physical barriers are most talked about in the disability literature as sources of everyday frustrations. Structures of rewards and punishments in society for the social identity of differently abled individuals are not even gleaned over. At times, it feels that atypical children are oblivious of peer achievements and an ostrich-like stance of wishing away problems shapes parental approach.

Maya seemed content watching the achievements and accolades bestowed on peers until her mother heard her mumble, 'perhaps I can be awarded for full attendance'. A school ceremony rewarded almost a 100 students for excellence in specific subjects, securing positions in sports, drama, math or science quiz and even recognition of 100 per cent school attendance. This last category spelt hope and possibility based on physical effort with no mental stress of reproducing facts in sequential order, all cognitive skills that challenged Maya. On hearing of Maya's comment and aspiration, the school principal was imaginative enough to introduce a category 'Mountain Climber's Award' that fulfilled her dream and would later serve to recognize many other individuals. The mother felt no qualms in sharing the child's dream with the principal.

It is only debate and discussion that will bring redressal and public attention to disabling social processes. Social, physical, natural, ideological and geopolitical environments need to be favouring universal design to validate all types of bodies and minds and not cater to unique contexts that marginalize atypicality. As facilitator in theatre workshops, there is a particular exercise of sharing personal moments. I cite one to focus on disability marginalization.

> 25 year old Music teacher Rahul growing up in Canada watched his sister who had a neuromuscular disorder being teased in school. He was pained that she was frequently subjected to being an object of ridicule causing immense emotional bashing. Such acts were often dismissed as merely 'unfortunate' with no punishment for the doer of pervert acts. Rahul dealt with the life events of his family by writing songs about difference and diversity. (Personal Narrative: Workshop on Special Needs 2004)

Disabling stories in everyday lives of individuals have to be shared as real contexts to influence social discourse and search for appropriate resolve.

Maya reported being accused of taking a boy's 10-rupee note. To the question by the family, 'Did you take it?' her hard stare and stupefied response shamed each family member. But the resolve she had for the problem was to just give a 10-rupee note and bring closure to the controversy. She did not want any public scrutiny, and deeply internalized absence of social support led her to push the controversy away from public gaze. She handed back the money in front of the whole class and the matter rested with no interjection either by the teacher or by other peers. The family respected Maya's decision and did not intercept. Personal narratives such as of Rahul have disturbing and disconcerting resonances of victimization of children in everyday encounters in inclusive settings. Certain issues make children more vulnerable in everyday routines. Evading of confrontation is a form of protecting verbal violence, yet siblings and families' beliefs and trust in children with limitations will evolve innovative ways to raise empathy and social justice.

Culture of Print Expertise

Maya was also being subjected to comply with academic standards to achieve certificates of academic acclaim and gain social position. The intensity in storing dense textual content becomes difficult to cope specially for a mind that is searching and struggling. We had tried different ways to foster basic literacy using 'focused content and reduced quantity' for assessment; however, structures of the public examination leave little scope for individualized assessment. Schools profess inclusion until class IX, after which keeping the fear of Public Board Examination wills off their social will. Maya left the school routine as a student to avoid continued rejection or experience her presence as a pressure by the teachers. 'Why political science? or Why in my class?' were statements from teachers who the mother considered to be change makers. The resistance to discrimination no longer seemed meaningful. Perhaps it was time to seek individualized learning spaces or moving beyond situations that trained for cognitive competence. Maya finished her class X and XII from the National Institute of Open Schooling.

Experiences with Professionals: Building Daily Rhythms

Different experts and friends provided options for everyday engagement. Maya needed a work routine, daily rhythms marking the 24-hour cycle like any other person. Maya worked in a variety of social contexts. Welcoming groups and individuals opened many doors with a little bit of knocking. A leading sociologist was working in communities researching health care systems and practices for well-being. She identified Maya's bilingual fluency as an asset that could be used gainfully for facilitating conversational English. Maya accompanied the team of researchers to resettlement colonies sharing her ability in easy use of two languages and in turn learning about diversity of social lives. Absence of competition and comparison and displaying only cognitive competence was relaxing. Interactions in new social geographies made it easy to strive for cognitive competence, especially with no prescribed texts with absence of specific assessment patterns. Though Maya enjoyed the work in communities, the logistics of travel time seemed very time intensive and had to be discontinued.

A more convenient and welcome opening was an offer to be teacher assistant in an inclusive public school. Regular working hours with little pressure to perform on any measures excited both Maya and her mother. In a span of six years, the field of inclusion seemed to have made progress in leaps and bounds. The school was visibly disability sensitive with social workers, ramps, elevator and toilets. Training and exposure of teachers to patterns in inclusion had sensitized teachers who served as appropriate mentors for Maya. The friendly group of colleagues engaged constructively facilitating her to be an efficient assistant teacher. Specifically assigned responsibilities comprised supervision of children's accuracy in recording homework questions with correct date. Tasks of distributing circulars, matching quantities for each class may be routine but required number correspondence, ensuring precise circulation without missing any group. Consistency in executing daily chores with commitment brought additional responsibilities of managing dispersal of primary section children to board homebound buses. Her self-esteem grew by leaps and bounds, further empowered by being given the position 'in charge of bus duty'. Such gestures fuelled more passion and ownership, influencing both confidence and cheer.

Employment did not deter Maya in working on her qualifications. After class XII through Open Schooling, she successfully worked towards a graduate degree from National Open University. The self-study was facilitated by support of tuition interventions. With each qualification, the school provided monetary benefits.

Presently, schools address the inclusion envelope by 'employing' differently abled persons as teacher's aide; however, none follows disability rights of appropriate remuneration. Parents provide sealed envelopes as fake salaries to the individuals. Parental compliance to such arrangements continues as dignified employment for atypical young adults are few as mentioned in the beginning. Systematic assessment of the contributions of teacher assistants in the classroom needs to be examined for appropriate positioning of the differently abled.

CONCLUSIONS

The experiences in this chapter have been described to critically examine the parental role in dealing with disability in society. The goal in using a personal narrative approach has been to contribute to emergence of disability studies on lived experience of dealing with real social barriers. The road boulders could be social insensitivity, professional apathy and dismissive attitudes and such obstacles have to be circumvented and not cause freeze frames of tragedy and parental icons of grief and inordinate amount of stress. The tenor of disability discourse stresses constructive spearheading by family. Support groups accentuate advocacy for ways to identify niches based on children's needs echoing research studies in other continents with similar repressive and prejudiced social climate as described here (Goddard et al. 2000, 281–82).

Educational institutions as microcosm of society reflect structural and socio-cultural dynamics that (re)produce or (re)construct forces of oppression or exclusion as reiterated by Disability Division Mission Statement (2017). Parental–child empowerment to negotiate on what 'I can do' than merely focus on memorizing chunks of print matter may ease journeys of differently abled individuals.

Societal assumptions, attitudes, dismissive stances and acts of omission and commission will be social realities unless replaced with enabling disability discourse. Social events, entrepreneurial initiatives or assisted independent living have to fire the imagination of parent support groups' contemporary disability discourse. Sharing experiences in formal conferences, institutions or parent organizations empowers atypical individuals, enhancing public visibility.

Innovative rhythms and stories of empowerment of diversity of skills will defy assumptions and eliminate prejudices that make different-abled vulnerable. Narratives of parents of differently abled children will contribute richly in understanding the challenges that disability studies need to address displacing notions of tragic and dysfunctional attributes often associated with differences in ability.

Stereotypes and deterministic certainty among professionals have irked parents. Waves of discontent impelled parental comradeship facilitating humour and laughter to critique. Admonishing assumptions, authority and isolation will emerge from ethnographic research that explores disability status in social contexts (Mehrotra 2005).

The different narratives may find more questioning of social barriers in an individual's evolving social presence influencing ability of the family to take bold decisions and act on individual experiences to open possibilities. Collaborations through disability dialogues may generate cooperation, creating positivity and enabling social milieu.

REFERENCES

Barbour, A. C. 1996. 'Supporting Families: Children Are the Winners!' *Early Childhood News* 8 (6): 12–15.

Cameron, S. J., A. Snowdon, and R. Orr. 1992, March. 'Emotions Experienced by Mothers of Children with Developmental Disabilities.' *Children's Health Care* 2 (2): 96–102.

Disability Division Mission Statement. 2017. 'Division of Disability at the Society for the Study of Social Problems', University of Tennessee, USA. Available at: https://www.sssp1.org/index.cfm/pageId/1351/m/464 (last accessed on 27 August 2017).

Finkelstein, V. 1993. 'The Commonality of Disability.' In *Disabling Barriers— Enabling Environments*, edited by J. Swain, V. Finkelstein, S. French and M. Oliver, 9–16. London: SAGE.

Goddard, J. A., A. Lehr, and J. C. Lapadat. 2000. 'Parents of Children with Disabilities: Telling a Different Story.' *Canadian Journal of Counselling* 34 (4): 273–89.

Gorman, J. C. 1999, January/February. 'Understanding Children's Hearts and Minds: Emotional Functioning and Learning Disabilities.' *Teaching Exceptional Children* 31 (3): 72–77.

Jeynes, W. 2012, July. 'A Meta-Analysis of the Efficacy of Different Types of Parental Involvement Programs for Urban Students.' *Urban Education* 47 (4): 706–42.

Lenny, J. 1993. 'Do Disabled People Need Counselling?' In *Disabling Barriers— Enabling Environments*, edited by J. Swain, V. Finkelstein, S. French and M. Oliver, 233–40. London: SAGE.

Mehrotra, N. 2005, February 5. Review of *Exploring Differences Women, Disability and Identity*, by Asha Hans and Annie Patri (New Delhi: SAGE). *Economic and Political Weekly* 40 (6): 65–72.

Parry, A., and R. E. Doan. 1994. *Story Re-vision: Narrative Therapy in the Postmodern World*. New York, NY: Guilford Press.

Simon, C. Cecilia. 2013, November 1. 'Disability Studies: A New Normal.' *New York Times*.

Slee, R. 2012. 'How Do We Make Inclusive Education Happen When Exclusion is the Political Disposition.' *International Journal of Inclusive Education* 17 (8): 895–907.

Smith, P. 1999. 'Drawing New Maps: A Radical Cartography of Developmental Disabilities.' *Review of Educational Research* 69 (2): 117–44.

Swann, M., Peacock, A., Hart, S. & Drummond, M.J. (2012) Creating Learning without Limits. Maidenhead: Open University Press.

White, M., and D. Epston. 1990. *Narrative Means to Therapeutic Ends*. New York, NY: W.W Norton and Company, Inc.

Chapter 12

Life-writing and Disabled Self in the Works of Oliver W. Sacks

Sandeep R. Singh

The term life-writing is not easy to define as it encompasses varied modes of self-narratives and it does not follow any one particular style, structure, theme, trope or literary genre. Several critics have attempted to define this form of writing by extending their horizons to all possible forms of self—confessional, experiential and recollective. Life-writing, as Zachary Leader defines it, 'is a generic term used to describe a range of writings about lives or parts of lives, or which provide materials out of which lives or parts of lives are composed' (2015, 1). Life-writing as a form therefore encompasses sketches, memoirs, vignettes, anecdotes, musings, confessions, biography, autobiography, memoir, testimony, letters, oral narratives, fictional and non-fictional interventions into narratives of everyday, (psycho)pathologically marked discourses, trauma narratives, confessional narratives (ranging from religious to online blogs) and narratives of marginality like illness or disability. However, the list of such writings is ever-expanding, especially now, with the advent of different forms of cyber technology and social media. As Leader states in the 'Introduction' to his edited anthology *On Life-writing* (2015, 1).

> Some writers on life-writing distinguish between shorter forms, conceived of as source material, and 'life-writing proper' or 'extended life

narratives' or 'formal biography and autobiography'; others distinguish between life-writing that is exemplary or formulaic, often associated with older periods, and the sort that seems or seeks to express more modern qualities: authenticity, sincerity, interiority, individuality.

The 'modern qualities' of life-writing that lend itself to the affective, has—as suggested by Leader—facilitated a premise for an engagement with the interiority of experience in the pursuit of an authentic subjectivity. The reiteration of an authentic subjectivity becomes crucial within the domain of hegemonic, violent and oppressive structures that enable the discourse of normativity. Therefore, life-writing as a form, since its inception, has engaged with the narratives of the afflicted and marginalized and this resonance of voices speaking from marginal and liminal spaces characterizes life-writing even today. Experiential accounts of battered and raped women, victims of the holocaust, homosexuals, slave narratives and people who suffered from the traumas of caste atrocities, racism, war and social exclusion have found voice in this form. Similarly, it is only after the 1980s that the narratives of the disabled—who have been 'For centuries.... oppressed and repressed... isolated, incarcerated, observed, written about, operated on, instructed, implanted, regulated, treated, institutionalized and controlled to a degree probably unequal to that experienced by any other minority group' (Davis 2013, xv)—began to emerge in the form of life-writing. Some examples of this are Hellen Keller's *The Story of My Life* (1903), Irving Zola's *Missing Pieces: A Chronicle of Living with a Disability* (1982), Fern Kupfer's *Before and After Zacharaiah* (1982), Lucy Grealy's *Autobiography of a Face* (1994) and Lennard J. Davis's *My Sense of Silence* (2000).

In her essay 'Coming to Terms: Life Writing—from Genre to Critical Practice' Marlene Kadar (1992, 12) argues:

> Life writing as a critical practice... encourages (a) the reader to develop and foster his/her own self-consciousness in order to (b) humanise and make less abstract (which is not to say less mysterious) the self-in-the-writing. Thus, there are many forms, or genres, in which a reader may glean this written self, but we usually think immediately of autobiography, letters, diaries, and anthropological life narratives, genres in which

the conventional expectation is that the author does not want to pretend he/she is absent from the text. Add to these original life-writing genres the fictionalised equivalents, including self-reflexive metafiction, and life writing becomes both the 'original genre' and critical comment on it, and therefore the self-in-the-writing. At its most radical, the critical practice of life writing enhances reading as a means of emancipating an overdetermined 'subject,' or various subject-locations.

While life-writing need not necessarily locate itself in the first-person experience, it does tend to adopt the first-person narrative. By attempting to perceive itself from a third-person perspective, it also tries to understand the 'other' from a first-person perspective. While engaging in each of these activities the narrator 'transgresses' the boundary between the 'self' and the 'other'. Thus, the engagement of life-writing as a genre would be to make the realm of the unexperienced real to the reader, and also conceive of the 'other' as a complete being in the world. In as much as this is concerned, Bakhtin's (1984, 68) notions of self and other dynamics, as articulated in *The Problems of Dostoevsky's Poetics*, are relevant:

> The consciousness of other people cannot be perceived, analyzed, defined as objects or as things—one can only *relate to them dialogically*. To think about them means to *talk with them; otherwise they immediately turn to us their objectivized side:* they fall silent, close up, and congeal into finished, objectivized images. (Emphasis in the original)

The experiential mode of discourse embodied in life-writing allows for the 'reader to glean' identities and communities beyond the familiar but also more significantly those that operate from the margins or spaces of liminality. As apparent in the Bakhtin quote, relating to the other prevents the other from becoming a mere objectivized persona. In as much as this is concerned, while one is addressing concerns of subjects who were sufferers of historical victimization—slaves, victims of the holocaust, untouchables, women, homosexuals and the disabled—who have been operating from the periphery of social normativity, life-writing accords them a mode of subjectivization. Further, life-writing allows for the self-consciousness of the subject who is also the other for the reader to permeate the self of the reader. In doing so, life-writing also enables for a potential engagement with, and counteraction of, dominant discourse.

The recounting of life stories whether in the form of oral narratives or biographies is influenced by both experience and peculiarities of genre. For instance, the American slave narratives of the early 19th century that were initially recovered in oral form and were documented towards the late 19th and the early 20th centuries provide a historiography of violence and pain through experiential narratives. However, the very genre of oral history lends itself to '… the search for a connection between biography and history, between individual experience and the transformations of society…' (Portelli 1998, 25). Thus, genre also plays a vital role in the realm of life-writing owing to the way it enables the representation of the self.

Derrida in 'The Law of Genre' argues 'Every text participates in one of several genres, there is no genreless text… yet such participation never amounts to belonging' (1980, 212). A text, while operating within a genre, is seemingly determined by it or, more specifically, the genre might, at a certain level, affect the narrative but, because for Derrida the law of the genre is transgressive, that is, the text operates within a genre through participation and transgression, the text also moves beyond genre confines. Life-writing like memoir, testimony, biography and oral narratives are therefore marked by genre 'demarcations'; however, narratives of self-consciousness allow for the articulation of subjectivities that move beyond the confines of genre. Derrida's position in the essay is also about what constitutes the 'inside' or the 'outside' of a text. This position is vital when, specially within the purview of life-writing, one is looking at experiential narratives articulating positions of the self inside the text being negotiated by the other outside the text. In connection with this idea, the chapter seeks to navigate the terrain of life-writing and disability discourse to question the means of subjectivization offered in the dialectics between abled-bodied others and the disabled self. This premise will be examined through the works of neurologist and writer Oliver W. Sacks (1933–2015). However, before such an examination, it would be helpful to trace an epistemology of disability studies.

It is in the early 1960s that disability studies began to emerge as a field of inquiry, the primary focus of which was to provide a position that came from a medical approach wherein matters related to cure and rehabilitation were given impetus. It was a discourse largely emerging from the perspective of an 'ableist' position which, to a great extent, undermined the voice of disabled individuals. In the late 1960s and 1970s, however, there was a slight shift in the existing discourse. During this period, disability studies departments were established in a few Western universities to study and challenge the existing medical model of disability. A critical framework was also being built to create a social model whereby an inclusion of persons with disability in the society could be made possible through a criticism of the social barriers that perpetuate disability. This was largely attempted by the disabled thinkers and activists themselves, who began to question the very notions of 'normalcy' and began to raise questions about who belonged where and how one had come to belong where one did. While the battle for survival and the demand for inclusion continued in this period, not many writings of the disabled self emerged.

Though disability studies emerged as both an academic field of inquiry and an area of political activism, it was only in the next decade that disability studies as a new discourse could 'claim space in a contested area, trace its continuities and discontinuities, argue for its existence and justify its assertions' (Davis 2013, xv). Thus, disability studies encountered another major shift wherein experiential narratives began to find a position of reckoning. Some of these narratives were written by disabled writers themselves, while most of them still remained to be the narratives written by the able-bodied others, who recorded the extracts of the lives of the disabled self through their engagement as caregivers, therapists and friends and family members, and who had direct access to the trauma faced by disabled persons and the coping mechanisms they developed to survive in this world. It is only in the last decade and a half that the proliferation of the experiential narratives of the self by the disabled themselves has gained momentum. The emergence of this self-narrative has facilitated disability discourse to enter into other disciplines like literature and cultural studies, psychology, gender studies, sociology, economics, political science and so on. On the one hand, disability studies engages with the questions of the body, identity, sexuality, normativity, poverty, accessibility, issues related to exclusion, rights and policies and so on through an epistemology of disability, and on the other through activism, self-representation, community and groups of disabled individuals under the rubric of call to action to achieve what has so far been denied for persons with disability.

Within disability studies, experiential narrative has created a special moment of consonance and dissonance which allows the able-bodied other to move away from the sympathetic moment of association to the empathetic moment of belonging. This specific relationship can only be established through continuous involvement with the disabled self and observing the challenges faced by them in adapting to a world which so far the 'other' has not been able to delve into. This form of involvement can be realized in the form of a parent, partner, caregiver, therapist, neurologist or counselor. It could also be a friend, a well-wisher or a teacher who observes one's life from close quarters. Jonah Lehrer (2007) in his article 'The Listener' suggests about Oliver Sacks that a neurologist has to be in constant connection with his patient to observe the slightest of changes that the patient experiences to mark her/his alternative ways of being. By which he means that a therapist or a neurologist cannot afford to disconnect with their patients at any time, lest they may miss out on the biggest leap that the patient may have taken in her/his recovery. Especially, when a therapist or a neurologist is converting a case study into a life narrative, these small but yet important details may represent a greater reality of the patient who otherwise cannot represent herself/himself. At this juncture, I would like to illustrate this point by providing what Hans Renders (2014, 174–75) has to say about a life writer, in comparison to an autobiographer:

> The Life Writer adopts the stance of a therapist. The subject is declared a sacred and infallible source. Every bit of information that the Life Writer obtains from the subject is considered exciting and worthwhile. The critical contextual analysis of research materials, so important for academic biography, is omitted. This cultural-historical confirmation of solidified victimization at its best is not only a fundamental watershed between biography and Life Writing, but also between scholarship and well-meant therapy.

It is in this milieu that I wish to explore the inter-relationship of life-writing and the narratives of illness and disability. As Renders points out, life-writing's primary preoccupation is not a deconstructive critique but the articulation of a narrative imbued with a potential sense of catharsis. This has to be read as a movement away from the restraint of normative discourse to alternate modes of articulation available outside of a conformity to definitive identities like victim or survivor. Therefore, life-writing of the disabled self enables a movement away from the patronizing tokenism that either extends sympathy or valorizes the disabled identity to allowing for a disability discourse to undercut the normative. For instance, Sara Newman (2011) in her essay 'Disability and Life Writing Reports from the Nineteenth-century Asylum' notes, historically, especially before the 20th century, issues of access to accommodation and education have constrained all individuals with disabilities, preventing most from acquiring the means to self-express and thus to present a public voice. Nonetheless, individuals with disabilities in past centuries have found ways to present their own perspectives on creativity, difference, identity, politics and other issues. The forms these earlier statements have taken, the individuals who succeeded in speaking and the stories thereby told offer significant insights into lives otherwise lost.

In his essay, 'Disability, Life Narrative, and Representation', Couser (2013, 456) argues that 'one of the most significant developments in life writing', within an American context (this is also largely applicable to most of the Western world), since the 1970s has been the 'proliferation of book length accounts (from both the first- and the third-person point of view) of living with illness and disability'. Life-writings engaging with disability can be traced from the Second World War. As Couser remarks, 'war both produces and valorises certain forms of disability; not surprisingly, then, disabled veterans produced a substantial number of narratives after the war' (2013, 457). Couser goes on to examine how 'the post-World War II cultural phenomenon was the generation of large numbers of narratives about a small number of conditions', in contrast, he argues that a 'complementary phenomenon has been the production of small numbers of narratives about a large number of conditions…' (p. 457). Couser very quotably puts it: 'As the twentieth century drew to a close... many disabilities came out of the closet into the living room of life writing' (p. 457).

It is in the interstice between the varied critical positions stated that I wish to locate the genre of life-writing through the works of Oliver W. Sacks, a neurologist and writer who gives experiential accounts of several diseases and disabilities through narrating the lives of his patients. Sacks' work reflects that he is concerned above all with the way in which individuals survive and adapt to different neurological diseases and conditions, and what this experience can tell us about the human brain and mind. Sacks' stories are based on neurological cases such as Tourette's syndrome, autism, Parkinsonism, musical hallucination, phantom limb syndrome, schizophrenia, retardation, Alzheimer's disease, and other disabilities encountered by him as a physician. His association with his patients has led him to study the medical history of some of these cases which he uses as a reference in order to present the case in consideration. In representing their neuro-pathological conditions, Sacks (1985), in his preface to *The Man Who Mistook His Wife for a Hat*, affirms that a neurologist cannot study any case without looking at the subjective experience of the diseased. It is this basic connection that Sacks as a physician establishes with his patients that allows him to heal his patients, letting them recover their 'sense of self'.

Thus, this chapter will now examine how the narratives of non-personal accounts of disability can be studied from the perspective of the able-bodied other through Bakhtin's analysis of the dynamics of the relationship between the self and the other. Bakhtin, in his *Dialogic Imagination: Four Essays* (1975) argues on the lines of how the self discovers itself from the experience of the other and how dialogicity between the two precipitates this action. It is through this interdependency of self and the other which is enabled by the dialogicity that exists between them that aids the constitution of the self from the perspective of the other. It is within these circumstances that Sacks' experiences with his patients create a moment of 'empathetic epiphany' in his writings. Hence, Sacks' narrative is marked by his uncanny ear for the consonances and dissonances of being. He believes 'we underestimate the power of listening'; he goes on to say, 'it is by listening to our patients that we can discover their humanity. It is the only way to grasp what they are going through' (Lehrer web).

It is through a close association of Sacks with his patients that the narrative of the self from the perspective of the other vis-à-vis the voice of the narrator emerges. Sacks, in his *Preface* to the original edition of the book *Awakenings* (1973, xviii), claims:

> My aim is not to make a system, or to see patients as systems, but to picture a world, a variety of worlds—the landscapes of being in which these patients reside. And the picturing of worlds requires not a static and systematic formulation, but an active exploration of images and views, a continual jumping-about and imaginative *movement*.

Sacks utilizes the narratives of his patients to create an arena where the disabled experience gets expressed. He explores an active image of an imaginative movement in describing their 'thoughtscape'. The term 'thoughtscape' is taken from Wittgenstein's Preface to his *Philosophical Investigations* (1958), wherein he talks about the necessity of depicting the landscape of the mind or thoughtscape by images and remarks to denote the most complex sufferings and the thoughts which are most difficult to grasp or express.

While Sacks focuses on the aspect of disability, he also gives us some of the other idiosyncrasies and positive approach that his patients have, with which they continue to live life and accept their disability. Sacks, in most of his stories, changes the names of his patients, the name and the location of the hospital where they live due to his professional constraints, but he does try to preserve the feeling of their lives, their characters, their illnesses, their responses and the essential qualities of their strange situation creating a landscape of their being. He also narrates the changes that disability brings in to the lives of his patients and how they apply themselves to a new mode of living. In appreciating the lives of his patients with imaginative lyricism, Sacks convincingly ushers his writings into the domain of life-writing.

The imaginative element in Sacks' narratives enhances the aesthetics of 'life cases' of the patients and assists in moving the 'cases' over the threshold of medico-pathological discourse into the realm of creative rendition. The imaginative element situates his writing in the purview of a semi-fictional mode that is, however, largely marked by the narratives focusing on the human spirit, 'preservation' of the 'self' and studying the identity of the patients to reflect upon the inner worlds that they create during their illness.

Sacks in *Awakenings* (1973), narrates the medical history of a group of patients who had contracted sleeping sickness (*encephalitic lethargica*) after the First World War. Sacks administered them with an experimental drug L-Dopa as part of the cure. This drug had an astonishing and immediate effect of 'awakening' these patients from their decades long sleep. Sacks chronicles the changes in the lives of his patients brought about by L-Dopa. The book also looks into the basic care and question of health. Sacks (1973, xxvii) states:

> [W]hen I came to Mount Carmel I did not just encounter 'eighty cases of post-encephalitic disease,' but eighty individuals, whose inner lives and total being was (to a considerable extent) known to the staff, known in the vivid, concrete knowing of relationship, not the pallid, abstract knowing of medical knowledge. Coming to this community—a community of patients, but also of patients and staff—I found myself encountering the patients as individuals, whom I could less and less reduce to statistics or lists of symptoms.

Sacks here seems allied to the notions of a Bakhtinian dialogic engagement between the patients and staff; this terrain of the self and other dynamics mediated through the genre of life-writing moved beyond the sterility of medical discourse and engaged with the human subjects participating (rather than 'objectivized') in them. 'So what one studied, was not just disease or physiology, but *people,* struggling to adapt and survive' (Sacks 1973, xxvii).

Sacks' third book, *A Leg to Stand On* ([1984]1998), is an autobiographical testimony of his experience after sustaining an injury in his leg. Sacks was gored by a bull in the mountains of Norway and had to face a period of recuperation, during which he experienced what it felt like to be a patient—Sacks claims that his injured limb felt like an alien appendage to his body. This book offers a unique perspective of a neurologist who has become the patient and simultaneously analyses one's identification with the body. Hence, it suggests that though Sacks' writings are based on his case studies, they do take up concerns which are not narrowed to the confines of illness and its cure. Sacks' writings address the emotional experiences of his subjects and their ways and means of adapting themselves in their sociocultural milieu.

Sacks' narrativizing the case studies of his patients has been criticized by critics like *The Nation's* columnist, Alexander Cockburn and disabled British academic Tom Shakespeare for depathologizing his subjects, by presenting their obscure neurological conditions in non-clinical language. Couser (2001), in a lecture titled 'The Case of Oliver Sacks: The Ethics of Neuroanthropology' presented by him at Indiana University on 24 October 2001, evaluates Cockburn and Shakespeare's arguments against Sacks. He addresses the questions of the ethics of representing the disabled experience in Sacks' writings about his cases. Couser in the first half of his lecture explores how some of the reviewers of Sacks' writings have been critical in their responses. He quotes Cockburn, according to whom Sacks' works are a high-brow freak show that invites his readers to gape at human oddities. Couser also highlights that reviewers of Sacks claim that he functions, '… as a genteel contemporary Barnum who displays his cases with often devastating (and generally irremediable) conditions that place them at the border of humanity as cautionary examples of calamities that might beset his audience' (Couser 2001, 2).

Couser's lecture also illustrates how Sacks, in studying people with 'neurological anomalies', makes an argument for the emergence of a community of the neurologically affected. This community identity diminishes the divide between the affected and the non-affected, between the patient and the physician, thereby enabling a levelling of the power hierarchy that makes the physician dominant and the patient subservient. In spite of these criticisms that are labelled on Sacks' work, I wish to locate his writings within the interstice of medico-humanistic concerns. By this, I imply that even though there is a divide between the physician and his patients that excludes the physician from the community that he engages with, he is nonetheless able to adequately bring out their subjective experiences and, in doing so, accords them with a space that counteracts the normative order by attempting to present the neurological disorders in the form of ethnography rather than pathology, creating what Margaret Rose Torrell (2011) claims as 'emancipatory disability community'. I believe Sacks' writing is also contributing to this group identity of the disabled community by providing representation to those who have been isolated from this 'emancipatory disability community'. Thus, in conclusion, I would like to put forth the point that Sacks, in creating an ethnographic mode of generating a disability discourse, manages to resuscitate disability discourse from the margins of scholarship and creates a space for it that challenges the normative. Simultaneously, he also succeeds in subversively normativizing discourses on disability by deliberately using the mode of the narrative to investigate his case studies. He removes his patients from the isolation of being othered by becoming the other voice that can articulate their disabled self. By narrativizing the case studies of his patients, he does not look at them merely as objects of medical study but also as subjects of an alternate experience. Sacks familiarizes his reader to the disabled experience through the narratives of life-writing that mediate an elimination of the divide between the able-other and the disabled self.

REFERENCES

Bakhtin, Mikhail Mikhailovich. 1981. *The Dialogic Imagination: Four Essays.* Translated by Caryl Emerson and Edited by Michael Holquist. Austin, TX: University of Texas Press.
———. (1972)1984. *Problems of Dostoevsky's Poetics.* Edited and Translated by Caryl Emerson. Minneapolis, MN: University of Minnesota Press.
Couser, Thomas G. 2001. *The Cases of Oliver Sacks: The Ethics of Neuroanthropology.* Poynter Center, Indiana University Foundation.
———. 2013. 'Disability, Life Narrative and Representation.' *The Disability Studies Reader,* edited by Lennard J. Davis, 456–59. London and New York: Routledge.
Davis, Lennard J. 2013. *The Disability Studies Reader.* London and New York: Routledge.
Derrida, Jacques. 1980. 'Law of Genre.' *Glyph* 7: 202–32. Available at: http://www.english.upenn.edu/~cavitch/pdflibrary/Derrida_LawofGenre.pdf (accessed February 15, 2016).
Kadar, Marlene. 1992. 'Coming to Terms: Life Writing—from Genre to Critical Practice.' *Essays On Life Writing: From Genre to Critical Practice,* edited by Marlene Kadar, 3–16. Toronto: University of Toronto Press.

Leader, Zachary, ed. 2015. *On Life-writing*. Oxford: Oxford University Press.
Lehrer, Jonah. 2007, October 29. 'The Listener: Brain and Behaviour.' *Seed Magazine.com*. Available at: http://seedmagazine.com/content/print/the_listener/ (accessed October 29, 2007).
Newman Sara. 2011. 'Disability and Self Life Writing: Reports from the Nineteenth Century Asylum.' *Journal of Literary & Cultural Disability Studies* 5 (3): 261–78.
Portelli, Alessandro. 1998. 'Oral History as Genre.' In *Narrative and Genre*, edited by Mary Chamberlain and Paul Thompson, 23–45. London and New York: Routledge.
Renders, Hans. 2014. 'Biography in Academia and the Critical Frontier in Life Writing: Where Biography Shifts into Life Writing.' In *Theoretical Discussions of Biography: Approaches from History, Microhistory, and Life Writing*, edited by Hans Renders and Binne de Haan, 169–75. Leiden and Boston, MA: Brill.
Sacks, Oliver. 1973. *Awakenings*. New York: A. A. Knopf. Rev. ed., 1990.
———. 1985. *The Man Who Mistook His Wife for a Hat*. New York: Simon and Schuster.
———. (1984)1998. *A Leg to Stand On*. New York: Touchstone (Simon and Schuster).
Torrell, Margaret Rose. 2011. 'Plural Singularities: The Disability Community in Life Writing Texts.' *Journal of Literary & Cultural Disability Studies* 5 (3): 321–37.
Wittgenstein, Ludwig. 1958. 'Preface.' In *Philosophical Investigations*. Translated by G.E.M. Anscombe (pp. vii–viii). London: Basil Blackwell.

Chapter 13

Blind Culture and Cosmologies
Notes from Ved Mehta's Continent of India

Hemachandran Karah

I squatted down on the narrow ledge between the streams and put a hand in each stream. The right stream felt glacial, and I could scarcely keep my hand in it. The left stream was thick and soupy, and felt almost tepid. I remember thinking that, in their way, the two streams were as different as *Daddyji* and *Mamaji* (Mehta 1984, 128).

INTRODUCTION

Ved Mehta (1934–) is a blind autobiographer and essayist. His autobiographical compendium, 11 books altogether, is known collectively by the series title *Continents of Exile*. Due to an idiosyncratic twist, Mehta's *Continents* signify much more than a mere geographical category. For example, consider this list: *India, America, Britain, psychoanalysis, The New Yorker* and *blind culture*. These are Mehta's autobiographical narrative domains and are fondly called by him as 'Continents'. As narrative clusters, *Continents* boast a rare capacity to host autobiographical recollections, standpoints, political commentaries and raw imprints of personhood. Naturally, they command a wherewithal to upholster a fuller critique of a knowledge system such as blindness. Now, one may believe that all the upholstering takes place within the Continent of blind culture. Perhaps yes. In fact, by the time the Continent evolves, so do meanings tied to the notion of blind culture. At one point, Mehta's narrative domain of blind culture takes to mainstream visual culture as its potent counterpoint. At others, it evolves as a sensory universe bereft of sight and a specialist institutional arrangement for the blind. And yet in others, it performs as a transformative literary endeavour, a psychoanalytic mode, an intermedial system of communication and a cosmology that lurks between the visible and the invisible. This essay concerns such cosmologies, which go on to populate Mehta's Continent of India.

Originally from the Punjab province in Pakistan, Mehta and his family migrated to India as refugees during the partition. Mehta received his primary school education at Dadar School for the Blind, Bombay, during the early 1940s. When he was 18 or so, Mehta flew to the United States, where he joined Arkansas School for the Blind (ASB). Mehta chose to remain in America ever since then. However, he continues to fall back on the memories of his childhood in India. Perhaps this was to step back a moment and review the nature of his connect with scopic worlds in America. In stepping back, Mehta also comes to terms with cosmologies of his childhood in India, which bring him visibility at one moment, and invisibility at others.

Disability studies scholarship is abound with commentaries concerning the notion of overcoming. A good many of them treat overcoming as a propensity to surpass, hide and disown one's disability. Such an impulse lavishes Mehta's oeuvre too. Nevertheless, he also takes to overcoming as a transition from cosmologies that restrain to those that enable a flourishing. For this reason, it may be interesting to observe how the protagonist of *Continents of Exile* trains himself to hop over a restraining cosmology because he is seen as its natural insider on account of a disability.

THE LEDGE AND THE TWIN COSMOLOGIES

The tiny passage cited initially in the chapter recalls an episode from Mehta's childhood in Punjab. It is all about a long-lasting and yet enduring memory of a moment on a ledge between two streams. For

Mehta, who is now a child, the stream on the left seems glacial and fast-flowing like *Daddyji*. The right one, like *Mamaji*, feels rather tepid and stagnant.

Let us fast forward a bit so that we can comprehend how a playful event like this can afford to haunt an adult writer-figure. Mehta, who is now a staff writer at *The New Yorker*, seeks recourse to the ledge, this time as a symbolic retreat. In this way, the ledge emerges as a sort of a space of reflection to handle seemingly opposite streams of thought, and the cosmologies that they flow into. Again and again, Mehta finds himself perching on such a writerly ledge so that he can remember with ever more sophistication the biographical profiles of *Mamaji* and *Daddyji*. From such an artistic pact unfolds sketches of Hindu cosmologies that both his parents dearly espouse. Let us begin with Mehta's narrative plunge into *Mamaji*'s cosmos. In *Mamaji*'s little world, Mehta is known as Vedi where he grows up.

THE COSMOS OF MAMAJI

To comprehend *Mamaji*'s cosmos, let us take stock of a feminine ethos unique to 19th and early 20th-century Punjab. *Mamaji* inherits a cosmos where a woman's identity is mainly grounded on her attainment of motherhood, even more than the familial positions that she was given to hold as a wife, daughter-in-law and a daughter (Malhotra 2002). Having secured her position as a mother and a *Pativrata* or husband-worshipping wife in an extended family set-up, *Mamaji* presents herself as a tireless primary caregiver for her blind child. *Pativrata* is a ritual tradition that is concerned with principles and practices of ideal conjugal life that is to be upheld by a devoted wife. A devoutful conjugal life is almost reassured by the ritual of *Kanya Dan* (virgin as gift). During a *Kanya Dan* ceremony, a bride is presented as a gift to the bridegroom (Malhotra 2002). Having been gifted to the family of *Daddyji*, *Mamaji* tirelessly serves the members of the household, especially the children who need more care such as Vedi. Although he enjoys this maternal care for longer periods than others, Vedi remains ambivalent towards the ideal of *Pativrata* that dominates the feminine world of *Mamaji*. For one thing he is reminded of the fact that the wedding is a distant goal in itself; and for another, he is ineligible to receive *Kanya Dan* like any other able-bodied Punjabi man. He may end up marrying a Westerner, or a Christian who has nothing to do with *Pativrata*. Not surprisingly, during his marriage to Lynn, an American, Mehta feels saddened by the fact that she is not like what *Mamaji* is for *Daddyji*, an ideal Hindu *Pativrata* wife.

In addition to the ideal of *Pativrata*, a significant thing that connects Mehta with his childhood mother is the practice of sensory training. *Mamaji* and her womenfolk provide the main environment for the education of the senses for their sons until they become men in their own right. The womenfolk are also primarily responsible for giving the boys a training in toilet habits, family customs and an optimal usage of all the senses. As a lonely blind child, Vedi has more and longer access to certain private spaces of the *Chaubara* (private room) which are either unavailable or inaccessible to other boys of his age. He listens to the gossip of the women; makes a sneak estimate of the contents of their jewellery cases; gets exposed to their overpowering emotional outflows as in breast-beating, wailing and weeping; surreptitiously makes a tactile mapping of their breasts and acquires rudimentary knowledge of the childbearing nerve that is located somewhere at the bottom of a woman's navel. He even happens to see with his fading eyesight, *Mamaji*'s ominous vagina as she is taking a bath. A visual experience of this kind is known as primal scene in classical psychoanalysis. If not for his long engagement with Freudianism, Mehta may not have recourse to this event, which may or may not be true in the first place. His reactions to these experiences oscillate between seeing *Mamaji* and her female surrogates as either good or bad mother types; say, ones whose breasts are nourishing and generous and those whose breasts are overwhelming.

Mehta's portraits of *Mamaji* as a bad or malevolent mother are intricately linked to the ways in which he remembers the remedial measures that she makes use of for curing his blindness. Unable to believe that her son will be blind for the rest of his life, *Mamaji* takes Vedi to hakims, astrologers, practitioners of Ayurvedic medicine and several other native healers to restore his eyesight. The native healers prescribe stinging eye drops that she administers in full faith. Besides performing rigorous penances and fasts, *Mamaji* forces her son to comply with native healing traditions that give him an ominous image of her as a bad mother. Also, her daily lessons in orientation and mobility include activities that are meant to improve his eyesight, which she mistakenly thinks that he possesses in certain measure. Noticing that Mehta turns his head to follow her movements, *Mamaji* subjects him to a series of tests that convinces her again and again that he is able to see after all. One such test involves switching on and off the electric light: after having discovered that Vedi is able to identify whether the light is on or off from the sound of the clicks, she does the clicking rapidly. This time also, Vedi gets it right as he had always done before (Mehta 1957). Strict disciplinary exercises of this kind convince Vedi that *Mamaji* is malevolent, although she remains benevolent to him all through.

Sketches of *Mamaji*'s benevolence and otherwise are intertwined with narrative accounts that centre on the myth of goddess Durga, who is an embodiment of both these traits. In the Punjab region, the pan-Indian goddess, Sakti, is worshipped and addressed by her devotees as *Seranvali*, the lion rider, or Durga (Erndl 1993). The goddess worship in Punjab is ecumenical in character and is open to all religious and caste groups. They believe that Durga's *Darshan* (sacred vision) is omnipresent and is realized through occasional demonstrations of goddess possession. Possession is described as any complete but temporary domination of one's body and consciousness by an alien power during which the person acts out the will of the power in dominance. An ordinary Punjabi participates in a goddess possession ceremony in order to gain special insights into the workings of the divine within the community. During the event of goddess possession, *Pavan*, or wind, takes control of the person in possession, making him or her rotate the head uncontrollably like an automaton. *Mamaji* is instructed by a woman who is possessed by such a *Pavan* to perform certain rituals in order to seek atonement for her son's blindness. As it is expected of her, *Mamaji*, to the utter discomfort of her son, performs all of the rituals with total faith and commitment.

In addition to divine materialism of goddess worship, the cosmos of Mehta's first identity as a blind child of *Mamaji* is populated by Hindu shamans, Moslem sorcerers, practitioners of Ayurveda, Hakims and astrologers. Such a population ensures that Vedi's blindness is treated not as an individual problem, but as a cosmic issue. One need only be a little familiar with Shamanism and Ayurveda to comprehend such a cosmic orientation within *Mamaji*'s life world. While Shamans are concerned about the spiritual equilibrium of an individual's cosmos, Ayurvedic practitioners focus on the wholeness of a person. For them, body, soul and mind are not discreet entities, but are integral constituents of one and the same person. Ayurvedic medicine is based on the theory of *Pancha bhuta*, according to which, the cosmos is made up of the elements of earth, fire, water, wind and the sky or the ether. Ayurvedic medicine also emphasizes the balance of the three bodily humours, the wind, the bile and the phlegm. Any disturbances associated with the act of seeing, for example, are attributed to imbalances in Alochaka bile in the eye (Kakar 1982). It is also notable that in Hindu tradition there are two bodies other than the gross physical body. They are the subtle body (*Linga Sharira*) and the causal body (*Korana Sharira*), the former being tied up with ego and the self and the latter with Karma as a metaphysical cosmic force. The principle of Karma determines one's individual status (disabled and otherwise) in the cosmic whole. To Mehta, such a karmic view appears restrictive because it is institutionally over-deterministic.

Having imagined blindness as a sort of a temporary invisible curtain of the eyes, *Mamaji* takes her blind son to astrologers and Shamans for a consultation. In one such a meeting with an astrologer, *Mamaji* is told that her son is blind because of a sin that she has committed in her previous birth or incarnation. After having made rigorous calculations on his charts, the astrologer prescribes a multitude of atonement rituals that call for scrupulous observance on the part of *Mamaji*. She is instructed to administer eye drops to Vedi and gently massage his eyeballs with warm water. *Mamaji* is also instructed to gently flog him in order to drive off the evil forces (Jinn) that caused the curtain of blindness to fall upon his eyes in the first place. As a ritual sequel, she is to place a piece of raw meat and a pair of eggs in a stipulated area of the town so as to entice the wayward demons away. Yet another ritual involves dropping golden eyeballs into the begging bowl of a leprous beggar; this time, on advice from a Moslem seer who suggests that Vedi is blind because he urinated on the grave of a Moslem Saint in Gujarat. *Mamaji*'s ritual performances do not stop there: Hakim, the practitioner of the Unani system of medicine, prescribes several doses of *Terminalia Chebula*, the pill of life, alongside mixtures of unpleasant medicinal salt compounds (Mehta 1979b). All these rituals inculcate in Vedi a standpoint that *Mamaji*'s feminine Punjabi cosmos will render him totally invisible. Naturally, little Vedi seeks solace via his brief stay at Dadar School for the Blind.

AN INTERREGNUM

Mehta's first identity as a blind child of *Mamaji* comes to an abrupt halt when he departs for Dadar School for the Blind with the injunction from *Daddyji* that he is a man from then on (Mehta 1982). Vedi joins the school when he is five and stays there until he is eight. The school catered solely for blind girls when it was founded in the year 1900, but by the time Vedi gains admission, it had become co-educational with a renewed system of integrated education in place. In an integrated arrangement of education as envisaged by Rasmohan Haldar, the then principal of the school and a father surrogate for Vedi, blind students are allowed to attend mainstream schools for sighted pupils on a part-time basis. As a Bengali Christian missionary who was trained at Perkins Institute in America, Rasmohan Haldar stands as an embodiment of modernity and progress. In this respect, he resembles *Daddyji* who is cosmopolitan in his outlook. It happens that Vedi is the only student who is from a well-to-do family; the rest are 'poor destitutes' picked up from the busy streets of Bombay by the Christian missionaries. Vedi also happens to be the youngest of all; some inmates appear to have much passed their adolescence; some are even partially sighted, like Abdul and Rajas.

As a member of a well-to-do family, Vedi is not permitted to go for chair-caning sessions since they are designed for blind pupils with little or no ambition for higher education. He is also prohibited from practising music lest the rough strings of the musical instrument callouses his Braille-reading fingers. Vedi finds a father surrogate in Rasmohan. He teaches Vedi to hold himself in an upright posture when he is walking; provides lessons in upper-class table manners; offers lessons in Braille and even writes letters of recommendation to the Perkins Institute for the Blind in America pleading his pupil's case for high-school education in that country. In this way, he resembles *Daddyji*, who is authoritative, disciplined, scholarly and yet approachable.

With his new identity as a member of the Dadar School, Vedi comes to an understanding that he is done once for all with the feminine servitude and illiteracy of *Mamaji*'s *Chaubara*. At one point, after having acquired some braille literacy through a Bible study course in the school, Vedi is almost carried away by the thought that he is a member of the Christian family that consists of Jesus, Mary and Joseph. He even imagines himself to be a member of a 'blind flock' that follows Jesus of Nazareth who leads them to the greener pastures located far away from Dadar School for the Blind. Thus, for Vedi, Rasmohan's Christian blind flock appears as a potential force that could lead him away from remembrances of penury, death, illiteracy, leprosy and blindness that dominate *Mamaji* and her cosmos of native healing traditions.

Although Dadar School for the Blind is remembered as a space of upward mobility by the narrator, he never reconciles himself to its opposite linkage with poverty and mendicancy. This becomes apparent when Ved Mehta, the interviewer-figure and a staff writer from *The New Yorker*, runs into Rajas, his childhood blind colleague at the Dadar School. Mehta realizes how much things have changed between them; he is no more able to reminisce with her in Marathi, her mother tongue and the language of their schooling. When he hears Rajas whine like a street beggar, Mehta flees, tumbling his way down the stairs, for her begging tone stirred up in him the old memory and an old fear that he will be a deserted sheep behind the fence (Mehta 1982). It is this fear of desolation that makes the blind narrator, be it during his childhood or otherwise, wary of *Mamaji*'s feminine cosmos.

DADDYJI AND THE VISIBLE COSMOS

Vedi's first-ever catapult into *Daddyji*'s visible cosmos transpires at the 'Dinner Table School'. The Dinner Table School is nothing but a conversation-based model of learning that *Daddyji* introduces to Vedi and his siblings at the dinner table. At the school, the children are introduced to the virtues of liberal education, as well as cosmopolitanism. Having travelled widely in the West, *Daddyji* coaxes his children to converse in English about the differences between Western and Indian styles of living (Mehta 1984). During these conversations, Vedi is almost taken on a voyage to Europe and America where people are better enlightened about the blind. With that passing note on Vedi's imaginary passage to the West, let us consider for a moment *Daddyji*'s legacy.

At a time when there was no dearth of female infanticide in Punjab, *Daddyji* is preceded by three stillborn female babies. After a careful scrutiny of his birth chart, the astrologers predict that he will grow up to be a wealthy man who will be fortunate enough to ride on an elephant. Indeed, he becomes the Director General of Medical Services in the Punjab province and rides an elephant in that capacity. Perhaps, he is the first Indian to gain membership in various British clubs in the Punjab province. Having gained a membership in the Arya Samaj like his ancestors, *Daddyji* denounces idol worship, astrology, Unani system of medicine and other native customs that he deems to be superstitious. As an Aryan and a Kshatriya, he prudently maintains his status as a man of the family, a north Indian, a Punjabi, a doctor Sahib, an aristocrat, educator and a leader.

As a doctor Sahib, *Daddyji* travels around the Punjab province to perform medical inspections. He is also the first person in the family to travel abroad for higher education; he acquires his advanced degrees in medicine from England and America. Mehta emulates his father as a globe trotter and even aspires further. He flies to America at the age of 17 for his high school education at ASB. Further, he chooses to do an undergraduate degree at Oxford so that he is able to get into the cosmopolitan circles of Oxford life. He joins Pomona College for a BA degree and Harvard University for a Masters in History for the same reason.

Mehta's conduct as a writer-figure also is in sync with the cosmopolitan ideals of *Daddyji*. Sometimes he appears like a tourist whose vocation is the consumption of the exotic, especially the spectacular. At others, he is an interviewer whose travel itinerary extends far and wide. Yet in others, he seems like a celebrity figure who has overcome all the limitations and parochialities of his childhood blindness. In *Walking the Indian Streets* for example, Mehta looks more like a sighted visitor from Oxford than a blind writer who needs assistance in reaching the exotic. After 10 years of study in England and America, Ved Mehta revisits his home in India in the summer of 1959. He is joined by his friend from Oxford, the poet Dom Moraes, and together they spend a full carefree month which he calls 'bummy' days in India and Nepal (Mehta 1971). At the end of his sojourn, Mehta interviews Jawaharlal Nehru, the then prime minister of India, with whom he has been in touch ever since his travel to America for schooling.

During his interviews, Mehta presents himself as someone who is very keen on the visual aspects of the situations of interviewing. He records in vivid detail the physical appearance of his interviewees, the costumes they wear and the ways in which they approach him as a blind interviewer. To access the minute details of the visual environments of interviewing, Mehta deploys facial vision, which is a skill that is associated with obstacle perception of the blind. When he is in his early 50s, Mehta becomes a proper householder like *Daddyji* with his marriage to Lynn, as well as his construction of his own 'palace on sand'. Thus, *Daddyji*'s resolve appears fulfilled: his son will be different from the rest of the blind in India who loaf around with their begging bowls and a staff in their hands.

Daddyji's cosmopolitan aspirations concerning his blind son, as well as Mehta's narrative enactments of them, derived their strength from Arya Samaj, an institution concerned with the revival of Vedic Hinduism. As an Anglo-Vedic Church, Arya Samaj was not anti-British in its approach. Instead, it was bent on restoring the sanctity of Hinduism based on its Vedic past (Rai and Śarman 1967). Founded by Swami Dayanand Sarasvati in 1875, Arya Samaj grew up as a reformist organization. In 1892, it split into two factions with meat-eaters forming one group and vegetarians the other, so, iconoclast as he was; *Daddyji*'s membership in the Arya Samaj was not compromised by his meat-eating habits. This is in concurrence with his principle of world citizenry and cosmopolitanism that when in Rome do as the Romans do.

Daddyji's special cosmos of Arya Samaj also contains certain 19th-century Punjabi Hindu ideals, such as *Arya Dharm* or virtue (living according to the rulings of the Karmic lifecycle), Hindu notions of masculinity or *Virya* and Kshatriya pride. Interestingly, Mehta's cosmopolitan narrative enactments are inspired by these ideals as well. For example, in its own right, Mehta's idealization of *Daddyji* in itself is closely connected to *Pitri Yajna* or devotion to one's parents, a practice recommended by Arya Samaj.

First of all, in all earnestness, Mehta idealizes *Daddyji* in the name of Sharvan, a legendary hero who is known for his unstinting commitment and devotion to his blind parents. So entrenched is the idealization that Mehta's autobiographical compendium begins and concludes with the portraits of *Daddyji*. In fact, *Continents of Exile* reads as a ceremonial offering of *Pitri Yajna* or the ritual of parental devotion. For this reason, *Daddyji* is always represented as an ideal son, perfect father, global citizen, courteous lover and an adorable husband. *Daddyji*'s love affair with Rasil, his paramour, receives only a posthumous treatment in *The Red Letters* (2004), and even then only as an instance of the differences between fiction and autobiography.

The idea of karmic life cycle is one more notion of *Arya Dharm* (Arya Samaj way of living) that Mehta is obsessive about as a blind autobiographer. There are four stages in one's life. They are *Brahmacharya* or student life, *Grihastha* or family life, *Vanprastha* or retirement from family life and *Sannyas* or sainthood (Rai and Śarman 1967). *Daddyji* completes his *Brahmacharya* life before he is 25 and goes on to the *Grihastha* way of life which he continues to cherish until he dies at the age of 91. Almost all of the volumes of *Continents of Exile* bear witness to *Daddyji*'s life situations in these two stages. The only flaw that emerges concerns his romantic involvement with Rasil. A second reason for idealizing *Daddyji*, in addition to *Pitri Yajna*, is that the blind narrator is pre-occupied with *Daddyji*'s successes as a captain of his destiny as against his own setbacks during the life stages. In *The Ledge between the Streams*, for example, one notices Vedi's concerns about his lack of formal education at the appropriate time period of *Brahmacharya*. When all his siblings are in Schools and Colleges, Vedi remains at home thinking about the dancing girls of *Hiramandi* at Lahore. His days of residential schooling at Dadar School for the Blind, Emerson Institute and St Dunstan's only give him a feeling that he is no match to his sighted siblings who are fortunate enough to further their career prospects in their *Brahmacharya* stage of life. Autobiographical volumes such as *Sound-Shadows of the New World, Stolen Light, Up at Oxford* and even *Face to Face* either speak about Mehta's extended student life or his failure to attain transition into the *Grihastha* stage of life, a blissful conjugal life with wife and children. Not until *Dark Harbour*, the penultimate volume of the series, can he celebrate success in having a home of his own with wife and children before he is 50, the age limit that forms the threshold to *Vanprastha*.

Vanprastha or the life of renunciation, I argue, is experienced by Mehta as a time of involuntary exile although he runs into it more often than not as a consequence of his failures in securing a *Grihastha* way of life. From this it does not follow that Mehta treats *Vanprastha* as a stage next in hierarchy to *Grihastha*; instead, he seems to discover in it regions of deprivation and discontent that he could despise and celebrate alike. Regions of deprivation and discontent, for their part, do not just lead Mehta into life situations that permit little or no mobility into the scopic, they also provide him a celebratory alternative space to the life of *Grihastha*. The protagonists of *Sound-Shadows of the New World, The New Yorker's Mr Shawn and the Invisible Art of Editing* and many other non-autobiographical volumes owe their allegiance to the life of writing and renunciation and certainly not to the familial and social.

The Karmic state of *Sannyas* and the life worlds that come with it are the ones that are most admired and the dreaded alike by Mehta. As a person who belongs to the school of adversity, Swami Sarasvati is acknowledged by the family of the Mehtas as a perfect saint or *Sannyasi* (Mehta 1979a). Carrying forward this familial belief, Mehta acknowledges sainthood as the ideal order of an imagined community of *Sannyasis*. Because of a rare predisposition to detach, a closed order of sage-like people come across as *Sannyasis* to the blind interviewer. In fact, some of Mehta's interviews come across as a holy pilgrimage. They facilitate a rare *darshan* of sages including the tutors at Oxford, theologians, the Mahatma, Mother Teresa and *The New Yorker's* Mr Shawn. However, an occasional physical proximity with *Chachaji*, a poor relation reminds Mehta that *Sannyas* is not an easy proposition after all. *Chachaji* appears different from everybody else among the Mehtas. The children look at him with amazement because he has six fingers on each of his hands. He is deserted by his wife and children and almost reduced to a mendicant or a dispassionate *Sannyasi*. Although Mehta fears such a life, he knows very well that *Chachaji* is well placed to cross the sea of Karma. Because of his blindness Mehta feels he has no option save for a life of penury of the kind that surrounds *Chachaji*, yet it is in this life of 'deprivation and discontent' that he discovers his own selves as a writer.

Streaks of *Sannyasi*-like bodily renunciation are in fact deep-rooted in Mehta's faith in the Hindu notion of *Virya*. The notion entails the containment of semen for gaining self-control, physical prowess and mental agility. In the popular Hindu imagination, *Virya* is seen as sexual energy that flows up and down through the spinal cord. When it flows down *Virya* becomes semen and, in its upward movement, it attains *Ojas* or the highest form of sublimation (Kakar 1989). The downward movement of sexual energy is debilitating; such states of folly are best avoided by keeping oneself away from carnal acts of any kind. Indian metaphysical physiology allows at least 30 days for the food to undergo various transformations before it becomes semen or male essence. Likewise, there are various metaphysical calculations that demonstrate the wastage that comes with semen discharge. It is claimed that the energy spent on a single act of copulation compares with the energy that is required to do 24 hours of concentrated mental activity and 72 hours of hard physical labour. In its state of *Ojas*, *Virya* facilitates *Brahmacharya* or the life of sexual abstinence and learning. Even outside *Brahmacharya*, conservation of *Virya* has the potential to affect one's pursuits in art, education and spirituality. *Virya* is also associated with enhancement of longevity, creativity and other vital faculties. Ancient sages of Tantric tradition argue for conservation of semen even during sexual union. They prescribed rituals to achieve orgasm through the mental instead of the carnal (Kakar 1990).

Daddyji's advice to Mehta about masturbation reflects these principles. In *Sound-Shadows of the New World*, *Daddyji* advises his son not to yield to temporary pleasures; instead, he should strive to gain permanent pleasures that are attainable by living a life of Karmic integrity in the Hindu life cycle. Within the time period of *Brahmacharya*, Mehta is expected to concentrate only on learning and not on temporary pleasures, such as dating, that are pursued only by labourers and vulgar members of American society. Professionals and men of letters do not indulge in such practices; Mehta should just follow their footsteps (Mehta 1985). As a dutiful student, Mehta is advised to refrain from masturbation. *Daddyji*'s expert medical opinion is that there are certain excretions, such as perspiration, urine and faeces, which need periodical discarding. On the other hand, secretions like semen and saliva are of great value to one's vitality, creativity and intellectual agility and should therefore be conserved. In short, Mehta is advised to concentrate on his education and aim for permanent pleasures in life. In this context, permanent pleasure comes across as a formidable step towards an attainment of cultural capital that is visibly celebrated. Temporary pleasure, on the other hand, seems like deeds of darkness and social retrogression.

Discussion concerning Mehta's quest for permanent pleasure and his battle against temporary ones will be incomplete if no reference is made to his involvement with Freudian psychoanalysis. After having repeatedly failed in his desperate quest for love and permanent pleasure in the form of conjugal bliss, Ved Mehta goes in for Freudian psychoanalysis with Robert Bak between the years 1968 and 1974. Reclining on the psychoanalytic couch, the analysand realizes that his failures in attaining *Grihastha* status are deeply entrenched in his Oedipal bondage with his mother. He is shaken with the Freudian insight that his non-acceptance of his blindness is connected to the castration complex that he has suffered since his childhood. He tries to reconcile himself to Bak's assertion that the love–hate relationship that he has with his women is influenced by the relationship that he had with his mother (Mehta 2001). Mehta does not accept such an insight as ultimate truth. He knows too well that Freudianism is a cosmos in its own right and a climate of thought. Nevertheless, Mehta continues to fall back on Freudian psychoanalysis because of a promise of permanent pleasure.

And, finally, Mehta's idiosyncratic experiences with all these four stages of life are enriched by Kshatriya pride that is said to be traceable in *Daddyji*'s family history as early as the Moguls. When Mehta is at Oxford, for example, he proclaims that he is a Kshatriya, the community that nourished great warriors and maharajahs of the past (Mehta 1993). With this proclamation, he handles not only the stigma that comes with his disability, but also his shaky social status amidst upper-class communities at Oxford. His Kshatriya pride gets greater appreciation in the Continent of America than it does in the Continent of Britain. In America, his mastery over the science and art of facial vision gets somehow linked to his Kshatriya heritage. Gwyneth Cravens, for example, finds it less surprising that Mehta is able to bravely find his way by using facial vision since he belongs to Kshatriya caste, the community of the warriors (Jaggi 2001).

CONTINENT OF BLIND CULTURE AND THE TWIN COSMOLOGIES: A CONCLUDING REMARK

As a narrative of overcoming, *Continent of India* draws on the writer's successful and yet strugglesome passage to America during the 1940s. From this story emerges the narrative domain of blind culture which remains conspicuously interlinked to competing Punjabi Hindu cosmologies. It may appear that Mehta privileges a cosmos that is favourably disposed towards a masculine dispensation. Perhaps this is a truism.

Nevertheless, Mehta's oeuvre highlights the import of cosmologies in the making of disability culture and one's location thereof. For example, Mehta describes a strand of blind culture which is nothing more than a shadowy region of visual culture. If you like, this was rather a fringe culture of the blind marked by social invisibility during the 1940s. The lepers, beggars and members of *Mamaji*'s *Chaubara* find themselves frequenting such a shadowy region.

Mehta's narrative domain of blind culture is not a negative construct altogether: it also entails a training of the senses other than sight. Such a training either takes the form of special education or caregiving where a million trials transpire in the name of sensory modulation. In a caregiving setting, such as the ones provided by *Daddyji* and *Mamaji*, blind culture also takes the shape of an idiosyncratic trope and symbolism that are in sync with ideologies such as *Arya Dharm* and goddess worship. This is comparable to the influences of Christian ethos on Vedi's Dadar School for the Blind.

Ved Mehta is ambivalent about a dip into blind cultures and cosmologies that influence the same. However, his oeuvre urges an understanding that the connect between both the phenomena is anything but negligible and linear. A third-world disability studies programme may benefit from such an insight.

REFERENCES

Erndl, K. M. 1993. *Victory to the Mother: The Hindu Goddess of Northwest India in Myth, Ritual, and Symbol.* New York: Oxford University Press.

Jaggi, M. 2001. 'Sight Unseen.' *The Guardian Profile*, London.

Kakar, S. 1982. *Shamans, Mystics and Doctors: A Psychological Inquiry into India and Its Healing Traditions.* Chicago: University of Chicago Press.

———. 1989. *Intimate Relations: Exploring Indian Sexuality.* New Delhi: Penguin Books India.

———. 1990. 'Stories from Indian Psychoanalysis: Context and Text.' In *Cultural Psychology: Essays on Comparative Human Development*, edited by James W. Stigler, Richard A. Schweder and Gilbert Herdt. Cambridge, UK: Cambridge University Press.

Malhotra, A. 2002. *Gender, Caste, and Religious Identities: Restructuring Class in Colonial Punjab.* New York: Oxford University Press.

Mehta, V. 1957. *Face to Face, an Autobiography.* Boston, MA: Little.

———. 1971. *Walking the Indian Streets.* London: Weidenfeld and Nicolson.

———. 1979a. *Daddyji.* Oxford and New York: Oxford University Press.

———. 1979b. *Mamaji.* New York: Oxford University Press.

———. 1982. *Vedi.* New York: Oxford University Press.

———. 1984. *The Ledge Between the Streams.* New York: Norton.

———. 1985. *Sound-shadows of the New World.* New York: Norton.

———. 1993. *Up at Oxford.* New York: Norton.

———. 2001. *All for Love.* New York, NY and Berkeley, CA: Thunder's Mouth Press/Nation Books. Distributed by Publishers Group West.

Rai, L., and Ś.-R. Śarman. 1967. *A History of the Arya Samaj.* Bombay: Orient Longman.

PART 4

Disability in Literature and Culture

Chapter 14

Disability across Cultures

Shubhangi Vaidya

INTRODUCTION: CONCEPTUALIZING CULTURE

This chapter aims at an examination of the category of disability through the lens of 'culture'. Culture is a concept that has a long and contested history. Anthropologists and sociologists have used it as a comprehensive term encapsulating both material and non-material artefacts, ideas and ways of living that mark a particular society or community as distinct. In this sense, culture includes the entire gamut of knowledge, beliefs, customs, ways of doing things and living in the world that human beings acquire by virtue of their membership in society. Culture is a learned system of meanings and behaviour transmitted inter-generationally. However, it is crucial to note that cultures are never static and constant, but ever changing and evolving, in response to both natural and human factors. Culture also involves the dimension of power and control; power relations shape what is considered appropriate or desirable and therefore 'normative'.

Culture involves both a sense of 'identity' and belongingness that reinforces group identity as well as a common attribute of shared humanity that unites the human species. In a globalized world order, marked by flows of human beings, ideas, capital, money and technology, culture is also characterized by hybridity and plurality.

Urbanization, migration, the communication revolution and changing geopolitical configurations have profoundly transformed the world we live in. It is against this backdrop that this chapter will examine the category of disability as an evolving construct shaped by local understandings and realities as well as global influences.

There will be a discussion of disability in a cross-cultural context with the help of selected examples, and it will highlight the importance of factoring in cultural values in disability management and rehabilitation. It will then discuss the emergence of a 'disability culture' through the formation of disability communities and their efforts to question and challenge their discrimination and exclusion. Finally, it will highlight how the experience of disability has resulted in the emergence of 'biosocialities' and solidarities based upon specific impairments in which alternative ways of living and being are foregrounded. Specifically, it will refer to Deaf pride and autistic neurodiversity and the challenges and contestations they pose to what is considered 'normative' and culturally competent. It will highlight the role of 'virtual' or online communities in creating new forms of community that transcend the confines of geography.

DISABILITY: A CULTURAL CONSTRUCT

The disabled mind and body have always challenged and disturbed the idea of what is 'normative' and within the bounds of culturally and socially desirable behaviour. Persons with disability are often identified as the 'other', whose position in human society is ambiguous and questionable. According to Devlieger (2005, 4),

> Disabled people are a reflection of their societies. In disabled people, people who identify themselves as non-disabled read who they are not. Disabled people however are not a new tribe. They live among us and the non-disabled are becoming more and more conscious of the fact that they too can and probably will be disabled for shorter or longer periods in their lifetimes. The disabled are same *and* different.

The 'sameness and difference' referred to by Devlieger are interpreted differently by societies and cultures across time and space.

Social and cultural practices and belief systems across the world and through history have sought to 'deal' with the non-normative body and mind in a variety of ways. Dalal (2002) points out that societies develop their characteristic patterns of coping with disability, depending on the way disability is understood and their resources identified. Disablement is socially constructed by drawing upon historical events, sacred texts and social institutions. In the Indian context, for instance, the Hindu notion of karma or the law of ethical or moral compensation that governs existence has a strong resonance with the cultural understanding of disability. Not only is disablement regarded as a retribution for misdeeds committed in past lives, but the consequent discrimination, marginalization and suffering is to be internalized and borne in a spirit of resignation to atone for previous sins and transgressions (Ghai, 2015). *The Mahabharata* and *The Ramayana*, which provide moral guidance and ethical role models to Hindus even to this day, are deeply ingrained in the cultural ethos and also provide interesting insights into the experience of disability. Ghai (ibid.) through her discussion on the characters of Dhritarashtra, Gandhari and Shakuni in the Mahabharata and Manthara and Surpanakha in *The Ramayana*, identifies the following themes: disability as a deficit of body and mind, an 'evil' that reflects a flawed or vicious character, a state to be feared and a condition of de-sexualization. She also draws attention to the idea of disability as 'punishment' through the story of Ekalavya in the Mahabharata. Ekalavya, the tribal youth who wanted to become a great archer, secretly practiced his craft and excelled in it. His 'transgression' of social hierarchies resulted in him being 'disabled' at the behest of the Guru Dronacharya whom he idolized. The idea of disability as a punishment for transgressing social/filial norms also comes through in the story of Ashtavakra in the Chandogya Upanishad, who is cursed, while still in the womb, by his father who is a learned sage, for interrupting his discourse to his disciples. He was born with eight deformities, but, eventually, proved himself to be a worthy son and a great scholar, bringing his dead father back to life. His repentant father releases him from the curse of his deformities, and he finally becomes perfect in body (Pal, 2013).

The Western constructs of disability and rehabilitation often do not sit easily with the local ideas about what constitutes (dis)ability and (in)competence, particularly in 'socio-centric' societies where group and community values hold sway over individuality and self-assertion. Cross-cultural studies on disability have yielded rich insights on how different societies and cultures conceptualize (dis)ability, personhood and social value.

At the same time, they also open spaces for accommodation and inclusion within the social matrix. The framing of disability within a Western rights-based paradigm that fails to account for local cultural constructs has resulted in the Disability Rights Movement (DRM) being dominated by elite, English-educated scholars and activists while local grassroots level-experiences and realities become marginalized.

A deeper understanding and engagement with culture would perhaps lessen the dichotomy between the ideal and the actual. At the same time, scholars and activists working in the field of disability studies can learn much from diverse cultural understandings that may also have humane and accepting ways of conceptualizing disability or difference.

DISABILITY IN A CROSS-CULTURAL PERSPECTIVE: SOME EXAMPLES

Anthropologists and sociologists have made a significant contribution towards understanding disability using cross-cultural data and the comparative method, and providing analyses that are 'historically informed, contextual and culturally specific' (Mehrotra, 2013: 115). One of the earliest anthropological discussions on the cultural construction of disability was given by the American anthropologist Ruth Benedict (1934), who placed the very notion of 'abnormality' under scrutiny. Benedict pointed out that it was culture that set the limits for what was considered acceptable or appropriate behaviour or normalcy for its members, and that these norms were variable across cultures. In the context of epilepsy, for instance, she showed how a condition that was considered as a disabling one in American society was actually considered a highly valued and revered state in some of the Native American communities that she studied. Similarly, many cultures regard extreme psychic manifestations as quite normal and desirable, and in fact even as signs of giftedness (1934: 60 cited in Staples and Mehrotra, 2016: 37).

Ingstad and Whyte's pioneering collection of papers *Disability and Culture* (1995) raised fundamental questions about the connection between disability and 'personhood' and culturally defined differences among persons. They ask: Are people with impairments impaired people? Are they valued differently than other members of society? Does being different mean being a 'lesser' human being?

The anthropological concepts of liminality and impurity have also been used to describe the socially ambiguous position of disabled people. In Jenkins' collection *Questions of Competence* (1998), which brings together cross-cultural studies on intellectual disability/mental retardation, the concept of 'competence' as differently understood and operationalized across cultures is highlighted. Competence, according to Jenkins, is 'the capacity or potential for adequate functioning-in-context as a socialized human' (1998: 1). These cultural understandings or 'local models' are confronted with and contested by global discourses and practices, as the world becomes a more interconnected place, and ideas are imported from the West to help 'solve' problems in diverse societies and cultures.

Ingstad and Whyte's (1995) edited volume, as mentioned earlier, was a very important contribution to the study of disability, even though they did not explicitly engage with the contributions of scholars in disability studies. The introduction to their later collection, *Disability in Local and Global Worlds* (2007), however, addressed this gap and acknowledged the contributions of disability studies especially the writings of key figures in British disability studies like the sociologists Barnes, Watson, Corker, Shakespeare and so on (Staples and Mehrotra, 2016: 38).

One of the very interesting papers in earlier collection by Devlieger (1995) examines how the Songye people the of Zaire in Africa attempt to answer the question 'why disabled'? Disability is not viewed in terms of the individual's own impairments or biomedical factors, but rather, because of wronged relationships with the environment, the family members and ancestors or, other explanations failing, with God. Certain disabilities may be seen as the consequence of violation of food or sexual taboos by the mother during pregnancy, that is, environmental factors: she may have consumed foods or meat that are expressly forbidden, resulting in the birth of a child with physical defects or 'habits'. Parents are blamed in such cases. Disability may also be regarded as a consequence of infringed relationships within the family, especially between parents and close relatives and between co-wives. Belief in the power of sorcery plays a very powerful role in Songye society and is believed to be particularly effective when the victim is vulnerable on account of family quarrels and weakened family ties. Sorcery is believed to 'cause' the birth of children with disabilities, especially in families that are prosperous and may incite jealousy, or in situations where co-wives are jealous or resentful of each other.

Disabilities may also be viewed as a consequence of displeasing or disrespecting ancestors. Improper distribution of the 'bride-wealth' that is given to the wife's family at the time of marriage may also be reckoned to be the cause of ill-feeling by a member of her family, and may be considered a reason for a child to have a disability or physical affliction.

Thus, we see that for the Songye, disability is not a biomedical category located in the affected individual, but rather a social and relational one, involving family relationships and social and community responsibilities. When it cannot be deciphered within this framework, it is attributed to God, whose will is unknowable. Devlieger (1995) highlights the need for community workers oriented in Western frameworks of rehabilitation/service provision, to work 'with', rather than against cultural beliefs and practices, and begin with an examination of how the local culture itself conceptualizes disability.

Jenkins' (1998) edited volume as mentioned earlier also raises the issue of cross-cultural understandings of mental (in)competence. Whyte's (1998) chapter draws upon discussions with 14 individuals and their families from the Nyole people of Eastern Uganda, who were thought to have 'mental problems'. Whyte discusses the essentially social nature of 'mental ability', which manifests in 'receptivity' and 'conversation'. A person's mental ability is found to be lacking if s/he does not follow the advice or counsel of others, and is stubborn or not able to understand and follow instructions. A person who is unable to follow or participate in a conversation, talks 'nonsense', is violent or who withdraws from interaction, is considered to be lacking in mental ability. While individual intelligence or cleverness is valued and highly regarded, social skills are at the heart of what is construed as 'competence'.

In his comparative analysis of (in)competence in America in the same volume, Devlieger (1998) highlights the role of culture and history in shaping notions of (in)competence and (dis)ability. He draws our attention to the 'division of life into a number of separate functional sectors: home and workplace, work and leisure, white collar and blue collar, public and private' in contemporary American society, which has profound implications for persons with disabilities, particularly intellectual disabilities. 'Local models of competence, as they apply to individuals in the United States, replicate deep cultural roots that both favour individualism and self-reliance, and encourage an ethic of avoidance, exemplified in the metaphor of space' (pp. 74–75).

The emphasis on self-reliance in contemporary American society shapes and limits the lives of persons with intellectual disabilities and makes them dependent upon service providers and systems put in place for them by bureaucratized institutions. Avoidance and making encounters predictable and understandable via 'mediators' are typical strategies to manage the 'difference' of intellectually disabled persons in American society.

In marked contrast, Devlieger presents a case study of a young woman in rural Zimbabwe, whose disabilities limit her participation in the 'outside' world, but who is nonetheless well integrated into the daily domestic round with her kin group. She participates in the household activities to the extent she can move around with other young women and is 'protected' by the community, who let her live her life in the way she wants and is most comfortable doing. She is not 'drawn' into some occupation as a young person in America might have been, in the belief that this would maximize her potential; rather, she is free to 'sort out' her own capabilities. 'Social integration and participation develop according to capacity' (1998, 73).

In another context, in the modern nation state of Israel, the 'disabled body' also becomes emblematic of the 'national body'. In their ethnographic study of adult persons with disabilities in an Israeli rehabilitation centre, Agmon and colleagues (2016) attempt to identify ingrained, culturally bound assumptions about disability. They highlight how contemporary Israeli culture with its emphasis on bodily health and perfection, constructs the new Jewish nation and the new Jews as 'the chosen ones'. This is in contrast to the enfeebled and disabled body of the Jews in exile. Disabled persons deviate from the idea of the 'worthy person' actively involved in nation building, and are thus devalued, infantilized and de-sexualized, treated as 'half persons' or children.

Back home, Nilika Mehrotra's work on disability in rural Haryana provides a nuanced understanding of the interplay between local cultural idioms and constructs and the role of state policy in making disability a part of the development agenda. Writing of the cultural perceptions of disability in Haryana, Mehrotra (2013) notes that persons with locomotor impairments or limb deformities are recognized as disabled in an agrarian society requiring manual labour. In other words, it is the capacity to perform agricultural and domestic work that is crucial to determine disability. Persons with disabilities are frequently viewed as erratic, hot-tempered and quarrelsome, and are the butt of ridicule and name-calling.

Regarding the local aetiologies of disability, Mehrotra (2013) identifies a number of culturally specific beliefs, including *hawa lagna* (being affected by 'wind' or sudden change in temperature), the will of God and the person's fate (*kismet* or *bhag*), the cosmic intervention of malevolent gods and goddesses who need to be appeased (e.g., *Shitalamata* and her association with potentially disabling diseases like chickenpox), breaches of social and ritualistic sanctions, including breaching sexual abstinence on proscribed days, 'pseudo-medical reality' or failed medical procedures by quacks and untrained people and possession by bad spirits.

Mehrotra points out that these multiple causal explanations reflect an understanding of the interconnections between the operation of fate, ritual obligations, the work of supernatural beings and medical negligence. They operate in a continuum and reflect the cognitive understandings of the people (2013, 136).

The above examples demonstrate how the disability experience cannot be conceptualized as a unitary one, but is embedded within layers of culture and local realities. Differential cultural understandings of what constitutes ability and disability is often observed to be at odds with the aims and objectives of developmental programmes which espouse a different definition of disability. Community-Based Rehabilitation (CBR) programmes which have particular Western-inflected understandings of what constitutes 'development' have often been critiqued for disregarding cultural specificities. Thomas and Thomas (1999) point out that in many developing countries, kinship networks based upon mutual obligations and expectations are more useful than formal services. Unlike in the West, the idea of 'individual rights' may not exist, and therefore planning individual-centric strategies for 'empowerment' based upon formal service provision may not work.

Elaborating the critical role of 'culture' in development, Coleridge (2000) cites CBR programmes in war-torn Afghanistan. The Comprehensive Disabled Afghans Program (CDAP) set up in 1995 by the UNDP and UNOPS began as a programme drafted by foreign experts with little local consultation on the ground. Coleridge problematizes the connections between culture, development and disability through an analysis of Afghan social structure, the overwhelming importance of Islam, the patriarchal family and seclusion of women and the revivalist tendencies that emerged due to social and political breakdown caused by armed conflict. Afghan attitudes towards disability cannot be oversimplified and dubbed as harsh or repressive, as disability, as in the case of much of South Asia, is subsumed within family coping and caring. The marginal position of persons with disabilities arises if they are unable to marry or contribute to the family. The very idea of individual 'empowerment' or 'enablement', which is a key component of CBR, is problematic in a setting where the extended family and community assume primacy in the life of the individual.

Miles' (2009) critical essay on CBR in Asia highlights the problematic and decontextualized application of Western ideas and concepts around disability to the Asian context in the 1980s. As he puts it, '... largely monocultural (or westernised), disability evangelists exported community slogans, muddled with the rhetoric of individual disability rights, to third-world countries having minimal formal service structures' (2009: 70). He highlights critical issues like the unequal distribution and circulation of information, the realities of grinding poverty and absence of services and the potential conflicts and discontinuities between traditional, modern and post-modern knowledge systems. He recommends the development of disability histories of South Asia as the 'fundamental research' on the basis of which culturally and conceptually appropriate disability services may be developed, and Western paradigms evaluated for their suitability and 'fit' with indigenous concepts.

Despite the growth world-wide of the DRM and disability studies, the condition of persons with disabilities continues to be mired in structural problems and conflicting understandings. In India, the gap between 'haves' and 'have-nots' is widening day by day and the rhetoric of the DRM has failed to touch the lives of the majority of disabled persons particularly in the rural hinterland. However, the category of disability is becoming a more recognized and salient one with the expansion of information, knowledge and awareness of rights and entitlements. Despite an urban, middle-class bias in disability studies and activism, there is a growing body of literature from South Asia that documents and analyses disability experience using the foundational ideas of disability studies. In the following section, we will review how disability as a category of social oppression and discrimination has brought together people and inaugurated a 'disability culture' across the world.

'DISABILITY CULTURE': NEW MOBILIZATIONS AND MOVEMENTS

Peters (2015) defines disability culture as 'the sum total of behaviours, beliefs, ways of living, and material artifacts that are unique to persons affected by disability'. She draws attention to its historical, sociopolitical and individual dimensions.

> Historical definitions of disability culture focus on art, poetry, language, and social community developed by disabled people. Definitions of disability culture that blend the social and the political focus on a minority-group distinction with common values of social and economic justice, radical democracy, and self-empowerment. Notions of disability culture

grounded in the personal and the aesthetic emphasize a way of living and positive identification with being disabled.

'Disability culture' emerged with the remarkable growth in 'disabled communities' in the 1970s, both in the West and in the developing countries. Peters (2015) gives the example of Zimbabwe where young people with impairments who were sequestered in residential missionary schools, away from their families and communities, built strong ties and support systems amongst themselves. 'Inmates' at a school in Nguboyenia started a social club and organized meetings and discussions that enabled them to become aware of the discrimination and injustice they all experienced. They launched a countrywide campaign and membership drive all over Zimbabwe and set up their headquarter in Bulawayo that they called Freedom House. This formed the basis of a shared community and a group identity that later became known as the National Council of Disabled Persons of Zimbabwe.

In the Indian context, a similar example may be given of the blind community. The residential schools for the blind played an important role in shaping the nature and scope of the advocacy movement in India. Chander (2013) elaborates on the role played by associations like the National Federation of Blind Graduates in 1970, which was renamed as the National Federation of the Blind (NFB) in 1972, in rights-based advocacy. The 1970s were also a period of political ferment in India, and socialist as well as radical Marxist movements were emerging on the ground. The NFB played a pivotal role in the 1980s in lobbying the State to ensure and implement the job reservation policy in Central Government Services and public undertakings for certain categories of disabled persons and achieved considerable success in terms of recruitment of blind persons in government jobs. The movement also played a key role in the formulation and passing of the first comprehensive rights-based law for persons with disabilities, namely, The Persons with Disabilities Act (1995).

Disabled people's movements in the developing world were closely tied to the imperatives of development, that is, provision of food, shelter, healthcare and education and the inclusion of persons with disability as integral to the process of development. Peters (2015) draws attention to the fact that the sense of community and coming together of disabled persons for political and social causes also had the effect of developing in them a sense of pride and affirming their confidence in their individual strengths. They attempted to articulate their understandings about their lives and bodies and share their unique perspectives through art, literature, theatre, film and other cultural forms.

Within the academy, disability studies scholarship has become a fertile ground for the flowering of disability culture. Academic networks and platforms, dedicated publications and journals and seminars and conferences are instrumental in generating new knowledge and perspectives on the historical and cultural evolution of disability and also in challenging and contesting prevalent ideas and theories. Disability studies perspectives have the potential for being fundamentally subversive, challenging and overturning received understandings about ability, normality, difference, worthiness and ultimately the value of life and humanness itself.

However, it is important to reiterate that this alternative vision of disability as a source of community and individual empowerment and the celebration of 'difference' as a valid and valuable way of being is also deeply entwined with class, gender and availability of opportunities. As Peters (ibid.) notes, the process of globalization has certainly made a big impact on the lives of persons with disability through medical and technological interventions such as electronic vision and hearing devices and communication via Internet. This has expanded opportunities to forge connections and communicate experience, and thus strengthen disability culture. However, the flip side is the digital divide, wherein persons with poor access due to their structural and geographical locations get further marginalized. Hence, globalization is a mixed blessing.

Another significant development is the huge advancement in the field of genetics and biomedicine, which has led to biological identities becoming the basis for social ones. People with rare medical or genetic conditions are able to connect with each other and form solidarities based upon biological or genetic identities.

The term 'biosociality' was coined by Rabinow (1996) in the context of the Human Genome Initiative, but it is currently used to connect the worlds of biology and technology with the social sciences. Interestingly, while the social model on which the edifice of disability studies and DRM were founded challenged the medical model which categorized individuals on the basis of their biological or physical impairments, biosociality uses the medical or genetic markers as sources of identity and group formation. 'Nature' and 'culture' thus seem to collapse into each other. Disability studies has to think through these developments in a nuanced and careful manner. On the one hand, community formation that results from the categorization of a certain condition or impairment can facilitate mutual support and collective advocacy for resources, particularly in the case of rare conditions which do not receive much public attention or governmental funding. On the flip side, a 'single disease/disability focus' can lead to fragmentation of the disability movement as these discrete groups may fail to engage with other disability communities over the common goals of non-discrimination, access and inclusion (Block et al., 2011).

In this connection, it would be interesting to briefly examine two impairment-specific communities that view themselves as distinct 'cultures': Deaf culture/Deaf pride and autistic neurodiversity communities. 'Deaf Pride' refers to a movement of self-assertion and celebration of identity of Deaf people in the United States and other Western nations who reject the notion of deafness as a lack or a disability and view themselves as a community with a distinct culture mediated through sign language. In 1972, Professor James Woodward, a sociolinguist, suggested using 'deaf' (written with a lowercase 'd') to refer to the audiological condition of deafness, and 'Deaf' (written with an uppercase 'D') to refer to Deaf culture. The emergent academic discipline of Deaf Studies, which examines (Padden and Humphries, 1990) Deaf experience, 'uncritically embraces the concept of a monolithic and universal Deaf culture' (Friedner, 2013: 246). A Deaf individual, says Friedner, is a member of a Deaf culture and the Deaf Community, communicates using sign language, sees the world through Deaf eyes and possesses Deaf pride. On the other hand, a 'deaf' person is one who has a medical condition or impairment and most likely does not use sign language. As Friedner informs us, the Deaf community in America has more or less successfully managed to secure for itself access to education in sign language, sign language interpretation and appropriate communication technologies. Deafness is regarded as the master identity that trumps all others and entails certain rights and entitlements predicated upon it. The Deaf pride movement has a global scope, as its proponents believe that due to communication barriers and the resultant alienation from hearing people including family members, Deaf people can seek and find companionship and belongingness with their own 'kind'. Breivik, the Norwegian Deaf Studies scholar, focuses on how Deaf people around the world are similar, and 'potentially and actually members of a transnational and translocal framework that overrides any local or national loyalty they may additionally possess' (Breivik, 2005: 12, quoted in Friedner, 2013: 257).

Autistic 'neurodiversity' is another interesting mobilization of individuals who identify themselves on the Autism Spectrum particularly Asperger's Syndrome. They hold that Autism is not a disability or disorder, but an expression of neurological difference or differently 'wired' brains (Runswick-Cole, 2014). The term 'neurodiversity' was coined by the Australian sociologist Judy Singer (1999) who argued that the 'neurodiverse' population also constitute a political grouping comparable with other identity groups, such as those based on class, gender, sexuality or race. Neurodiversity advocates actively affirm and celebrate their biological uniqueness or difference from the so called neurotypical (NT) or 'normal' people, and therefore resist and reject the search for a 'cure' for autism. They also reject the 'people first' language of the disability movement, preferring to call themselves 'autistic persons' rather than 'persons with autism' as they believe their autism is an integral part of their identity (Runswick-Cole, 2014).

Advocates of neurodiversity view autism as a distinct 'culture', much like the Deaf culture does. In this context, Davidson (2008: 793) notes that even though the very notion of culture is complex and contentious, persons on the Autism spectrum indicate that 'autistic differences in perception and "processing" tend to involve Other ways of being-in-the-world, separate senses of selves and space that give rise to distinctive cultural experience, and so also, cultural expression'.

One of the core 'difficulties' experienced by persons on the autism spectrum is social communication and expressive language. However, the Internet revolution and the possibilities for virtual communication, unmediated by problematic social conventions that many persons on the autism spectrum find hard to deal with, has opened up the world for autistics as never before. Davidson (2008: 792) quotes Singer (1999) who affirmed that 'the democratization of information flow which is the Internet has promoted the emergence of new ways of self-identification for autistics' (Singer, 1999: 64). Singer quotes the journalist Harvey Blume who stated that, 'The impact of the Internet on autistics may one day be compared to the spread of sign language among the deaf' (Singer 1999: 67). Nearly two decades later, the import of this statement is quite clear, as the Internet has indeed proved to be the most fertile site for creating and sustaining an 'autistic culture' that transcends geographies. The difficulties and unpredictability of face-to-face communication for persons with autism has been well documented, and a range of narratives by persons who self-identify as autistic has shed light on the way they experience the world (see Davidson, 2007, 2008). The world of computers seems ideally suited to their style or being-in-the world, and has opened up spaces for them to engage with others and make their reality visible.

CONCLUSION

This chapter has traced multiple dimensions of the relationship between disability and culture. Disability is a ubiquitous feature of human existence and, unlike other categories like gender, caste and class, is highly fluid and unpredictable. Cultural imaginations and constructions of the impaired body and mind provide rich insights into the manner in which humans negotiate the existential frailty of the body and find explanations for the fundamental questions and crises that affect us all. At the same time, the attempts of marginalized people to make sense of their own conditions and challenge received notions are the drivers of social and cultural change. The changing understandings of the body, ability and competence also reflect material historical realities. The ideas of biosociality and neurodiversity problematize and disturb the binaries of nature and culture, normal and abnormal, ability and disability, thus adding a new dimension to the ongoing debates and discussions around disability studies.

REFERENCES

Agmon, Maayan, Amalia Sa'ar, and Tal Araten-Bergman. 2016. 'The Person in the Disabled Body: A Perspective on Cultures and Personhood from the Margins.' *International Journal for Equity in Health*. doi:10.1186/s12939-016-0437-2 (accessed September 14, 2017).

Benedict, Ruth. 1934. 'Anthropology and the Abnormal.' *The Journal of General Psychology* 10 (1): 59–82.

Block, Pamela, Eva L. Rodriguez, Maria C. Milazzo, William S. MacAllister, Lauren B. Krupp, Akemi Nishida, Nina Slota, Alyssa M. Broughton, and Christopher B. Keys. 2011. 'Building Pediatric Multiple Sclerosis Community Using a Disability Studies Framework of Empowerment.' In *Disability and Community*, edited by Allison C. Carey and Richard K. Scotch, 85–112. Bingley: Emerald Group Publication.

Chander, Jagdish. 2013. 'Disability Rights and the Emergence of Disability Studies.' In *Disability Studies in India: Global Discourses, Local Realities*, edited by Renu Addlakha, 61–77. New Delhi: Routledge.

Coleridge P. 2000. 'Disability and Culture.' In *Selected Readings in CBR*, edited by M. Thomas and M. J. Thomas, 22–41. Bangalore: *Asia Pacific Disability Rehabilitation Journal*. Available at http://english.aifo.it/disability/apdrj/selread100/index.htm

Dalal, A. K. 2002. 'Disability Rehabilitation in a Traditional Indian Society.' In *Selected Readings in Community Based Rehabilitation: Series 2. Disability and Rehabilitation in South Asia*, edited by Maya Thomas and M. J. Thomas. Bangalore: Asia Pacific Disability Rehabilitation Journal. Available at: http://english.aifo.it/disability/apdrj/selread102/contents.htm

Davidson, Joyce. 2007. '"In a World of Her Own…" Re-presenting Alienation and Emotion in the Lives and Writings of Women with Autism." *Gender, Place and Culture* 14 (6): 659–77.

———. 2008. 'Autistic Culture Online: Virtual Communication and Cultural Expression on the Spectrum.' *Social & Cultural Geography* 9 (7): 791–806. doi:10.1080/14649360802382586.

Devlieger, Patrick J. 1998. '(In)competence in America in Comparative Perspective.' In *Questions of Competence: Culture, Classification and Intellectual Disability*, edited by Richard Jenkins, 54–75. Cambridge: Cambridge University Press.

———. 1995. 'Why Disabled? The Cultural Understanding of Physical Disability in an African Society.' In *Disability and Culture*, edited by Benedicte Ingstad and Susan R. Whyte, 94–106. Berkeley, CA: University of California Press.

———. 2005, October 14–16. 'Generating a Cultural Model of Disability.' Paper presented at the 19th Congress of the European Federation of Associations of Teachers of the Deaf (FEAPDA), Geneva, Switzerland.

Friedner, Michele. 2013. 'Identity Formation and Transnational Discourses: Thinking Beyond Identity Politics.' In *Disability Studies in India: Global Discourses, Local Realities*, edited by Renu Addlakha, 241–62. New Delhi: Routledge.

Ghai, Anita. 2015. *Rethinking Disability in India*. New Delhi: Routledge.
Ingstad, Benedicte, and Susan Reynolds Whyte. 1995. 'Disability and Culture: An Overview' In *Disability and Culture*, 3–32. Berkeley, CA: University of California Press.
———. 2007. *Disability in Local and Global Worlds*. Berkeley, CA: University of California Press.
Jenkins, Richard, ed. 1998. 'Culture, Classification and (In)competence.' In *Questions of Competence: Culture, Classification and Intellectual Disability*, 1–24. Cambridge: Cambridge University Press.
Mehrotra, Nilika. 2013. *Disability, Gender and State Policy: Exploring Margins*. Jaipur: Rawat Publications.
Miles, M. 2009. 'Community, Individual or Information Development? Dilemmas of Concept and Culture in South Asian Disability Planning.' In *Disability and Society: A Reader*, edited by Renu Addlakha, Stuart Blume, Patrick Devlieger, Osamu Nagase and Myriam Winance, 65–85. New Delhi: Orient Blackswan.
Pal, Joyojeet. 2013. 'Physical Disability and Indian Cinema.' In *Different Bodies: Essays on Disability in Film and Television*, edited by Marja Evelyn Mogk, 109–30. Jeffersons, NC, and London: McFarland and Company, Inc., Publishers.
Padden, Carol and Humphries, Tom. 1990. *Deaf in America: Voices from a Culture*. Harvard: Harvard University Press.
Peters, Susan. 2015. 'Disability Culture.' *Britannica Online Encyclopedia*. Available at: https://www.britannica.com/topic/disability-culture (accessed September 17, 2017).
Rabinow, Paul. 1996. 'Artificiality and Enlightenment: From Sociobiology to Biosociality.' In *Essays on the Anthropology of Reason*, 91–111. Princeton, NJ: Princeton University Press.
Runswick-Cole, Katherine. 2014. '"Us" and "Them": The Limits and Possibilities of a "Politics of Neurodiversity" in Neoliberal Times.' *Disability & Society* 29 (7): 1117–29. doi:10.1080/09687599.2014.910107.
Singer, Judy. 1999. '"Why Can't You Be Normal for Once in Your Life?" From a "Problem with No Name" to the Emergence of a New Category of Difference.' In *Disability Discourse*, edited by M. Corker and S. French, 59–67. Buckingham: Open University Press.
Staples, James, and Nilika Mehrotra. 2016. 'Disability Studies: Developments in Anthropology.' In *Disability in the Global South*, edited by Simon Grech and Karen Soldatic, 35–49. Switzerland: Springer.
Thomas, Maya, and M. J. Thomas. 1999. 'Influence of Cultural Factors on Disability and Rehabilitation in Developing Countries.' *Asia Pacific Disability Rehabilitation Journal* 10 (2). Available at: http://www.dinf.ne.jp/doc/english/asia/resource/apdrj/z13jo0400/z13jo0403.html (accessed September 4, 2017).
Whyte, Susan Reynolds. 1998. 'Slow Cookers and Madmen: Competence of Heart and Head in Rural Uganda.' In *Questions of Competence: Culture, Classification and Intellectual Disability*, edited by Richard Jenkins, 153–75. Cambridge: Cambridge University Press.

Chapter 15

Corporeality and Cultural Difference

Shilpaa Anand

Is disability a universal concept? This chapter will explore the diverse ways in which corporeal (mind–body) conditions are comprehended, discussed and acted upon in distinct cultural contexts. For the purposes of this chapter, 'corporeal/ity' refers not only to the physicality of the body but to a complex composition of physiological, intellectual and emotional aspects of human beings. The use of 'culture' and 'cultural' refers to ways of going about the world as well as ways of knowing the world. The aim of this chapter is to discuss how normative ideas about corporeality develop in distinct cultural contexts. For instance, under what conditions does blindness come to be known as a disability? While we cannot deny that there are sightless people everywhere in the world, we cannot be sure that the social and cultural meanings attached to being sightless are the same everywhere. So too, the way societies respond to sightless people is likely to be determined by the ways in which that society composes knowledge about being sightless and goes about being sightless. Drawing on historical and anthropological studies, the chapter will investigate culturally different ideas about corporeality, systems of treatment, personhood, ethical action, social interaction and social exclusion.

NORMATIVE NOTIONS ABOUT THE CORPOREAL

Certain cultural contexts, such as the Western one, are primarily dominated by normative ideas that contain binaries such as health/ill-health, whole/part, good/evil and so on. Meanings of corporeality depend on the standards that are established. Standardizing is a way in which knowledge about the world is produced and acted upon in such contexts. One example would be the way in which skin conditions such as leprosy are considered impure within enduring Judaic-Christian traditions. This means that anyone with leprosy would have been socially excluded within the history of development of Judaism and Christianity. Connotations of impurity include ideas about what is good and what is evil. We may comprehend this by thinking of instances from the New Testament of the Bible where people with leprosy were thought of as impure and as requiring healing. The leper's body was an important site where the contest between religions was dramatically played out. Christian missions that settled in India brought with them a story of leprosy that was plotted within a narrative that typified the leper as the innocent sinner, a reprobate who had no role in being cast as such. The narrative also projects the idea that Christianity would save the leper through a programme of salvation that would ultimately become a crucial tool for conversion of natives into the new religion. What is significant about this emplotment, something that is often forgotten, is that leprosy was presented as a 'problem' that needed solving, an idea that may or may not have been present prior to missionary intervention. Another significant aspect of the plot was the casting of other religions and their customs as being villainous to those affected by leprosy. A third feature of the leprosy story is that leprosy served as the stage on which the presentation of Christianity as a reformed and continually reforming religion could be performed. Medieval/early Christian characterization of leprosy as an evil condition and the leper as one who was despised and ostracized was shunned in the later Christian rendition that was prevalent in colonial India. The link between the missionary approach to the disease and the (then) new public health discourse was strong. Hospitals and asylums run by the Mission to Lepers received funding from the British government in India, thus supporting wholeheartedly the missionary initiatives.

Significant actors of the British Empire Leprosy Relief Association (BELRA), such as Rev. Cochrane, were informed by and invested in Biblical notions of leprosy and applauded the transition the religion had made from severe Old Testament beliefs to the New Testament practices of bringing salvation to the leper:

> It has happened that God in His mercy has overruled the mediaeval misunderstanding regarding leprosy and used it for His glory. Through it He has wrought a marvellous work, leading His Church into fresh avenues of service among people who, the world over, were utterly despised and rejected... God reveals to men from time to time human injustices which must be put right, and through His servants He issues the challenge that these things must not be. (Cochrane 1961, 22)

The public health view of leprosy, in its attempt to provide a rational aetiology of the disease, presented an 'orientalized' picture of leprosy that succeeded in further moralizing the emergence and existence of the disease in India:

> Leprosy may be regarded as a malady of uncivilized or partially civilized races, and its chief predisposing causes comprise personal uncleanliness, overcrowded and dirty dwellings, combined with a dietary that is deficient in quality or insufficient in quantity.... The eradication of the native filthy habits and customs which predispose to, and assist in spreading, leprosy is recognised to be a matter attended with many difficulties; it would therefore seem that the hope for the future must lie in the education of the rising generation in the elements of personal and domestic hygiene. (*The Lancet* 1913, 1557)

It is not hard to detect the moral tone that guards this seemingly scientific 'public health' discourse in the report above. Evidently, medical concepts and moral connotations had become so deeply intertwined that the more scientific of interventions had to be ushered in by those actors who were in fact working as social reformers and political activists.[1] So, we see in the encounter between British colonialism and the Indian context, in colonial India, normative notions about

---

[1] Reprinted/adapted with permission from: *Interrogating Disability in India: Theory and Practice* by Nandini Ghosh. Springer, Cham. COPYRIGHT (2016) Springer Nature.

leprosy guarded by moral ideas took root and medical notions about leprosy were suggested as interventions that would remove the moral stigma attached to it within the Christianized view of the disease. Both the moral and the medical interventions suggest that corporeal conditions within the Western knowledge framework are normative in nature—leprosy is standardized as a moral problem and later leprosy is standardized as a medical problem. Concepts of the normal and abnormal emerge in contexts where knowledge of the world is normatively composed. Normalcy is a standard and desirable state and is determined by all those conditions that are outliers or 'abnormal'.

Let us look at another cultural context to understand what a non-normative way of thinking about corporeal conditions looks like. In the case of Greek antiquity, a corporeal condition, let us say, the absence of the loss of a limb, would be treated differently based on the context in which the individual became limb-less. The names used for deafness, blindness and limb-loss are multiple within the ancient Greek context. Every manifestation of the same impairment was treated differently based on a variety of factors such as heredity, ritual aspects and other features that are not familiar within the Christian West. While Aristotle's view that deformed infants had to be killed has become popular within contemporary histories of disability, it would be significant to note that this may not have been his view about all deformed babies (Rose 2003). The point of argument here is that knowledge about deformity or what we now call disability was not produced in a normative (standardized/universal/generalizable) manner but was related to context-sensitive factors. In the ancient Greek context, one would find men with impairments who were part of military forces (Rose 2003, 43–44). One also knows that women were thought of as 'deformed' men because they did not have the same physical traits as men. So, what is debatable here is whether the concept of 'deformity' is the same concept that we know from the modern West, or does this English translation of the concept erase the cultural specificities that the concept for corporeal difference obtained within the context of Greek antiquity?

STANDARDIZED NORMATIVE 'TREATMENT'

Institutionalized care within the Western context draws our attention to another aspect of how normative notions about disability emerge historically. Anglo-American notions of corporeal difference are determined by institutions of care that developed to address certain conditions and in turn established these corporeal conditions as normative kinds. The case of leprosy serves as a good instance. Leprosy colonies of the medieval period in Europe developed at the outskirts of the town because leprosy-affected people were excluded from civil and social interaction. With the emergence and establishment of Christianity, leprosariums were instituted for the homing and treatment of people affected by the disease, as acts of charity. Some such institutions, those affiliated with the Roman Catholic church were known as lazar houses, named after the patron saint of leprosy, 'Lazarus the beggar'. Theories of contagion that had developed with advances in medical knowledge also impacted the instituting of such measures. People affected by leprosy moved from the outskirts of the town to the innermost centres of the town because the task of addressing leprosy and those who were leprosy-affected became an important focus of the development of religious practice. As a result, leprosy became a normative condition whose knowledge became specialized with the progression from notions of impurity to theories of contagion in the period of the emergence and establishment of Judaism and Christianity as well as development of medical knowledge. Similar histories of asylums have also been traced which show how the development of institutional care of insanity simultaneously resulted in the establishment of knowledge about psychiatric conditions.

One of the most significant outcomes of such institutional development of corporeal conditions is that they standardized the treatment of people with similar kinds of corporeal 'symptoms'. Diagnosis and classification of conditions led to the discourse of disability developing by focusing on addressing the condition and disregarding its antecedents. One finds that the present-day discussion about disability is dominated by information and conversations about treating disability, about addressing blindness, leprosy, lameness and deafness for instance. Are there no other ways of talking about and acting upon corporeal differences?

RECONCEPTUALIZING 'TREATMENT'

If we return to the instance from Greek antiquity discussed earlier, we find that the naming and classification of different corporeal conditions was based on distinctive antecedent features. This way of knowing corporeal conditions which was dominant in antiquity, later becomes subordinated to normative classifications of diseases, impairment and disabilities. Other cultural contexts retain, though in a subordinated manner, ways of knowing corporeal conditions based on antecedent factors. For instance, among the Songye of the Zaire region of Africa, it is not so much the similarity of impairment or corporeal conditions that determines classification but causal factors. Devlieger (1995) finds that in Songye society categories of 'abnormality' include 'ceremonial' children, 'bad' children and 'faulty' children; these categories impact the social status of children. Ceremonial children are considered as having special powers and occupy a higher status in society. They may be categorized as such because of the conditions of their birth—being born with the umbilical cord around the neck, being born with a hand on the cheek or being born feet or hands first. Bad children are those who are thought of as supernatural and as beneath the status of being human. In our present-day categories, this category would include hydrocephalic children, those of short stature and those affected by albinism.

The third category of children, 'faulty' children include those who are known to have 'not only an imperfection of the body but also a distorted relationship' (Devlieger 1995, 96). The birth of such children results in the family trying to find the person causing the fault; the notion of the fault is not located within the individual's body but at the level of interpersonal relations. The way engaging with these so-called faulty children is by searching for the cause or fault in a relationship within the family that led to their birth. The object of the attention in these situations within Songye society draws attention away from the person with the corporeal condition and is directed elsewhere.

In another departure from classifying corporeal conditions based on symptom and subsequent treatment, Ayurveda and Siddha traditions could be of interest. Ayurveda and Siddha conceptualize the human body as 'a system of relationships defining functions which manifest themselves through the structures' (Jayasundar 2012, 42). In Ayurveda, a function is constituted by collective effort of numerous factors, including structures (as in biomedicine), biochemistry, electric and magnetic activities and the mental and emotional status of a person. For instance, these systems do not assume the duality of mind and body or conceive of the body in terms of separate systems such as the skeletal system, the endocrine system and so on. A function, in Ayurvedic terms, reflects the entire system of a human being where a variety of components work together to constitute it (Jayasundar 2012). Siddha practice does not regard disease in terms of organs affected, so the concept of organ is not a useful entity within the Siddha tradition. In Siddha, different substrata of the body are composed by substances that nourish them, be they items such as food and water that nurture the earthly or gross parts of the body as well as subtle substances like prana (the concept of air circulating through hollow channels of the body) and thoughts and intellect (Sujatha 2012). Ayurveda uses the concepts of *vata*, *pitta* and *kapha*, the *tridoshas* (three elements), that refer to 'a set of parameters which include functions like movement, transformation and support and growth, respectively, and other physico-chemical and physiological parameters contributing to these functions' (Sujatha 2012, 43). The *doshas*, however, literally mean 'that which can become impaired and also [have] the potential to impair other tissues' (Sujatha 2012, 43). These *doshas* include physiological as well as psychological functions. The concept of health within this system of medicine is not linear (as in biomedicine) and refers to homeostasis or fine balance among the doshas. Thus, 'disease' as well is a result of imbalance in the doshas.

'Diagnosis' in Ayurveda consists of an assessment of any deviation from the state of equilibrium of *doshas*; the impaired *dosha* must be identified. 'Diagnosis' here includes the evaluation of the inherent mental and physical constitution of the patient, age, occupation, the season in which the 'disease' has manifested itself, the immediate living environment of the patient including the weather, the food habits of the patient and so on. Ayurvedic 'diagnosis' is aimed at knowing the root cause of the disease condition. As the method of treatment is tailor-made for a specific patient, it is important to know all these factors; sensitivity to context is of prime importance (Jayasundar 2012). Ayurvedic diagnosis also pays keen attention to cause of the 'disease', why something is happening to the patient, rather than merely knowing the symptoms or what is happening to the patient. These treatment traditions provide personalized treatment to each patient, thus not repeating the same method of treatment even for two people who may have the same symptoms and the same 'impairment'.

Siddha tradition believes that the only source of knowledge for treating the living human being is the living human being; 'one can never study the flow of prana in a body that is devoid of prana' (Sujatha 2012, 86). Siddha practitioners believe that cognition is something that everyone is capable of because they include perception and inference (Sujatha 2012). So also, as in Ayurveda, knowledge of the 'disease' is based on how the patient experiences their ailment (Bode 2012). The context is important to 'diagnose' the disease as well as the information given by the patient; both contribute to this process of diagnosing in ways that are different from the biomedical system. These systems then deploy narratives of the patients to develop the treatment. In a work by Mishra and Chatterjee (2013), the editors discuss the significance of narratives in non-biomedical treatment practices. The volume of essays draws on studies of narratives of practitioners of different medical and treatment systems as well as the patients. Though the introduction to the book acknowledges its debt to the emergence of illness narratives within biomedical practices as a guiding framework (Mishra and Chatterjee 2013), it becomes clear as one reads through the essays how and why narratives are intrinsically part of these treatment traditions.

Ayurveda and Siddha systems, as also bone-setting traditions, depend heavily on the knowledge that a person has of themselves and their bodily functions; therefore, the narratives of patients play a vital role in developing the treatment. Treatment in Ayurveda is denoted as *chikitsa*, which includes procedures 'aimed at removal of disease-causing factors' as well as repair of imbalances (Jayasundar 2012, 51). The root causes and not surface-level symptoms are the focus of treatment—another reason that the narratives of patients form the corpus of knowledge which also forms part of the treatment. Siddha and Ayurvedic practices address the patient in context. To know the context of the patient, these systems need the active participation of the patient to inform them of their contexts in terms of environmental factors, daily activities and bodily functions. This gives the practitioners a sense of minute changes in the routines of the person, including why they may have done something differently on a particular day. Details like this invariably involve a narrative that describes the social context of the person being treated. Treatment in turn is developed to address the specificities of the individual's condition in context, thereby giving us a different theory of individuality, one where the treatment is individuated, not the person. What this demonstrates is that the context and the individual are contiguous; the separation between the two does not exist in the conceptualization of 'patient', 'disease' and 'treatment'.[2]

Treatment, as in the case of *nirvicikitsa*, a form of addressing the external is prevalent within the Jaina tradition. In a kind of 'practice of the self', this *chikitsa* requires that a person overcome their disgust or repulsion that may be caused by another person's disfigurement. The practice of '*nirvicikitsa*' would enable one to feel no revulsion at the sight of disease, deformity or disfigurement of any kind in another human being. The Jaina form of indifference adhered to the idea of detachment which meant 'all passion spent and all compassion absent' (Miles 2000, 607) and thus diverges significantly from the modern-day disability activism that emphasizes compassion which is framed within the human rights discourse. It is a practice of studied indifference that one adopts to improve oneself. This concept helps us see that ways of addressing corporeal difference may include a method that primarily focuses on the transformation of one's mindset or affective responses but results in the by-product that may impact the social status of the one affected by a 'disabling' condition.

SOCIAL CONTEXTS OF CORPOREAL DIFFERENCE

Let us consider that within the ancient Greek context, a deaf child would most likely have been considered as intellectually unstable, if at all normative notions applied. Given that teaching-learning as well as social interaction employed oral–aural methods and Greek society held in high regard the philosophical orientations of individuals, those who were deaf became excluded from the intellectual realm (Rose 2003). Contextual categorization of corporeal difference is a robust indicator of the way in which cultures organize their sense of corporeality—which faculties are prioritized over others and which faculties are involved in meaning-making about the world.

---

[2] Reprinted/adapted with permission from: *Interrogating Disability in India: Theory and Practice* by Nandini Ghosh. Springer, Cham. COPYRIGHT (2016) Springer Nature.

Another such instance is offered in the case of the appearance of Shah Daula's *chuhas* in the *dargahs* of pre-Partition India/Pakistan. '*Shah Daula's chuhas*'[3] (literally 'the mice of Shah Daula'), were a category of microcephalic youth prevalent in the Indo-Pakistan region between the 17th and 19th centuries. Asylum registers and psychiatric case notes of the time ran concurrent to the reports that appeared in the *Indian Medical Gazette*. Based on these institutional records, psychiatry scholars classified the *chuhas* as a culture-specific form of mental derangement. Published in 1912, Overbeck-Wright's book, *Mental Derangements in India: Their Symptoms and Treatment,* acted like a handbook of psychiatric diagnoses along with case notes from asylums.[4] A major section of the book catalogues a list of conditions that are indexed as Indian forms of mental derangement. Overbeck-Wright was the superintendent of the mental asylum in Agra and may have been considered an authority on Indian strands of mental conditions. By the time he published his second book on the same subject, *Lunacy in India* in 1921, an updated version of the previous book, he also held positions in scholarly bodies such as 'Member of the Medico-Psychological Association of Great Britain and Ireland' and was 'Lecturer on Mental Diseases to King George's Medical College, Lucknow' and was a lecturer in the Agra Medical School as well.

Overbeck-Wright (1912), in a chapter titled 'Brief Discussion of the Main Differences between European and Indian Psychoses', under the subheading 'Psychoses Peculiar to India', commented on the absence of variation in the 'mental diseases' of the 'Eastern and Western races' and proceeded to name 'Shah Daula's mice' as one of the 'very few forms' that was peculiar to India. He describes them as a category of

---

[3] The phrase 'Shah Daula's *chuha*s' has been spelled variously as 'Shah Dowla's chuas', 'Shah Daulah's chuas' and so on. This chapter adopts the spelling 'Shah Daula's *chuha*s' in keeping with the phonetic transcription of the Urdu word '*chuha*' meaning rat or mouse. However, where the components of the phrase have been spelled differently in various historical records and scholarly accounts as 'Shah Dowla' in some cases and as 'chua', the spellings used in those accounts have been retained in the references and within quotation marks as necessary.

[4] Overbeck-Wright (1921) followed this book up with an updated version in 1921 titled *Lunacy in India*. The description of Shah Daula's *chuha*s is retained as is in the second book, showing that he found little that was new to add to his previously existing account.

'microcephalic imbeciles of comparatively uniform type' (p. 99) that were found in large numbers in the Punjab region. The *chuhas*, as per his account, were hired out to *faquirs*[5] at the shrine who took them around for begging. His position as an official of the mental asylum enabled him to document, as follows, the physical and mental capacity of the *chuhas*:

> A large percentage of them appear, however, to be deaf and dumb, and strabismus is common among them, indicating probably some error in refraction or other visual defect. They are capable of being taught simple employments, and are by no means immodest or indecent, and as a rule show none of the revolting tendencies or depraved appetites so commonly seen among other types of imbeciles. (Overbeck-Wright 1912, 100)

Overbeck-Wright's descriptive account speculated that the *chuhas* may have predominantly 'sprung from the lowest classes' (Overbeck-Wright 1912, 100) and recorded the different theories of origin associated with the *chuhas,* including the one about infertile mothers coming to the shrine to fulfil vows that would help them bear children. He retained the other popular theory as well, about the use of iron clamps to change the shape of children's' heads in their infancy so that they would serve as companions to alms collectors at the shrine. In relation to the third theory of mental influence on pregnant mothers having caused the birth of *chuhas*, Overbeck-Wright suspects that women staying at the shrine for a few days were given access to one of the male microcephalics by the 'guardians of the shrine' so that they may give birth to a *chuha* and thus 'maintain the reputation of the tomb' (1912, 100). Overbeck-Wright's account confirms microcephaly as a kind of psychiatric condition, but also highlights cultural variance as a striking feature of the phenomenon. While the medical records dismissed the cultural specificities of the shrine and the *chuhas*, psychiatry ascribed a higher status to them. It is perhaps due to Overbeck-Wright's account that later histories of the *chuhas* (e.g., Miles 1996) owe the identification of the shrine as a site of healing and institution of care.

While the official colonial documents of the time and region focus on the microcephaly of the *chuhas*, closer reading of literary and cultural

---

[5] A religious ascetic who is known to live only on alms.

narratives of the prevalence of the *chuhas* reveals that the more critical issue may have been about the infertility of the mothers who came to the shrine. If at all one had to learn something about how 'disability' was conceptualized within that context, in that time, we may learn that the women who came to the *dargah* faced the threat of social exclusion by them being branded as childless within their social worlds. Flora Annie Steel's short story, 'Shah Sujah's Mouse'[6] (1893) is about how a *chuha* from the shrine of Shah Shujah, who was wandering and begging for alms, rescues the narrator's lost child. Flora Annie Steel, a British woman who lived in Punjab, wrote extensively about local people in her fiction and non-fiction work. She was, we are told, invested in educational reforms in the area and had interacted with the women in the region. Her story is not bereft of orientalist overtones like those in the medical reports. She likens the *chuhas* at the shrine to the biblical Samuel in the temple. The story is narrated from the point of view of a British mother of a young child who is in India[7] with her husband because of his official service in the colonial government. Written in a sentimental vein, the story captures the emotions of a mother's love and loss of her child. Sonny is lost and found later by the *chuha* only to die later because of a severe fever. The story relates the affection that Sonny develops to the mute *chuha* who could draw all the squirrels in the garden to him by whistling a tune.

The story dwells on the social ostracism faced by women who were unable to bear children, which remain under-emphasized in the archival and medico-psychiatric records (Ewens 1903; Lodge Patch 1928; Overbeck-Wright 1912). This fictionalized account, commenting on the differences between the colonial-official conceptualization of the *chuhas* and the local ones sharply draws into the picture the figure of the *chuha*'s mother: 'These mouse-like ones belong to Shah Shujah's shrine, because they are the firstlings of barren women made fruitful by the saints' intercession. Therefore, from their birth they bear the token of the mother's vow, dedicating them to his service' (Steel 1893, 79–80).

---

[6] Shah Sujah is either another name for Shah Daula that was prevalent locally or may be accepted as a fictionalized name used by the author for Shah Daula.
[7] Pre-partition India.

Saadat Hasan Manto's short story, first written in Urdu, titled *'Shah Dule ka Chuha'* (literally 'Shah Daula's mouse') was later translated into English (Manto 2008) with the title 'The Mice of Shah Daula' and takes as its central theme the suffering infertile mother who had visited the shrine in the hope of a boon of fertility. Salima, the young woman, is distraught because of her inability to bear a child. Not only Salima, but also her mother and her mother-in-law were as troubled. Salima, the protagonist who is keen to undertake any action if it enables her to bear a child, agrees to visit the shrine of Shah Daulah though her friend has warned her that as per the customs of the shrine, the woman seeking the boon of fertility must submit her firstborn to the service of Shah Daula. Being unable to have a child, consumed Salima's life. She has also been warned that the child born to her may have a very small head, but that does not daunt her. In fact, she believes that it would not matter whether the child had crossed-eyes or a flat-nose; she would not love it less because of that.

At the shrine, Salima encounters Shah Daula's *chuha*. At first, she shudders at the sight of the human *chuha* who physically manifest signs of 'mental enfeeblement' with a leaking nose and strange behaviour. Soon the antics of the *chuha* make Salima laugh for a moment before she dissolves into tears at the thought of how this child may be the victim of exploitation at the hands of the shrine keepers. As the story progresses, we find that Salima submits her first-born, Mujib, to the service of the shrine, under pressure from her friend to keep the promise she had made at the shrine. Mujib, it must be noted, is not a *chuha*, not microcephalic, but owed to the shrine because of the promise made by Salima. On returning home, Salima contracts, as a result of her grief, a delirious fever due to which she dreams that Shah Daula was a 'large mouse gnawing, with its razor edged teeth, at her flesh' (Manto 2008, 91). She hallucinates that her son enters a mouse hole and while she pulled at his tail, larger mice grab his snout so firmly that she cannot pull him out. The hallucinations multiply and she sees in her fevered state, the girl *chuha* from the shrine, mice everywhere in the house and herself as a *chuha* of the shrine. All these episodes end in inconsolable tears.

In due course Salima has another child, a girl and later two boys. When she visits the town of the shrine for a wedding, she goes in search of her Mujib but on not finding him convinces herself that he may have died. Salima, on returning home, organizes a memorial for her son and obtains some closure on the matter. Then, one day she meets him. He is the *chuha* performing antics on the street to collect alms, brought around by one of the shrine keepers. She recognizes him because of the unmistakable mark on his cheek and is overjoyed. She rushes into the house with him, embraces him and tells him she is his mother. He responds with more antics, unaware of what had caused her emotional outburst. Salima, in a last bid to own the son she had once lost, tries to buy him from the keeper but in the interim, her Mujib runs off, nowhere to be found.

Manto's (2008) location and perspective as a writer are different from Steel's (1893). His fiction, primarily his short stories, is critically acclaimed for its insightful and ironic vignettes of pre-Partition and Partition India. What his story uncovers for us is the extent to which the phenomenon of the *chuhas* is intertwined with the disabling experiences of the mothers who dedicated their children to the shrine. Inhorn and Bharadwaj (2007) in their paper titled 'Reproductively Disabled Lives: Infertility, Stigma, and Suffering in Egypt and India' allege that infertility is managed differently within the rights discourse in the Euro-American context. The presence of reproductive-rights discourse manifest in these parts is bolstered by the idea that individuals have a choice in reproduction which may not be prevalent in non-Euro-American societies, 'becoming a parent is rarely a choice for most men and women in non-Euro-American societies, where reproduction, both biological and social, is a cultural imperative, and where parenthood, for both women and men, is an integral aspect of adult personhood' (Inhorn and Bharadwaj 2007, 79). Inhorn and Bharadwaj (2007) also argue that infertility has not been 'conceptualized, theorized, or politicized as a form of bodily disablement' within the disability rights discourse. They add:

> [I]n many non-Euro-American societies, individual agency is often subsumed within larger collectivities such as the family, and thus strategies of everyday resistance are not openly political within cultural constraints framing and offering differing opportunities for action and expression. (Inhorn and Bharadwaj 2007, 79)

In Salima's case, we see that the subject of childbearing is shared by many of her family members; she is, in a way, a 'familial body' (Cohen 1998). Being infertile was a socio-corporeal phenomenon that may have well resulted in these women becoming mentally distressed.[8]

CONCLUSION

Cultural contexts are dominated by certain ways of knowing one's world and oneself. These dominant ways of knowing (episteme—conceptual) and ways of going about (discourse and action) may be referred to as cultural configurations. Historical and anthropological inquiries have argued that disability as a concept emerges under certain cultural and epistemic conditions peculiar to Euro-American West and cannot be assumed to be universal over time or across geographical regions and cultural contexts (Devlieger 1995; Ingstad and Whyte; Rose 2003; Miles 1996, 2000). The contextual emergence of the concept refers to the way impairments came to be problematized[9] (Foucault 1990) as belonging to a moralized domain due to historical and epistemic circumstances. It could further be argued that the development of disability studies as a field of study has, by extension, been dominated by *this* concept of corporeal difference and only minimally engaged with or described other culture-specific concepts of corporeal difference.

REFERENCES

Bode, Maarten. 2012. 'Ayurveda in the Twenty-first Century: Logic, Practice and Ethics.' In *Medical Pluralism in Contemporary India*, edited by V. Sujatha and Leena Abraham, 59–76. New Delhi: Orient Blackswan.

---

[8] Reprinted/adapted with permission from: *Bioarchaeology of Impairment and Disability: Theoretical, Ethnohistorical, and Methodological Perspectives* by Jennifer F. Byrnes and Jennifer L. Muller. Springer, Cham. COPYRIGHT (2017) Springer Nature.

[9] The concept of problematizing used here invokes Michel Foucault's use of it in his *A History of Sexuality*. Sexual activities in the context of Greek antiquity were not problematized within the moral domain. They were conceptualized within the framework of ethical action. Extending this distinction to the focus of this chapter, it could be posited that corporeality as well as corporeal difference in distinct cultural contexts may be problematized differently and not only in terms of Anglo-European-American framing of it as inherently carrying moral value.

Cochrane, R. G. 1961. *Biblical Leprosy: A Suggested Interpretation*. Tyndale Press. Available at: October 30, 2017. Available at: https://biblicalstudies.org.uk/article_leprosy_cochrane.html (accessed May 9, 2018).
Cohen, Lawrence. 1998. *No Aging in India*. New Delhi: Oxford University Press.
Devlieger, Patrick. 1995. 'Why Disabled? The Cultural Understanding of Physical Disability in an African Society.' In *Disability and Culture*, edited by Benedicte Ingstad and Susan Reynolds Whyte, 94–106. Los Angeles, CA: University of California Press.
Ewens, G. F. W. 1903. 'An Account of a Race of Idiots Found in the Punjab, Commonly Known as "Shah Daula's Mice".' *Indian Medical Gazette* 38 (9): 330–34.
Foucault, Michel. 1990. *A History of Sexuality: Volume II*. New York: Vintage Books
Ingstad, Benedicte, and Whyte, Susan Reynolds. 2007. *Disability in Local and Global Worlds*, 78–106. Berkeley, CA: University of California Press.
Inhorn, Marcia C., and Aditya Bharadwaj. 2007. 'Infertility, Stigma, and Suffering in Egypt and India.' In *Disability in Local and Global Worlds*, edited by Benedicte Ingstad and Susan Reynolds Whyte, 78–106. Berkeley, CA: University of California Press.
Jayasundar, Rama. 2012. 'Contrasting Approaches to Health and Disease: Ayurveda and Biomedicine.' In *Medical Pluralism in Contemporary India*, edited by V. Sujatha and Leena Abraham, 37–58. New Delhi: Orient Blackswan.
Lodge Patch, C. 1928. 'Microcephaly: A Report on "the Shah Daulah's Mice".' *Indian Medical Gazette* 63 (6): 297–301.
Manto, Sadat Hasan, ed. 2008. 'The Mice of Shah Daulah.' Translated by Aatish Taseer. In *Manto: Selected Stories*, 89–95. Noida: Random House India.
Miles, M. 1996. 'Pakistan's Microcephalic *Chuas* of Shah Daulah: Cursed, Clamped or Cherished?' *History of Psychiatry* 7 (28): 571–89.
Miles, M. 2000. 'Disability on a Different Model: Glimpses of an Asian Heritage.' *Disability and Society* 15 (4): 603–18.
Mishra, Arima, and Suhita Chopra Chatterjee. 2013. *Multiple Voices and Stories: Narratives of Health and Illness*. Hyderabad: Orient Blackswan.
Overbeck-Wright, A. W. 1912. *Mental Derangements in India*. Calcutta: Thacker, Spink and Co.
———. 1921. *Lunacy in India*. London: Bailliere, Tindall and Cox.
Rose, Martha L. 2003. *The Staff of Oedipus: Transforming Disability in Ancient Greece*. Ann Arbor, MI: The University of Michigan Press.
Steel, Flora Annie. 1893. *From the Five Rivers*. London: W. Heinemann.
Sujatha, V. 2012. 'The Patient as Knower: Principle and Practice in Siddha Medicine.' In *Medical Pluralism in Contemporary India*, edited by V. Sujatha and Leena Abraham, 77–99. New Delhi: Orient Blackswan.
The Lancet. 1913. 'The Leprosy Problem.' *The Lancet* 182 (4709): 1556–57.

Chapter 16

Interrogating Normalcy, Decolonizing Disability
Corporeal Difference in the Post-colonial Indian English Novel

Someshwar Sati

INTRODUCTION

Many of us have been studying and even teaching post-colonial Indian English fiction for quite some time now, little suspecting that this corpus of literature abounds in representations of disability. Desai (1980), Rushdie (1981), Kanga (2008) and Sinha (2007) have all produced narrative gems on the subject. Obviously, the social marginalization of disabled people has not resulted in their representational erasure, at least not within the pages of the Indian English novel. While the Indian English novelists are conscious of disability being a prime structuring category of social relations, the phenomenon, as a materially embodied experience of human diversity, is yet to become a part of the institutionalized critical tradition on this corpus of literature which, during the past couple of decades, has been obsessed with marginal subjects and their subjectivities. Race, gender, ethnicity and caste are the axes around which this tradition has, of late, revolved. What is absent from the rich and diverse contributions made by the field towards the academic decoding of marginalized subjects and their subjectivity is a sustained and substantive engagement with the representation of disability in various post-colonial modes of literary and cultural articulations. With the professed intention of addressing, or at least beginning to fill up the above gap, this chapter critically examines the representation of disability in the post-colonial Indian English novel in Desai's *Clear Light of Day* (1980), Rushdie's *Midnight's Children* (1981), Kanga's *Trying to Grow* (1990) and Sinha's *Animal's People* (2007). Although all these texts defy simple answers to the questions of how power operates within our society and structures normative hierarchies of ability, they, perhaps with the exception of Kanga's novel, provide provocative instances of the transgressive potential of the representations of disability. This set of texts, when read together, illuminates the various ideological processes through which the subjectivity of persons with disabilities are discursively constituted and negotiated within the pages of this corpus of literature. How does the Indian English novel represent disabled people? How do these representations shape the world they inhabit and define their relations with the non-disabled community? What form of agency or autonomy do these representations impart to the disabled subject? Do these representations cement long standing ableist constructions of disability or do they open up new discursive spaces from where these conceptions can be problematized and interrogated? In short, how can we comprehend the cumulative effects of these representations on the way we understand, perceive and respond to disability and the disabled population? Answers to the above questions will give us a sense of what is at stake in these culturally specific representations of disability which emerge at the contested boundaries of ableism, nationalism, globalism and modernity.

With the professed intention of introducing the uninitiated scholar to the key debates in the field and providing the initiated one with a fresh perspective for future research, this chapter is a brief survey of some of the principal representations of disability in the post-colonial Indian English novel and the critical tradition on them—a critical tradition, however meagre, that over the years has moved from reading these representations allegorically in metaphorical terms to seeing them as fascinating commentaries on the materially embodied experience of disablement.

THE PROSTHETIC ALLEGORY

Let us open the discussion by asserting what today has become a kind of academic truism, particularly within the disability studies circle. Literary cultures, across the globe, have over the ages appropriated the experience of disablement in their narratives as potent metaphors evoking states of lack, damage, helplessness, destitution, depravity and dependency. According to Mitchell and Snyder, disability in these narratives operates as 'a crutch on which the narratives "lean for their representational power"' (Mitchell and Snyder 2000, 49). This observation gathers great relevance in the context of post-colonial writing. Clare Barker (2012), in her seminal study of the representation of disability in the post-colonial novel reveals that this corpus of literature, as an effective mode of articulating post-colonial national identity, displays a peculiar discursive dependency on the trope of the impaired body. This, to her, is hardly surprising as disability is 'a metaphor with a specifically post-colonial resonance' (p. 2). The figure of the disembodied body, according to her, lends itself persuasively as a 'straight forward symbol for a nation or culture emerging from a damaging colonial experience' (p. 3). The impaired bodies that crowd post-colonial fiction, in this sense, can be read as 'witnesses to the (epistemic) violence of colonialism itself' (p. 3). Disabled characters, as she further notes, are frequently used by post-colonial literary artists 'to embody both the post-colonial nation state's potential for a radical difference and its supposed fragility' (p. 2).

Predictably, the post-colonial Indian English novel shows a peculiar fascination for disabled characters and the critical tradition on this corpus of literature, swayed by the metaphorical resonances of the experience of disablement tend to read the phenomenon allegorically. Morton, in his reading of *Midnight's Children* for example, while dwelling on the novel's staging of a national allegory and its overarching critique of post-colonial national culture and history, presents the ever disintegrating body of the novel's semi-grotesque protagonist narrator Saleem Sinai as an analogy of 'the fragmentation of the post colonial body polity' (Morton 2008, 51). *Midnight's Children,* with its focus on the staging of the national allegory does undoubtedly invite the reader to interpret disability metaphorically. But, as Barker points out, 'just as integral to his story is an account of Saleem's life as a disabled child' (Barker 2012, 2). Throughout the narrative, he constantly draws the reader's attention to his cucumber nose, deformed face and bandied legs. As the plot of the novel unfolds, he even becomes deaf in one ear, loses his memory—albeit temporarily—and is even castrated. As the narrator of his own story, Saleem perceives his ever-disintegrating body in dysfunctional terms, and shares with the reader the anxieties and exclusions that his non-normative corporeality generates. For instance, after his father's brutality damages his ear, Saleem tries to hide his loss and observes:

> My parents, who had become accustomed to facial birthmarks, cucumber-nose and bandy legs, simply refused things in me; for my part, I did not once mention the buzzing in my ear, the occasional ringing bells of deafness, the intermittent pain. I had learned that secrets were not always a bad thing. (Rushdie 1981, 169)

Thus, integral to *Midnight's Children* is a committed engagement with disability as a materially embodied experience of corporeal difference, with profound social and political consequences to questions of identity and agency.

Morton (2008), however, says precious little about the experiential aspect of Saleem's life as a person with multiple disabilities and simply refuses to engage with the materially embodied experience of disablement as an ontologically and socially contextualized phenomenon. Nor does he impart to disability any form of politicized agency. Such an uncritical disengagement from the materially embodied experience of disablement is not exclusive to Morton. This critical practice also manifests itself in the writings of a number of postcolonial critics like Neil Kortenaar (1995), Jon Mee (1998) and other leading post-colonial critics. In the light of the above, Barker poignantly observes that the 'symbolic readings of *Midnight's Children* problematically sideline its keen interest in the material nature of embodied experience' and 'obscures Rushdie's exploration of the human body' (Barker 2012, 2). She further adds that 'without attention to the narratives of physical and cognitive difference, post-colonial criticism effectively erases disability from view precluding its analysis as a socially significant phenomenon or a politicized aspect of identity' (p. 3).

For this reason, the rather rampant critical orientation to read disability metaphorically is an unfortunate one and the tendency to overlook the materially embodied experience of disability becomes yet another academic manifestation of what Michael Biwawi calls the politics of disavowal; which he associates with the psychological distance that most people place between themselves and disability. This problematic location within which disability finds itself in the academia is a telling indictment of a literary institution in which the phenomenon is still to become a part of its intellectual consciousness.

The current chapter stands behind Barker's unpacking of the materially embodied experience of corporeal difference that undoubtedly unsettles the privileged status granted to the metaphor in canonized readings of *Midnight's Children*. Accordingly, it seeks to look upon disability as an ontologically and socially contextualized phenomenon and understand it as a politicized aspect of identity. Before discussing Barker's reading of *Midnight's Children* in detail, however, there is a need here to make certain preliminary and elementary observations about representation of disability in fiction and how this representation relates to the constitution of disabled identity in relation to the narrative of the nation.

OTHERING IMPAIRMENT

Lennard Davis, Rosemarie Garland Thomson, Ato Quayson, David Bolt and other disability studies scholars recognize the experience of disablement as being integral to a structure of power in which normalcy enjoys the status of an assumed ideal of order. They, in their own respective ways, strike at the very root of this order, critically outlining and unpacking the hegemonic structures of ableism, notions of normalcy and the various processes of categorical othering through which the hegemonic structures of power is reproduced and propagated. This section, through a close textual reading of Desai's *Clear Light of Day*, uncovers the discursive manoeuvres through which the subjectivity of the so-called normal and its categorical other, the corporeally different, and the disjunction between the two have been framed within the pages of the post-colonial Indian English novel. It reads this novel as an over-determined ableist discourse based on a rather rigid polarity between the non-disabled and the disabled. This polarity needs to be decoded because it has played an important role in the construction and maintenance of the power hierarchies of ability not only within the world of the text but also within the world at large.

Clear Light of Day chronicles the reunion of two sisters at their family home in Old Delhi and explores the underlying tension in their relationship as they struggle to understand each other and reconcile their differences. While the elder Bim prefers to cling on to traditional cultural ideals and exhibits a passive resistance to change, the younger Tara is more open to modern influences and happily embraces Western cultures and values. As the two sisters negotiate the old and the new cultural norms, left out from their altercation is their autistic brother Baba. What is striking about the narrative of the Das family is that the autistic Baba, despite being an integral member of that family, has been silenced. While his sisters narrate their own respective tales, the story of their autistic brother is never told firsthand. We come to know about him only through the narration of his sisters. Baba's memories in fact become the absent centre around which Bim and Tara weave their family's past. More importantly, the sisters, through their narrative, bestow upon Baba a sense of identity through a relentless process of othering in which his disabled body is necessarily perceived in terms of lack. The two sisters are constantly evaluating their brother within the narrow standard of a non-disabled identity. Obviously, Baba is always found wanting, leaving him and his subjectivity open to denigration. Tara's story, for example, focuses on her brother's blatant incapacity to perform office work and she compares him with an amputee. Baba's corporeal difference is here appropriated by his sister to reinforce the assumed ideals of an ableist order and shore up the boundaries of a non-disabled identity revealing the constructed nature of disability and by extension of normalcy itself. Rosemarie Garland Thomson uses the term 'nonnate' to denote 'the veiled subject position of cultural self, the figure outlined by the array deviant other whose marked bodies shore up the normate's boundaries' (Thomson 1996, 8). The concept of the normate, according to her connotes 'the constructed identities of those who, by way of bodily configuration and cultural capital they assume, can step into a position of authority and wield the power it grants them' (Thomson 1996, 8). Both Bim and Tara step into a position of authority in relation to their disabled sibling and wield the power that this authority grants them over him. The two sisters portray him as dependent on them, and it is this dependency that justifies Bim's sacrifice. She decides not to get married so that she could stay back and take care of her autistic sibling. She often describes him as a lovable burden and the recipient of their dual care. Baba is also seen by them as incapable of striking a sense of communion in public spaces. In the climatic episode of the novel, while listening to a music performance, Baba's body is rendered completely passive and his face is described as grave as an image cast in stone (Desai 1980, 182). It is this sense of being cast in stone that becomes the defining image of his identity in the novel.

The impulse of two non-disabled sisters to narrate their story, and by extension the stories of their family, underlines the way the non-disabled world defines the normal and the abnormal, and underscores the disjunction between the two. Both Bim and Tara's perception of Baba's disability is necessarily evaluative and one should not shudder to say, pejorative. This brief plot outline of Desai's novel reveals that Baba's disabled subjectivity is discursively constituted within the narrative through a systematic process of silencing and exclusion and calls express attention to a wider ableist ideological machinery that excludes and marginalizes the disabled body within the national discourse.

This invisibility of people with disability within the Indian nation had, in fact, been inscribed way back in 1950 when the Indian Constitution was framed. While the foundational legal document of independent India abolished untouchability and forbade discrimination against Indian subjects on grounds of religion, race, language or sex, it chose to completely overlook disability as an identity marker (Baquer and Sharma 1997, 15). As a consequence, disability remained the least identifying grounds for social discrimination in post-colonial India. To make matters worse, people with disabilities were not even counted in the national census prior to 1981. The Indian state thus even fails to acknowledge the marginality of disability within the Indian society. In this context, Ghai poignantly observes that in India, 'a culture that valorizes perfection', people with disabilities have always 'been invisible, both physically and metaphorically' and that wherever they are present, 'disability represents horror and tragedy' (Ghai 2002, 89–90).

CENTRING CORPOREAL DIFFERENCE

The publication of *Midnight's Children* in 1981 saw the post-colonial Indian English novel mounting an intellectual challenge to the way disability had hitherto been represented in this corpus of literature. If *Clear Light of Day* reproduces and propagates the idea of the norm, Rusdhie's novel problematizes the same. If the former represents the disabled figure through a character who is marginalized and silenced, the latter sees its multiply disabled protagonist narrating not only his own story, but, also that of his nation. Born at the midnight hour of India's independence, Saleem is handcuffed, as it were, to history, fate and destiny of a newly born nation. In Rushdie's hands, his non-normative corporeality becomes the vehicle through which the novel explores the history of post-colonial India. It is significant to know that Saleem interweaves accounts of his disability with the stories of a thousand and one other children of his kind, all of whom possess unique abilities and therefore, extraordinary bodies. Rushdie (1981), to his great credit, moves the figure of the disabled subject from the margins of the nation, where Desai had firmly lodged it, to its very centre and transforms disabled identity from an individual identity to a collective one.

More importantly, *Midnight's Children* tends to expand the conventional meaning of disability and incorporate within its semantic purview virtually any distinctive physical characteristic and not only those that impose limitations on human functioning. According to the magic realist logic of the text, the historic moment of Saleem's birth endows him and hundreds of other children like him with fantastic forms of embodied and cognitive difference. In a sense, Rushdie (1981) disturbs and complicates the supposed hierarchical binary relation between 'the normal and disabled' by conceptualizing disability within what Barker calls a discourse of 'exceptionality', that is, by presenting a corporeally different subject as endowed with extraordinary bodies that need to be understood in terms of ability, capacity and wonderment (Barker 2012, 4). According to her, social devaluation is not necessarily the only response to corporeal difference. 'While disabled difference, she argues 'may attract social disadvantage and prejudice, it also generates valuable experiences, insights and often unexpected modes of access to cultural discourse and critique' (Barker 2012, 4). The midnight's children conference comprises individuals with a variety of non-normative physical features. We come across 'bearded girls, a boy with a fully-operative gill', 'Siamese twins with two bodies dangling off a single head and neck' and so on (Rushdie 1981, 275). Significantly, these non-normative physical characteristics are immediately mapped onto, or rather, explicitly linked with the possession of extraordinary powers. These exceptional cognitive potentials range from Saleem's very own telepathic powers to the super-normative skills of time travel, flight and lycanthropy possessed by the other children. Each one of these skills would put the idealized abilities of any uniformly disciplined and statistically normal body to shame. Peopled thus by characters with non-normative physical features and potentials, *Midnight's Children* reconceptualizes the notion of the corporeally different body from being an emblem of lack to becoming a kind of difference that symbolizes an exceptionality that 'marvels'. Accordingly, the children are repeatedly referred to in the text as marvellous, magical, fantastic and fabulous. The narrative, however, goes on to draw attention to the social and political consequences of their corporeal difference and exceptional ability particularly in the context of allegorical history.

The children of midnight, in Barker's reading, have access to both the midnight hour of India's independence and the proclamation of the Emergency and their experiences of these events generate an ambivalent narrative of national signification in which the secular vision of the Indian nation is both celebrated and critiqued (Barker 2012, 127). While, at the moment of Independence, the magical powers of these children are linked to the emancipatory possibilities opened up by an inclusive and tolerant Nehruvian paradigm, under the Emergency, the accommodation of difference promised by the idealist secularism proves to be unattainable as the magical powers that the children possess are normalized and surgically castrated under Mrs Indira Gandhi's imposition of a state-sanctioned notion of Indianness. During the Emergency, corporeal difference is officially seen as an anomaly to be remedied as the state mobilizes a vocabulary of eugenics to erase difference from the national stage evoking the vulnerability of the disabled Indian citizenry. As the novel moves from Nehru's secular vision to Mrs Gandhi's despotic one, disability becomes a powerful trope to represent the tension between a heterogeneous and homogenous national identity. According to Barker (2012, 128),

> If the essential ideological premise of Nehruvian secular pluralism was the conviction that what defined India was its extraordinary capacity to accumulate and live with differences, then the engagement with multiple differences enabled by the children generates a wholesale interrogation of the postcolonial nation's ability to live up to this promise and incorporate profound difference into its identity.

As normalcy is posited as the unrealized but frightening and rapidly crystallizing vision of a paranoid, power-hungry state, the text seems to mobilize a vocabulary of castration to underscore the children's vulnerability as disabled citizens of India. They become 'midnight's children, who may have been the embodiment of the hope of freedom', but now ought to be finished off (Rushdie 1981, 442). The disturbing representation of the once-exceptional and now-sterilized children raises a pertinent question: to what extent can the state go to impose normalcy upon its citizenry? However, the eradication of the corporeally different bodies from the space of the nation fails. At the end of the novel, Saleem's disintegrating body scatters among the multitudinous crowd and his presence remains, gesturing towards the survival of a heterogeneous citizenry of an inclusive nation. Significantly then, the novel ends by bringing to the fore Saleem's adopted son, the Ganesh-faced Aadam, whose complex embodiment captures the ambivalence and uncertainty associated with the fallout of the Emergency on India's future. We cannot but agree then with Clare Barker that Rushdie's overarching critique of national culture finds expression through a social and political commentary on materially embodied experience of these corporeally different children (Barker 2012, 2).

In this way, disability in Rushdie's hands serves a critical political and ideological purpose at a particular moment of national crisis in the post-colonial history of India. Barker's reading of *Midnight's Children* provides us with a provocative instance of the transgressive potential of disabled characters. Attempts have also been made to uncover the liberatory and transformative potential of disabled characters even within ableist narratives like *A Clear Light of Day*. Cindy Lacom, for example, locates the transgressive potential of the autistic Baba on the margins of the text. In her reading, she explores the ambivalent role that Baba as an autistic subject plays in the narrative 'both as sites of transgression and as repositories for cultural tensions in a postcolonial world' (Lacom 2002, 142). As already mentioned, while Bim embraces Indian cultural values, Tara is deeply influenced by Western ones. As Baba is left out from the altercations between the two sisters, he represents 'the... dream of detachment from postcolonial negotiations of power' thus exempting himself 'the anguish caused by such altercations' (p. 142). Lacom locates in the brother a 'fluid movement between symbolic identity categories' (p. 142). Baba, through his silence, simultaneously rejects both 'Bim's passive resistance to change... [and] Tara's internalization of Western values' (p. 143), disengaging himself from Indian and colonial influences. However, his act of transgression takes place exclusively within a symbolic semiotic order, having little to do with the materially embodied experience of disablement. The inherent suggestion here being that those who do not speak the dialect of the nation are dangerous and their threat to nationhood needs to be contained and silenced. Significantly, the final image of Baba in the novel is that of a face engraved in stone. If Desai's novel represents the silencing of the disabled subject within the rhetoric of the nation, *Midnight's Children* leaves us with an optimistic future in which the disabled subject though threatened, survives.

If the present and the previous section chronicle the ways in which Rushdie (1981) and Desai (1980) have used disability to reflect upon the various aspects of disability subjectivity and its relationship with national discourse, the following sections meditate upon the discourse of global modernity and its relationship with disability and disabled subjects in the context of the rhetoric of human rights. For this purpose, we shall now turn to Anand (2015) and her critical explorations of the representation of disability in the post-colonial Indian English novel. If Barker presents *Midnight's Children* as an overarching critique of national culture and deciphers Rushdie's novelistic strategies to destabilize the hegemony of normalcy, Anand in her writing reflects upon the notion of disability as a global developmental category and further problematizes the relationship between a disabled subject and a modern one.

GROWING GLOBAL

On 16 December 2016, the Indian Parliament passed the Rights for Persons with Disability (RPD) Bill. Thanks to this historic piece of legislation, disability in India has today become a thriving developmental category that speaks the language of human rights and empowerment. The passing of the RPD bill was indeed a great moment of triumph for the disabled community in India. It, however, was the culmination of larger global processes particularly those initiated by international organizations. The United Nation's declaration of the 1980s as the International Decade of Disabled Persons made disability into a subject of governance the world over. Schemes were devised and partnerships with international Non-Governmental Organizations (NGOs) were developed by various national and state governments across the globe for the rehabilitation, education, employment and empowerment of persons with disabilities. While the well-intended liberal humanist and socialist consciousness operating behind these much desired initiatives and interventions need to be applauded and even welcomed, there is a need here to sound a note of caution and acknowledge the possible pitfalls of global developmental disability agenda. Commenting on this issue, Shilpaa Anand (2015, 252) poignantly observes

> As services initiated by international as well as local NGOs increased and became widespread, a normative notion of disability also developed. The NGO discourse of disability presented a disabled person who was deprived economically, socially and culturally, and therefore also politically, due to his or her impairment. The NGO's support then would offer medical aid, social status and political voice to the people who had faced deprivation and stigma. In a more contemporary context, the NGO provides support to those who embrace a social identity of disability, one that is grounded in the liberal-human rights discourse and espouses the emancipatory rhetoric of pride and identity... The disability movement in the West is based on living independently, taking pride in being disabled and being different, attacking disability discrimination and in reclaiming an otherwise denigrated classification.

This developmentalist understanding of disability, Anand notes, force fits people into categories of classifications developing a normative notion of disability in which disabled people are seen as necessarily being socially, culturally, economically and politically deprived on account of their impairment. Such a discourse structures the phenomena within normative bounds and tells us how to belong in a disabled community. Operating from within such an understanding of the global disability rights movement, the present chapter goes on to explore Kanga's *Trying to Grow* and Sinha's *Animal's People* with the view of decoding and problematizing the global rhetoric of human rights and its constitution of disabled subjectivity. While the ensuing reading of Kanga's novel reveals that Brit Kotwal, who suffers from brittle bone syndrome, happily embraces a modern disabled subjectivity: one defined by the global rhetoric of human rights, Sinha's novel interrogates the basic fundamental tenets of this subjectivity.

Born and brought up in a highly Westernized Parsee family living in the upmarket neighbourhood of Colaba in Mumbai, Brit's struggle with osteogenesis imperfecta is cushioned by his overprotective parents Sera and Sam who are always on a lookout for a cure for their son's medical condition; who are always prepared to take great care of their son, keeping him from falling and breaking his bones by manoeuvring his wheelchair around difficult paths and even carrying him in their arms if and when necessary; and who never miss an opportunity to take him out to dinners, movies and other forms of pleasurable excursions. But in all this, the disabled protagonist literally has no agency. He says little and is never really consulted. His life seems to be dictated by the whims and fancies of his family and well-wishers. Apprehensive that he will find it difficult to cope with the hostile world outside, his parents even confine him to the enclosed space of his family's apartment from where he watches the world go by. However, his middle-class upbringing and liberal humanist education helps him become a writer, allowing him to own an altered disabled friendly accommodation where everything, including the kitchen, is accessible from his wheelchair. Clearly, he grows up into a disability subjectivity where being disabled has prosthetic and material connotations, linked to education, employment and the availability of an accessible disabled-friendly apartment.

Kanga, who is himself disabled and a voice in the disability movement in the West, through his novel, narrates a normative marginalized experience of being disabled. Brit Kotwal embraces, as Anand suggests, 'the contours of disability subjectivity and all its modern emancipatory rhetoric because it is there for him to embrace' (Anand 2015, 254). She adds that 'his growing into disability modernity is the same kind of transformation that is the experience of the West, where modernity is a temporal phenomenon' (p. 254). There is here an implicit awareness that the political motivation of a global rhetoric of human rights and its talk of empowerment and emancipation is to propel the third world onto a path of economic and social reform modelled on the West, which in turn pushes the third world onto a subaltern subject position. No wonder the parents of the novel's protagonist are never tired of proclaiming their undying love for Britain, even naming their child Brit: recognizably the short form of 'British'. But we should not forget that disability is not a universal phenomenon and it needs to be contextually understood. Its experiences vary from place to place and therefore the phenomenon needs to be deciphered in keeping with the differing experiences of modernity with different parts of the globe. How should we then understand disability in an Indian context?

LOCALIZING THE UNIVERSAL

In an attempt to address the above question, we should draw inspiration from contemporary researches on disability historiography carried out by academics like Miles (2001) and Buckingham (2011), who in their projects jostle with the problem of articulating non-Western experiences of disability in an academia whose primary conceptual framework is Western. While Miles tries to understand the phenomenon within a South Asian context, Buckingham places disability within the context of India. Anand, in her writings, attempts to carry the above project into the academic field of literary studies. In order to understand how the post-colonial Indian English novel offers resistance to and even problematizes the Western theorizations of disability, she turns to a reading of Indra Sinha's novel.

Indra Sinha's *Animal's People* is based upon the aftermath of the tragic events of the 1984 Bhopal gas tragedy in which the malfunction of the union carbide plant resulted in the unwarranted emission of methyl isocyanide and other poisonous gases killing thousands and leaving many others disabled for life. *Animal's People* chronicles how the inhabitants of Khaufpur (the city of fear), Sinha's fictionalized version of Bhopal, launch a popular movement which demands justice and compensation from the Indian government and the multinational company which owns the plant. Narrated by one of the victims of the tragedy, Animal, a 19-year-old boy who walks on all four as a result of the gas leak, this novel offers resistance to various hegemonic discourses of disability that seek to diagnose, define and classify the phenomenon. The narrator protagonist, throughout the narrative, for example, strategically claims and displays his animality as a means of asserting an ambiguous subjectivity that lies well beyond all contemporary normative categories like religion, caste and modernity, which segregate humanity into types and identities. The novel, in effect, underscores the uselessness of these categories for persons impaired by the gas leak and exposes these categories as necessarily evaluative. But most importantly the novel, as Anand suggests, interrogates the human rights rendering of disabled people as 'specially-abled' (Anand 2015, 251). Read from this perspective, at the heart of Sinha's plot is the figure of the human rights activist Zafar, who ceaselessly strives to frame Animal's experience as a disabled person within a normative global developmental phraseology of the especially abled. He repeatedly draws the Animal's attention to his entitlement to human dignity and respect. The latter, however, offsets such a developmentalist conception of his subjectivity and foregrounding his bestiality, exposes the moral claims of such global rhetoric as hollow. Animal simply fails to understand why his identity should be force fitted into categories and classifications and why he should claim a rather denigrated and marginalized subjectivity. In this sense, Animal stands in a sharp contrast to Brit Kotwal by questioning the very fundamental tenets of a global developmental agenda and, by extension, the human rights movement. After all, disability is not a universal phenomenon—its conceptualization is dependent on culturally specific social and economic contexts.

Keeping this in mind, it would be dangerous to conceptualize the phenomenon within a universal epistemological framework. Anand, for example, in her reading of *Animal's People,* foregrounds how disability in the Indian culture is differently conceptualized from its Western counterpart. In the West, disability that is monstrosity is largely an ocular phenomenon. But in Sinha's novel, the protagonist's bestial bodily form is hardly started at. This, according to her, is because the connection between staring and disability is weak in the Indian context. She adds that 'while modern Western notions of disability are founded on an ocular-centric conceptualization of monstrosity, abnormality and consequently disability, disability's globalization may develop differently in keeping with the experience of modernity in different cultural contexts across the world' (Anand 2015, 251).

However, given the hegemonic sway that English, as a world language, holds over the economy of publications and the circulation of knowledge in India today, the critical discourse most easily available to our scholars in the field of disability studies would be the American and British ones. Western theoretical formulations are therefore expectedly being assimilated by our scholars in their attempt to understand the Indian experience of disablement. But the critical discourse produced in the West has been produced within a cultural and epistemic context exclusive to the West. It would therefore be problematic to assume the universality of these paradigms and mechanically reproduce them to understand disability in an Indian context. After all, disability intermingles with culturally specific elements to generate diverse forms of signification in different geographical locations and cultural contexts. The availability of a critical discourse on disability from an Indian perspective is, however, limited. How should we then go about decoding the experience of disablement in an Indian context? This is a question that haunts most disability scholars in India today. In an attempt to address the above question, the present article has sought to draw attention to the various complexes, both conservative and progressive, representations of disability in the post-colonial Indian English novels and make a case for culturally specific readings of disability with the aim of stimulating and facilitating further research in the area.

REFERENCES

Anand, Shilpaa. 2015. 'Disability and Modernity: Bringing Disability Studies to Literary Research in India.' In *South Asia and Disability Studies: Redefining Boundaries and Extending Horizons*, edited by Shridevi Rao and Maya Kalyanpur, 247–62. New York: Peter Lang.

Baquer, Ali, and Anjali Sharma. 1997. *Disability: Challenges vs. Responses*. New Delhi: Concerned Action Now.

Barker, Clare. 2012. *Postcolonial Fiction and Disability: Exceptional Children, Metaphor and Materiality*. London: Palgrave Macmillan.

Bolt, David. 2012. 'Social Encounters, Cultural Representation and Critical Avoidance.' In *Routledge Handbook of Disability Studies*, edited by Nick Watson, Alan Roulstone and Carol Thomas, 287–97. Abingdon: Routledge.

Buckingham, J. 2011. 'Writing Histories of Disability in India: Strategies of Inclusion.' *Disability and Society* 26 (4): 419–31.

Davis, Lennard J. 1995. *Enforcing Normalcy: Disability, Deafness, and the Body*. London: Verso.

Desai, Anita. 1980. *Clear Light of Day*. New York: Penguin Books.

Ghai, Anita. 2002. 'Disability in the Indian Context: Postcolonial Perspectives.' In *Disability/Postmodernity: Embodying Disability Theory*, edited by Mairian Corker and Tom Shakespeare, 88–100. London and New York: Continuum.

Kanga, Firdaus. 2008. *Trying to Grow*. New Delhi: Ravi Dayal, Penguin Books.

Kortenaar, Neil. 1995. '*Midnight's Children* and the Allegory of History.' *Ariel: A Review of International English Literature* 26 (2): 42–62.

Lacom, Cindy. 2002. 'Revising the Subject: Disability as "Third Dimension" in "Clear Light of Day and You Have Come Back"'. *NWSA Journal* 14 (3): 138–154.

Mee, Jon. 1998. 'Itihasa, thus it was: Mukul Kesavan's looking through Glass and the Rewriting of History.' *Ariel: A Review of International English Literature* 29: 145–61.

Miles. M. 2001. 'Studying Responses to Disability in South Asian Histories: Approaches, Personal, Prakrital and Pragmatical.' *Disability and Society* 16 (1): 143–60.

Mitchell, D., and Sharon Snyder. 2000. *Narrative Prosthesis: Disability and the Dependencies of Discourse*. Ann Arbor, MI: University of Michigan Press.

Morton, S. 2008. *Salman Rushdie*. Basingstoke and New York: Palgrave MacMillan.

Quayson, A. 2007. *Aesthetic Nervousness: Disability and the Crisis of Representation*. New York: Columbia University Press.

Rushdie, Salman. 1981. *Midnight's Children*. New York: Vintage.

Sinha, Indra. 2007. *Animal's People*. London: Pocket Books.

Thomson, Rosemarie Garland. 1996. *Extraordinary Bodies: Figuring Disability in American Culture and Literature*. New York: Columbia University Press.

Chapter 17

Jataka Katha Goes On
Materiality as Metaphor

Santosh Kumar

INTRODUCTION

The parables of *Jataka Katha* and *Panchatantra* are not only the source of amusement but also of moral lessons during our childhood. These parables are dished out to Indian children as bedtime stories narrated by our grandmothers as well as in the form of children's literature which can be bought from a vendor in a moving train to any pedestrian roadside bookseller in India. The popularity of these texts is so high that even small stories are printed on high-quality paper. The huge publication makes it available to all kind of readers. The readers read the parable to enjoy and imbibe the moral lessons. Some parables, however, preach the normativity and cultural superiority of abled society. The readers who imbibe the moral lesson also inculcate the normative thinking through these parables.

One such parable is *The Blind Men and The Elephant* listed as Type 1317 in Folktales of Aarne-Thompson-Uther (Ashliman 2014). There are five variations of this parable: First, *Udana* (Buddhism), *Sanai*, second, *The Enclosed Garden of the Truth* (Sufism), third, Ramakrishna's *All Faiths lead to God: Four Blind Men and an Elephant* (Hinduism), fourth, John Godfrey Saxe's *The Blind men and an Elephant: A Hindoo*

Fable and fifth, Leo Tolstoy's *The King and The Elephant*, with the moral: The people who saw the Judas Tree. There is also a *Jaina* version of the story (Ashliman 2014). The fluidity of this parable across religions suggests that all religions preach their moral lessons through parables. The multiple and continuous representation of this folk parable through history just does not end there. The synchronic spread of the parable suggests its currency in those days across religions and regions. This parable has its modern treatment as well, in which the literary representation of this parable has been extended into the field of philosophy and science as well. The modern understanding of the parable has provided insight into the relativism, opaqueness or inexpressible nature of truth. This parable has modern treatment as well. It has been treated as an analogy for the wave–particle duality in physics (for detail, see Bohm 1951, 26), whereas in biology, the way the blind men hold onto different parts of the elephant has been seen as a good analogy for the polyclonal B-cell response (for detail, see Lederman and Margolis 2008).[1]

This parable has its genesis in the Indian subcontinent, and like other 'winged words of wisdom' it spreads not only in all the religious belief systems of India but also in other parts of the world. This parable has been accounted to illustrate a range of truths and fallacies in different time and context. However, the broad understanding of the parable implies that one's subjective experience can be true, but such experience is inherently limited by its failure to account for other truths or a totality of truth. This chapter will be concentrated on the literary representation of disability in folklore. The parable depicts the (in)famous story of four visually impaired men who wanted to know what could an elephant be. It turns out to be quite funny as they all give their own versions of description of the elephant according to the parts which they get to touch. But this story has been represented time and again to highlight the 'limitation' of the blindness to know the nature of truth. However, the characterization of blind persons in the parable to show the 'inability' to know all the dimensions of truth

---

[1] https://en.wikipedia.org/wiki/Blind_men_and_an_elephant

is ironical in itself, as it undermines the abilities of the blind person. It is interesting to note the equation between the nature of truth and trope of blindness which has been parallel structured.

The role of metaphor becomes significant in the construction and representation of disability. The metaphor of disability travels far and wide. Metaphor has been one of the most useful literary devices to express our thoughts through analogy. It is used by people in the common moment of daily life to express their feelings and ideas to other people. However, the journey of the metaphor needs to be scrutinized as advocated by Sontag (1977) in terms of 'illness is *not* a metaphor, and that the most truthful way of regarding illness—and the healthiest way of being ill—is to resist such metaphorical thinking'. A set of proverbs and parables are considered as the genre of literary representations which depict this metaphorical thinking. This chapter works on this formula and adapts to the analytical lens of applied semiotics that allows the examination of the term 'disability' which comes to interplay with cultural notions and human role determinations (Rogers and Swadener 2001, 4). To illustrate this, a popular *Jataka* folktale of *The Blind Men and The Elephant* and its recurring representations as a parable narrative in the medieval India and its adaptation as cartoon representation in modern time (Kumar 2016) has been taken into consideration. A brief account of this parable in different religions is described in the introduction, while three instances of its recurrences in two media: one in a contemporary essay on the importance of philosophical approach to sciences; and two, political cartoons in the context of Indian politics have been taken into consideration to illustrate the reinforcement of stereotype associated with blindness.

In the process, the chapter brings the multi-model analysis in which the focus shift from 'language' to 'semiosis' and perceives sociolinguistically informed semiotics as the disciplinary space (Kress 2009; Scollon and Scollon 2003, 2004) to unravel the implicit normative and ableist thinking about disabled people that prevails in day-to-day life. It is also being proposed that the disciplinary spaces such as linguistics, semiotics and media studies should also be informed from disability studies.

CONSTRUCTION OF DISABILITY IN FOLKLORE

Disability has been explored in the cultural construct in Indian context (Anand 2013; Baquer and Sharma 1996; Bhatt 1963; Ghai 2015) which suggests that disabled people were treated differently historically. Ghai (2015) provides a framework to examine the metaphorical representation of disability in the parable for the cultural landscape of disability in Indian context. This framework is useful because the categories of disability inform the stereotypes and prejudices about disability prevalent in the contemporary societies. In the cultural construction of disability, it is seen as a 'failure' and a personal tragedy.

THE POWER OF LANGUAGE

The philosophical underpinning of this chapter lies in the intimate relationship between language and power in the construction of knowledge. In the construction of knowledge, the dominant groups often express their superiority and normative worldview. Foucault (1980, 93) puts it 'The dominant groups perpetuate their privileged positions and exercise their power "through the production of truth"'. This can be understood within the framework of genealogy as the constitution of and relationship between knowledge, discourse and power that can be accounted for the production of truth and factuality (Kumar 2016). The legitimacy of the truth as absolute can be questioned as it operates in relation to action of power. The 'wisdom' and 'truth' expressed about disabled people in general and blind people in particular in the parable attain particular significance in this perspective. The historical analysis which is guided by genealogy helps not only to discover the roots of our identity but also to commit itself to its dissipation (Foucault 1972, 162). Hence, the analysis of parable related to blindness becomes problematic, as they are oriented to and revealing of particular, often dominant, versions of knowledge.

The linguistic-anthropological tradition offers a linguistics of communication in which denotational and propositional meanings of words and sentence take back seat, while the connotational significance of sign, that is, indexicality gets more attention in communication (Blommaeart and Rampton 2011). The theoretical framework of applied semiotics allows the semiosis of sign exchanges across and between disciplines to highlight how 'disability' acts, as it pertains to human interaction and discourse, as a created state, status, symbol, process, construction, definition and metaphor (Manning 1987, 55 cited in Rogers and Swadener 2001, 4). Lakoff and Johnson (1980, 5, cited in El Refaie 2003, 76) describe 'metaphor' as 'understanding and experiencing one kind of thing in terms of another'. This allows us to examine the 'The strong thesis' about metaphor is that all knowledge (or language) is metaphorical (Lakoff and Turner 1989 cited in Indurkhya 1994). However, cognitive theorists present a contrastive view that 'metaphor is a property of thought rather than of language and that it is about understanding and experiencing one kind of thing in terms of another' (Lakoff and Johnson 1980, 5, cited in El Refaie 2003, 76). This view entails that the underlying mechanisms of metaphor exist in the mind independently of language and the use of metaphorical language is surface realization of a particular way of thinking (El Refaie 2003, 76).

In Disability studies, Mitchell and Snyder (2000, 47–48) in their exposition of 'narrative prosthesis' propose that 'disability also serves as a metaphorical signifier of social and individual collapse'. They further ponder upon the concept of 'materiality of metaphor' as the metaphorical use of disability:

> Physical and cognitive anomalies promise to lend 'tangible' body to textual abstractions; we term this metaphorical use of disability the *materiality of metaphor*....

Mitchell and Snyder (2006, 205) explore that 'The perception of a "crisis" or a "special situation" has made disabled people the subject of not only governmental policies and social programs but also a primary object of literary representation'. The parable in the question also conforms to the representation of blind particularly in its various adaptations.

PREVALENCE OF PARABLE

This section deals with the prevalence of proverbial thoughts in the vicious cycle of talk and text through media representation. Media constructions have the potential to influence the perceptions and thereby the attitudes of the audiences towards disability (Haller 1999; Hunt 1966; Morris 2001; Shakespeare 1999; cited in Bendukurthi and Raman 2016, 2). Barnes (1992, 5) observes that—the impetus for the project stems from a growing awareness among disabled persons that the problems they encounter are due to institutional discrimination and that media distortions of the experience of disability contribute significantly to the discriminatory process. Thomas (2001) considers that the semiology of cultural production offers the requisite apparatus for methodological analysis.

This parable is taken into consideration in line with Mitchell and Snyder's (2000) analysis of 'artistic innovation that entrenched disability's association with corruption'. The authors note:

> The beautifully rendered figures in The Blind Leading the Blind, for example, dramatise a biblical allegory that equated a lack of sight with wayward leadership. On the back of the wood panel upon which The Cripple was created, Brueghel sardonically scribbled,—Cripples go and be prosperous!‖ This contrasting deployment of disability—as a device of artistic innovation that entrenched disability's associations with corruption—serve as a parable for many of the representations of disability traced in the book. (p. 5)

Similarly, the parable *The Blind Men and the Elephant* from the perspective of the Mitchell and Snyder (2000) framework, where the deployment of disability—as a device of creative metaphor is associated with 'ignorance' and 'half-knowledge' and its echo in all variants serves the reasons to take the parable for analysis as cases of reinforcement of disability metaphor. The other reason is its continuous contemporary ubiquity in different genre of literature.

REINFORCEMENT OF STEREOTYPE

The reinforcement of stereotypical representation of disability follows a restrictive pattern that hinders humane aspect of disability as Mitchell and Snyder (2000, 17) note that—'disability was viewed as a restrictive pattern of characterisation that usually sacrificed the humanity of the protagonists and villain alike'. To take this premise as a point of departure, it is significant to raise the question why disability is viewed as a restrictive pattern and what is its source. It seems that the parable and proverb about disability act as catalysts to form a restrictive pattern when they are depicted in the form of cartoon or other visual media.

Though this is part of every edition of *Jataka Kathas*, its reference can be found in one of the essays of Bahm *The Mother of the Sciences* in his *Philosophy: An Introduction* (1964). This essay is meant to inculcate the basic philosophical understanding of science among the future graduates who come from diverse background. Bahm (1964) while stressing the importance to holistic perspective of philosophy argues authoritatively:

> Who has not heard the story of the blind men of Burma who visited the elephant? Upon returning from their venture, they compared views about the nature of the beast. Said one, who had felt the elephant's legs, an elephant is like a tree. Another had grasped the tail, and reported him to be like a rope. The trunk was traced by a third, who insisted it was much like a serpent. A fourth, who had stretched himself on the elephant's side, likened him to a barn.

The authoritative style of narrative which begins with, 'Who has not heard the story of the blind men of Burma…' suggests the didactic function a folktale carries with it. Bahm (1964) makes an analogical statement about scientists which is problematic from the point of view of disability studies:

> Whenever a scientist insists that the whole universe is like the part which he investigates, he may be compared with a Burmese blind man.

Bahm (1964) with all contour of authority makes a stereotypical analogy, nonetheless his idea of functions synthesis played by philosophy.

The fluidity of the parable can be located in the other example of the parable's recurrence in the regular feature of Cartoonscape by Surendra in *The Hindu* (2011) with reference to the Indian National Congress (INC) party's aggressive campaign for the then upcoming assembly polls of 2012 in Figure 17.1. In his depiction, Surendra, the cartoonist, symbolically sketched Bahujan Samaj Party's (BSP) electoral

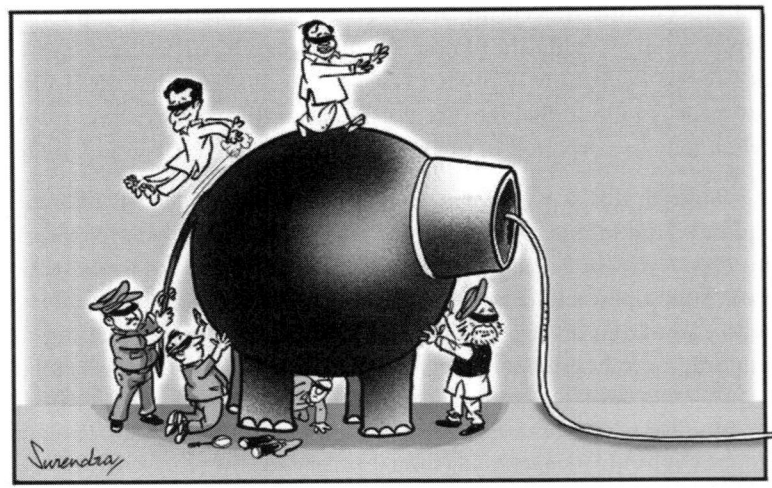

Figure 17.1 Use of parable to show six Congress leaders trying to decipher BSP's election symbol and all of them are blindfolded

symbol 'elephant' being visited by four blindfolded INC party leaders and an administrative staff and a police officer making it a group of six. The parable cartoon succeeded in depicting the political scenario of the electoral politics in which the INC leaders along with bureaucracy were trying to decode or understand the policies and popularity of BSP in order to defeat them in the election. The cartoon achieves two purposes as it signifies the absolute mandate and popularity BSP got in last election under the leadership of Ms Mayawati who holds the reins of Dalit politics in the central part of India. The cartoon also depicts the 'inability' of INC to read the game properly. The depiction of BSP's symbol elephant which is visited by blindfolded Congressperson becomes the link between the famous *Jataka katha* of Buddhism, Jainism, Hinduism and Sufism, and Bahm's analogical mention of the allegory. Note that the omission of the INC president Ms Sonia Gandhi is missing in the whole episode. The omission of Ms Gandhi is interesting, as it suggests the cartoonist's deliberate intention to match the structure of the original parable in which only male blinds are represented.

Coming back to the circularity of parable pictorial representation, a similar cartoon by Keshav, another regular cartoonist, of *The Hindu*

(2015) appeared in Cartoonscape in which he depicted the phenomenon 'Victory of AAP', written on an iconic Gandhi *topii* 'cap' bore by an elephant. The cartoonist achieves success in depicting the phenomenal victory of the Aam Aadmi Party (AAP) bore by the elephant, signifying the landslide victory of new political outfit promising an alternative politics. However, because of the knee-jerk shock of political defeat, the leaders of different political parties wearing black spectacles, instead of blindfolding as done by Surendra, are trying to figure out the elephant in Figure 17.2. However, this parable was depicted in a political cartoon after the massive win of AAP in Delhi which showed the proverbial elephant is being groped by the members of the rival parties.

It is interesting to note the similarities with which this cartoon has been drawn by Keshav, the regular cartoonist at *The Hindu*, in which four rival leaders bearing black spectacles, with one of them holding the white cane, remind one easily the old parable evoking the same sentiment. There was another occasion a similar cartoon by Surendra, a cartoonist at *The Hindu*, was published in which characters were slightly changed for the sake of contextuality. However, it is important to note

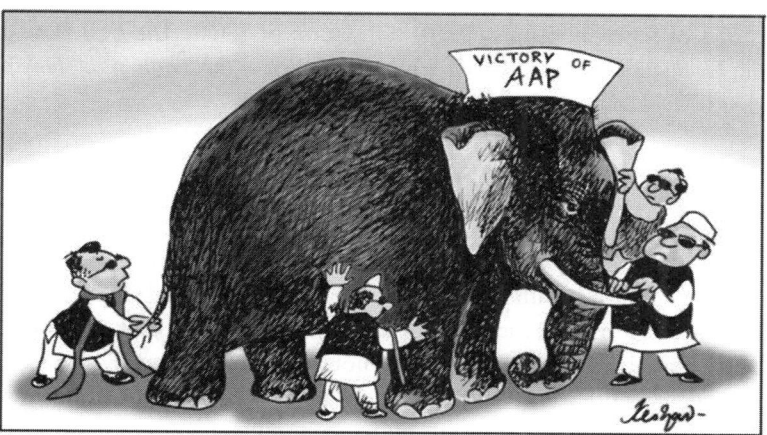

Figure 17.2 Victory of Aam Adami Party's win is shown through parable where four other party leaders are trying to understand the elephant wearing black spectacles and one of them is also carrying white cane

that the equation between the nature of truth and trope of blindness remains the same in all versions of this parable. Rogers and Swadener (2001, 4) argue that although humans use signs and symbols to represent understandings, in some cases, these over-represent, or over-determine, how an individual is known in the world. The various occurrences of parable also suggest that how blind people and blindness, if over-represented, contributed in the formation of stereotypes about them.

Similarly, in the Buddhist text of *Udana* or The Solemn Utterances of Buddha, this parable is used to describe 'sectarian quarrel' (Strong 1902), while in the Jaina tradition, Acharya Mallisena (13th century) in his *Syādvādamanjari* uses the parable to argue that immature people deny various aspects of truth; deluded by the aspects they do understand, they deny the aspects they do not understand. Due to extreme delusion produced on account of a partial viewpoint, the immature deny one aspect and try to establish another. This is the maxim of the blind (men) and the elephant (Dhruva 1933, 9–10). The other rendition of the parable such as in Sufi, Sanai has two morals to end the retelling of parable, one is by Rumi, the 13th-century Sufi poet, who eloquently ends his poem by stating 'If each had a candle and they went in together the differences would disappear' (Wikipedia), while the other moral is part of J. Stephenson's (1910) translation of Sanai, *The First Book of the Hadiqatu'l-Haqiqat: Or the Enclosed Garden of the Truth of the Hakim Abu'l-Majd Majdud Sana'i of Ghazna*, as follows:

> Everyone had seen some one of its parts, and all had seen it wrongly. No mind knew the whole. Knowledge is never the companion of the blind. All, like fools deceived, fancied absurdities.

There is a clear conflicting interpretation of the moral in the above renditions. However, it is important to note that the plot of Rumi's poetic rendition in his Masnavi does not depict 'blind men' as character; instead, it is titled *The Elephant in the Dark* in which not blind men but normal people with vision go to see the elephant in a dark room (Arberry 2004, 5–9). In Sanai, stereotypical moral statement is made not against the nature of truth but 'ability' of the blind, 'Knowledge is never the companion of the blind. All, like fools deceived, fancied absurdities'. It clearly sets a prejudicial equation of blind persons with universal quantifier 'all'.

DISCUSSION

The analysis of cartoons which depict blindness as incomplete requires more explanation in terms of the role of stereotype in life. Garland-Thomson (1997, 11) observes that stereotypes in life become tropes in textual representation. Hence, proverbs and idiomatic expressions about disabled persons are examples of stereotypes of life which are plying as tropes in proverbial representations. It seems quite clear that the representation of disability in general and blind in particular in the above vicious cycle of representation does not even connote the experiences of disability in social or political terms.

As outlined in the Prevalence of Parable, the recurrences of the parable can be taken in the framework Mitchell and Snyder (2000), where the deployment of disability—as a device of creative metaphor is associated with 'ignorance' and 'half-knowledge', and its echo in all variants serves the reasons to take the parable for analysis as cases of reinforcement of disability metaphor. Moreover, there appears to be a connection the way this equation may have got influenced by the cultural artefact such as proverbs (Kumar 2016). For example, there is a proverb in Hindi which expresses this connection in 1:

(1) *andhaa be-iimaan*
 'The blind man is unbelieving'.

Fallon ([1886]1998, 11) gives a narrative for this proverb which is related with

> a blind man at a feast, suspecting that other guests might be eating with both hands, began to do likewise. It then occurred to him that they might be eating with their mouths too. So he applied his mouth to the dish as well. Finally he thought that the others might be running away with their dishes so he took his dish and run away.

It seems that there has been a tendency to refer blind person in stereotypical way as (2) shows in which blind is considered *be-iimaan* 'dishonest' while deaf is considered as *bahishtii* 'heavenly':

(2) *andhaa be-iimaan, behraa bahishtii*
   'Blind is faithless, deaf is heavenly'.
   (The deaf man hears no evil.)

Fallon ([1886]1998, 11) paraphrase this proverb as, 'The deaf man hears no evil' hence he is heavenly while blind remains 'faithless'. The parable also signifies 'inability' of the behaviour of experts in fields where there is a deficit or inaccessibility of information and the need for communication in which respect for different perspectives can be accommodated. It is important to note that though this parable may be used for 'abled bodied' subjects' inability, however the trope of blindness remains intact; it is where the business of reinforcement of negative attitude operates. It is important to note that in all its reproduction, the characters remain the same, that is, blind persons.

In the semiotic analysis, 'preference for wholes, structures, or forms [which] means that semiotics is de-centered in the sense that language provides the roles or voices with which one speaks' (Lemert 1987, cited in Manning 1987, 31). In the above representation of blind person, there is a lack of whole structures as it is presented by 'majority'. Rogers and Swadener (2001, 4) argue that 'Disability is a plastic, changing, and variable notion that nevertheless has too often been represented as dichotomous stable notions: "ability" at one end of the polarity with "disability" as an uncompromising concept of less than able, less than whole, less than complete'. The parable and its various recurrences present blindness in that dichotomous notion that not only establishes but also reinforces the binary of ability versus disability. Moreover, these over-representation creates a narrative which does not allow us to measure the 'true complexity of all lives and the actual effort and progress of some lives' (Rogers and Swadener 2001, 7), because it just focuses on typical stories and notes the indexical markers of a commonality of lives.

Mitchell and Snyder (2006, 205) contend that centrality of disability works on representational strategies such as 'materiality of metaphor' which establishes a conundrum, while stories rely upon the potency of disability as a symbolic figure, they rarely take up disability as an experience of social or political dimensions. The analysis of the reoccurrence of a parable in which blindness has been used as a 'discursive dependency' in Mitchell and Snyder's (2000) formulation in the form of cartoon and explained them in terms of representation of disability in the media.

The stereotypical assumptions about disabled people often take references from folklore, as Barnes (1992, 5) states that 'Stereotype assumptions about disabled persons are based on superstition, myths and beliefs from earlier less enlightened times'. The analysis of the parable and its representation in cartoon show that the beliefs about disabled persons are prevalent in the society. The examination also suggests the various ways that propagate these biased beliefs which are maintained and passed from generation to generation. They become inherent to our culture and persist partly because they are constantly reproduced through the communications media. Barnes (1992, 5–6) observes that 'We learn about disability through the media and in the same way that racist or sexist attitudes, whether implicit or explicit, are acquired through the "normal" learning process, so too are negative assumptions about disabled persons'. Moreover, this interpretation of the parable is problematic from the point of view of disability studies for two reasons: one, the trope to drive the interpretation is the depiction of blind characters; second, the depiction stereotypes disabled person in general and blind in particular negatively. Rogers and Swadener (2001, 8) rightly point out, 'The current use of language that simplifies, or reduces the reality of people, who do not have lives described by existing development frames, also does not recognise the actual activity of everyday life'.

CONCLUSION

This paper presents an analysis of *Jataka* parable and its recurrences in the course of time. The reason is its continuous contemporary ubiquity in different genre of literature. A brief account of understanding of this parable in different religions has been taken in which three instances of its recurrences in two media: one in a contemporary essay on important of philosophical approach to sciences; and two, some political cartoons from the context of Indian politics. It is found that the parable had its genesis in Indian subcontinent and like other 'winged words of wisdom' spread not only in all the religious beliefs systems of the medieval India but also in contemporary India. The parable has been accounted to illustrate a range of truths and fallacies in different time and context. The broad understanding of the parable implies that one's subjective experience can be true, but that such experience is inherently limited by its failure to account for other truths or a totality of truth. The analysis suggests how the parable and its various adaptations as a cultural text reproduced and reinforced cultural notions of blind person in particular and disabled person in general.

As I am to conclude the chapter, I wish the cycle of over-representation of parable will stop some time; however, this parable is too powerful to get into oblivion of the mass imagination. This parable again appears as the Government of India rolls out the much anticipated goods and services tax (GST Bill), touted as the biggest reform in the history of taxation in India, so the creative imagination of some of the critics of the government got unlocked. Figure 17.3, by Surendra published on 2 July 2017 in *The Hindu*, captures the inability of the opposition to understand that the GST Bill gives the latest recurrence of the famous *Jataka Kathas* of an elephant and four blind men. This leads to a kind of unconventional to conclude this chapter with recurrence

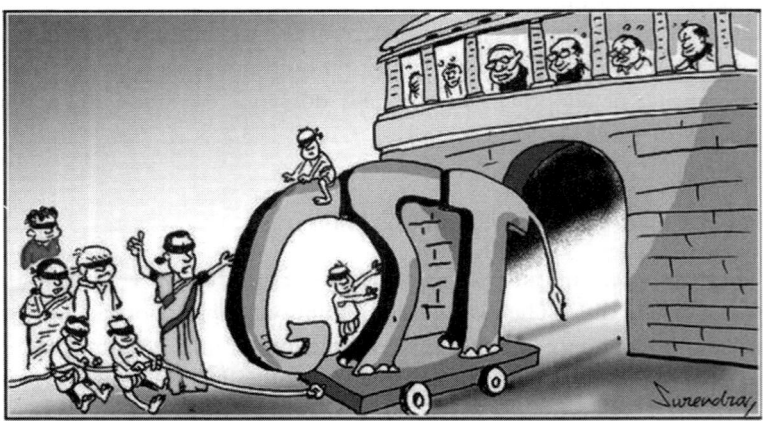

Figure 17.3 *Implementation of GST is shown by parable. The cartoonist sketched GST as an elephant which is being groped by leaders of opposition parties and people who are blindfolded while leaders of the government is looking at from the balcony of Parliament*

of parable; however, it cannot be helped as the convention of *Jataka Katha* goes on...

REFERENCES

Anand, Shilpaa. 2013. 'Historicising Disability in India: Questions of Subjects and Method.' In *Disability Studies in India: Global Discourse, Local Realities*, edited by Renu Addlakha, 35–60. New Delhi: SAGE Publication.

Arberry, A. J. 2004. '71—The Elephant in the Dark, on the Reconciliation of Contrarieties.' *Rumi—Tales from Masnavi*.

Ashliman, D. L. 2014. 'The Blind Men and The Elephant' Type 1317 in Folktales of Aarne-Thompson-Uther. Available at: http://www.pitt.edu/~dash/type1317.html (accessed on 9 May 2018).

Bahm, A. J. 2001. 'The Mother of all Sciences.' In *Improve your Writing*, edited by V. N. Arora and Lakshmi Chandra. New Delhi: Oxford University Press.

Baquer, Ali, and Anjali Sharma. 1997. *Disability: Challenges and Responses*. New Delhi: Concerned Action Now.

Barnes, C. 1992. *Disabling Imagery and the Media: An Exploration of Media Representations of Disabled People*. Belper: British Council of Organisations of Disabled People.

Bendukurthi, N. and Raman, U. (2016). 'Framing Disability in the Indian News Media: A Political Economy Analysis of Representation.' *Journal of Creative Communications* 11(2): 135–153.

Bhatt, Usha. 1963. *The Physically Handicapped in India: A National Growing Problem*. Bombay: Popular Book Depot.

Blommaert, J., and B. Rampton. 2011. 'Language and Superdiversity.' *Diversities* 13 (2): 1–21. Available at: http://newdiversities.mmg.mpg.de/?page_id=2056

Bohm, David. 1951. *Quantum Theory*. New York: Dover Publications.

El Refaie, Elisabeth. 2003. 'Understanding Visual Metaphor: The Example of Newspaper Cartoons.' *Visual Communication* 2 (1): 75–95.

Fallon, S. W. (1886)1998. *A Dictionary of Proverbs, Sayings, Emblems, Aphorisms*. Edited and revised by R. C. Temple with the assistance of Lala Dihlavi Faqir Chand. New Delhi and Madras: Asian Educational Services.

Foucault, Michel. 1972. *The Archaeology of Knowledge*. New York: Pantheon.

———. 1980. *Power/Knowledge: Selected Interviews and Other Writings*, 1972–1977, edited by Colin Gordon. New York: Pantheon Books.

Garland-Thomson, R. 1997. *Extraordinary Bodies: Figuring Physical Disability in American Culture and Literature*. New York: Columbia University Press.

Ghai, Anita. 2015. *Rethinking Disability in India*. New Delhi: Routledge.

Hakim Abu l-Majd Majdud Sanai. 1910. *The First Book of the Hadiqatu'l-Haqiqat: Or the Enclosed Garden of the Truth of the Hakim Abu'l-Majd Majdud Sana'i of Ghazna*. Translated by J. Stephenson. Calcutta: Baptist Mission Press.

Haller, B. A. 1999. News Coverage of Disability Issues: Final Report for the Center for an Accessible Society. Available at: from http://www.accessiblesociety.org/topics/coverage/0799haller.htm

Hunt, Paul. 1966. *Stigma: The Experience of Disability*. London: Geoffrey Chapman.

Indurkhya, Bipin. 1994. 'The Thesis That All Knowledge Is Metaphorical and Meanings of Metaphor.' *Metaphor and Symbolic Activity* 9 (1): 61–73.

Keshav. 2015, February 16. 'Cartoonscape.' *The Hindu*. Available at: http://www.thehindu.com/opinion/cartoon/article6898856.ece (accessed on May 9, 2018).

Kress, Gunther R. 2009. *Multimodality: A Social Semiotic Approach to Contemporary Communication*. London: Taylor & Francis.

Kumar, Santosh. 2016. 'A Sociolinguistic Study of Stereotypes, Prejudices, and Discrimination against Gender and Disability in Talk and Text.' PhD thesis, Centre for Advanced Studies in Linguistics, University of Delhi.

Lederman, Michael M. and Margolis, Leonid. 2008. 'The Lymph Node in HIV Pathogenesis'. *Seminars in Immunology*, 20 (3): 187–95.

Mallisena. 1933. *Syādvādamanjari*, 14: 103–104. Translated by A. B. Dhruva. pp. 9–10.

Manning, P. K. 1987. *Semiotics and Fieldwork*. Newbury Park: SAGE.

Mitchell, D., and S. Snyder. 2006. 'Narrative Prosthesis and the Materiality of Metaphor.' In *The Disability Studies Reader*, edited by L. Davis, 205–16. 2nd ed. New York: Routledge.

Morris, J. 1991. *Pride against Prejudice: Transforming Attitudes to Disability*. Philadelphia: New Society.

———. 2000. *Narrative Prosthesis: Disability and the Dependencies of Discourse*. Ann Arbor, MI: University of Michigan Press.

Rogers, L. J., and B. B. Swadener. 2001. *Semiotics and Dis/Ability: Interrogating Categories of Differences*. Albany, NY: State University of New York Press.

Scollon, R., and S. Scollon. 2003. *Discourses in Place: Language in the Material World*. London: Routledge.

———. 2004. *Nexus Analysis: Discourse and the Emerging Internet*. London: Routledge.

Shakespeare, T. 1999. 'Art and Lies? Representations of Disability on Film.' In *Disability Discourse*, edited by M. Corker and S. French, 164–72. Buckingham: Open University Press.

Sontag, S. 1978. *Illness as Metaphor*. New York: Farrar, Straus and Giroux.

Strong, D. M. 1902. *Udana or the Solemn Utterances of Buddha*. London: Luzac & Co.

Surendra. 2011, July 16. 'Cartoonscape.' *The Hindu*. Available at: http://www.thehindu.com/opinion/cartoon/article2230940.ece (accessed May 9, 2018).

———. 2017, July 2. *The Hindu*. Available at: http://www.thehindu.com/todays-paper/tp-national/article19196660.ece/alternates/FREE_660/ALL1News02ARGTK2146N43jpgjpg (accessed May 9, 2018).

Thomas, L. 2001. 'Disability Is Not So Beautiful: A Semiotic Analysis of Advertisements for Rehabilitation Goods.' *Disability Studies Quarterly* 21 (2). Available at: http://www.dsq-sds.org/article/view/280/309 (May 9, 2018).

PART 5

Disability, Family Epistemologies and Resistance to Shame within the Indian Context

Chapter 18

Disability, Family Epistemologies and Resistance to Shame within the Indian Context

Shridevi Rao

The term 'disability' and its claims for a universal epistemology have been the subject of much discourse in recent literature (Grech 2015; Kalyanpur 2015; Kalyanpur and Rao 2015; Titchkosky and Aubrecht 2016). Fostered by globalization and the rapid exportation of 'geodisability templates' (Campbell 2015, 75) from the Global North, disability as a construct has been assumed to have a universal epistemology that crosses geopolitical boundaries (Campbell 2011, 2015; Grech 2015; Kalyanpur and Rao 2015). The emerging scholarship on the disability experience in the Global South as well as the new quandaries arising from the exportation of disability-related ideologies and practices to the Global South draw attention to the deep dissonance that exists between these borrowed Northern templates of disability and the Southern contexts to which they are transported (Grech 2015; Kalyanpur 2014, 2015). This scholarship draws attention to the epistemological roots of the term 'disability' and the problems associated with using it as a global template to engage in a discourse on human differences (Anand

2015; Grech 2015; Kalyanpur and Rao 2015). It underscores the importance of recognizing, understanding and valuing the existence of local epistemologies of disability that capture contextual understandings of human differences (Addlakha 2013; Anand 2015). What do we mean by local epistemologies of disability? How do they manifest themselves? What constructs do they embrace? One way to explore local epistemologies of disability is through the perspectives of families of children with disabilities.

This chapter draws on the findings of a qualitative study that focused on the perspectives of Bengali families of children with disabilities and their experiences in enhancing the inclusion of their children within their families, neighbourhoods and communities. The study was guided by the following questions: How do Bengali families perceive disability and what language and frameworks do they use to communicate their understandings of disability? How do families perceive the identity of their child? What strategies do families use in order to facilitate the inclusion of their children in their families, communities and neighbourhoods? Findings from this study that focus on parents' use of language as well as their constructions of 'normality' have been discussed elsewhere.[1] This chapter, in particular, focuses on how families use the collective identity of a family to resist pressures to feel 'shame' and relent to the pejorative identities imposed on their child. The families' perception of the child as an integral member of the family, their use of the 'family policy', along with constructions of the child that focus on the humanness of the child helped not only resist pejorative labels but also educate extended family members and the community on ways to accept and include their child.

FAMILIES AND DISABILITY EPISTEMOLOGIES IN THE GLOBAL SOUTH

While the discourse on disability in the Global North, particularly the experiences and perspectives of families of children with disabilities,

---

[1] Findings from this study that focus on the families' use of language, their constructions of 'normality' and their approaches to inclusion have been published in *Disability and Society* (Rao 2001, 2006) as well as in the book titled *South Asia and disability Studies: Redefining Boundaries and Extending Horizons* (Rao 2015a).

has grown to embrace a more complex and nuanced understanding of the disability experience (Biklen 1992; Biklen, Ferguson and Ford 1989; Ferguson, Ferguson and Jones 1988; Harry 1992; Kalyanpur and Harry 2012; Rao 2000; Turnbull and Turnbull 1986), relatively less is known about the experiences or perspectives of families of children with disabilities from the Global South and how they construct disability. The use of borrowed and outdated templates from the Global North has resulted in the tendency to approach local interpretations of disability through deficit-based lenses that rely overwhelmingly on the medical model (Titchkosky and Aubrecht 2016) and grand narratives of the constructions of disability in the Global South. Professional epistemologies of disability tend to be predominantly privileged in these accounts (Titchkosky and Aubrecht 2016). What is often overlooked in this simplistic rendition families' views is that within the current context of globalization, constructions of disability are dynamic and multifaceted with biomedical frameworks existing alongside the more traditional views (Maudslay 2014). Family's attitudes towards children with disabilities and the ability to cope with stress have also traditionally been presented as major barriers to supporting and including children or youth with disabilities (Annapurna 1997; Gupta and Singhal 2005; Peshawria et al. 1998; Shanmugavelayutham 1999). Very little is known about how disability is constructed within the context of collectivist societies in the Global South where an individual's identity is closely tied to the family or community. While perceptions of disability that are tied to collectivist orientations are acknowledged to some extent, they are often deemed to be negative. For instance, earlier literature as well as recent literature describes the existence of shame and embarrassment and how this is exacerbated by a cultural emphasis on conformity to behavioural norms and expectations (Srinivasan and Karlan 1997). Although this might be the case in some instances, not much is known about the ways in which families mobilize collectivist orientations to resist the pressure to feel shame. How do families construct and present the child's identity as a member of a family or member of a community to resist the imposition of pejorative identities?

A small cluster of qualitative studies since the 1980s have focused on how families in some areas of the Global South, such as India, interpret and understand the construct of disability as well as their experiences with schools and educational systems (Appleby 1983; Kalyanpur 1994; Rao 2001, 2006). Findings from some of these studies indicate that some families may approach human differences in ways other than the typical lenses used in the medical model or the constructs used in the Global North. These findings are of particular relevance in the context of the current times, where scholars are drawing attention to the problematics of using terms such as 'disability' or inclusion in the Global South regardless of context (Anand 2015; Hodkinson and Devarakonda 2009; Kalyanpur and Rao 2015, 2015a; Richard 2014; Singal 2006) and the need to work through the 'contextual complexities and dilemmas' that comes with attempting to implement northern templates of disability and inclusive education (Maudslay, 2014, p. 423). More recent literature draws attention to the need to understand disability, inclusion and notions of inclusivity that are tied to collectivist frameworks of the community and family (Muthukrishna and Ebrahim 2014; Rao 2015b) and reiterates the importance of understanding the complex facets of the constructions of disability in the Global South (Gurung 2015; Grech 2015; Hammad and Singal 2015; King and King 2014). This literature also emphasizes the point that underlying the decision to export templates of inclusion is the problematic assumption that inclusion or inclusivity does not exist within the local contexts to which these templates are exported. Local understandings of disability, including the language used to refer to disability, are closely related to indigenous approaches to inclusivity.

METHOD

Data for this study were collected through the use of qualitative methodology where the focus is on the subjects' frame of reference (Bogdan and Biklen 2006; Flick 2002) and the insider's perspective (Fetterman 1988). Eight families participated in this study. The families lived in the city of Calcutta [now known as Kolkata] located on the east coast of India. All the families spoke Bengali, the language predominantly spoken in Calcutta. Four families selected for this study were from the low-income group, and four families belonged to the middle-income group. Five families had children with significant disabilities; three families had children with mild disabilities. All the children had pronounced difficulties in the areas of language and speech and were described by professionals as having moderate to severe degrees of 'mental retardation'. Data were collected through the use of in-depth interviews and participant observations. Field notes were recorded after each observation. Most of the interviews in this study were fully taped. Although interviews were also conducted with other family members and professionals, this chapter focuses primarily on the data that predominantly emerged from the mothers. Names used for the mothers in this chapter are pseudonyms. Analysis was inductive and based on the grounded theory and constant comparison method (Glaser and Strauss 1967).

FINDINGS

The following section describes how families constructed their child's identity and how these constructions resisted the pressures to feel ashamed of their child. The families' perceptions of the child were anchored in both collectivist notions of identity and a recognition of the child's individuality and humanness. They saw the child as a valued member of the family as well as an individual human being with his or her own strengths. The child's membership in the family brought with it an access to the responsibilities, privileges and protections that are typically given to members of the family. Perception of the child as an individual stressed the humanness and abilities of the child. This chapter describes both of these aspects.

THE CHILD AS A MEMBER OF THE FAMILY

For the parents and other family members, the child was an intrinsic member of the family. The children were viewed as a favourite grandson or granddaughter, as a niece or nephew, rather than a child with a disability. Mrs Dutta feels very moved when she talks about how her mother treats her son. Her mother never fails to bring some gifts for Joi, cash or otherwise, as is customary during festivals. Mrs Dutta feels that Joi's identity as a grandson is not overlooked just because he cannot speak or even ask his grandmother for a gift, as children sometimes do. The mothers felt that this kind of unconditional support was crucial:

> If we are all going in a car with friends or family members, he may want to go to the bathroom, we stop the car. With eating, he cannot eat by himself and he needs help. Nobody asks questions, 'Why does he have these inconveniences?' or 'Why are you all taking him out like this?' (Mrs Basu)

A crucial aspect that contributed to this support was the family policy and the ways in which it resisted the imposition of a pejorative identity on the child.

'Whoever comes to this house has to understand and come!': The family policy.

> I have seen when I have gone to some houses, they will keep their child locked in the balcony. That I should tie her because people have come. I can never do it. Whoever comes to this house has to understand and come that in this house there is a child like this (*janbe je erokhom ekta baccha ache*). (Mrs Som)

The 'policy' in the Som family is that people who come to their house have to accept Sharmi for who she is and build a relationship with her. Sharmi sometimes pinches, bites or pushes other children. While Sharmi's behaviours might be perceived as challenging, they see no reason to make amends for Sharmi, justify, or apologize for their daughter's presence in the house. Studies on Indian families have documented the strong sense of family solidarity, collective orientation, interdependence and reputation within the families (Ananth 1981; Balachandran 1985; Ross 1961, Sinha 1984–1985; Tuli 2012). Actions of every family member have an impact on the way the total identity of the family is perceived thus leading to a family member's actions being perceived as bringing shame to the family. While this sense of group identity might lead to avoidance of public disclosure and a sense of shame, it could also culminate in the family ensuring that none of its members is portrayed in negative or discrediting ways. This was strongly visible amongst the families in this study.

Similar to the Som family above, each family had a strong family 'policy'. This policy protected the child with a disability from being labelled or perceived in ways which were essentially pejorative to his or her identity. Debayan is a very important person in his house. Always well dressed in a crisp white kurta, he is often the first person to greet the guests. He is talked to and talked about with a lot of affection and respect by his family especially because he is the oldest son and the *dadamoni* (the big brother) of the family. The Basu family has a very strong policy about the way they want Debayan to be treated and so they set a strong example to others:

> I feel we parents have to be strong about certain things (*ami bhabhi amader parents der kichu kichu jinish e strong hote hobe*). Whether it is friends or relatives, if they come home and see we are behaving well with him then they will give him a lot of importance, and they will also behave well with him. That is why we follow that policy very much. (Mrs Basu)

The roots of the family policy emerged from the family's identity as a group and its efforts to retain its cohesiveness as a group. The mothers felt that if the family itself started portraying their child negatively, and focused only on the child's disabilities, they would make it harder for other people who have little or no relationship with their child to accept their child. The mothers believed that discussing family matters with an outsider threatened the cohesion of the family. Mrs Ganguly views such outsiders with great suspicion:

> There are a lot of bad type of people, they will talk about other people 'Oh your daughter-in-law is like this, or you are doing like this, this has happened in your family'. Such discussions happen often amongst relatives. These are all ways of breaking a family.

The family policy served as a means for the family to present a cohesive united front to the external community in order to protect its relationships from being threatened and the family being fragmented. Accepting the labels and the concomitant pejorative identities that come with them was considered by the mothers as a way of giving an 'upper hand' to the outsiders. Instead, the mothers focused on the crucial role that the family as a whole plays in resisting labels.

'Daughter is ours, why should we talk ill about her?': Labels as giving outsiders an upper hand.

For the families, talking about their child in negative ways signified giving the upper hand to outsiders who would then start defining the child in the same pejorative terms to the whole community. Mrs Ganguly does not let her relatives have the upper hand with regard to her daughter. She does not let them talk about her daughter in a way which is disrespectful:

> Five people will say five different things, I never listen to that. They will say, 'No she is foolish, not as cunning as you (*oh boka, tomar moton chalak noi*)'. I tell them, 'She is my daughter, I know her well (*amar baccha ami to jani*)'. Don't talk like this!

Mrs Ganguli's emphasis on the last sentence is especially significant. It is the mother who has the 'upper hand' by virtue of her close relationship with the children, not the outsiders. Thus, if the mother rejects the labels, she takes the control away from the outsiders and keeps secure the relationship with her child and the harmony within the family. Thus, family members never volunteered a specific label for their child to the public. The Noshokors believe that by doing so they would be insulting their own daughter and themselves:

> We don't tell anyone anything. Why should we say all this to others? Daughter is ours, why should we talk ill (*or ninde kano korbo*) about her, why should we say she is 'dumb' or 'cannot talk?' (*kano bolbo, oh boba, kotha bolte parena?*)

The discussion of the family policy would be incomplete without looking at its relationship to 'shame' which is the other side of the coin. When a family member's actions are perceived to reflect on the moral identity of the family as a whole, the issue of 'shame' comes in. Within the Indian cultural context, the collective identity of the family often brings with it implications of shame (Ananth 1981; Ross 1961; Saraswathi and Dutta 1988). Often, such family members are disowned from the family or hidden (Giel et al. 1983; Miles 1986). Other times even if the repercussions are not so severe as locking up the person, they could mean embarrassment for the family (Gandotra 1985; Raka 1989) and avoidance of social ceremonies or other social gatherings which could bring unwarranted inquiries about the child (Devkumari

1986). Families may not disclose they have a member with a disability especially when they have a daughter of a marriageable age. If they did so, the daughter's chances of getting married would diminish (Miles 1986). The cultural pressures to perceive these children as bringing shame to the family were evident in the initial attempts of the families in this study to take their children out into the community. It was through a strong family policy and a sense of group identity that the families challenged these pressures to feel ashamed.

Usually, a very calm and collected person Mrs Noshkor's voice steadily rises and she gets furious when she talks about the ways in which people imply that she should be 'ashamed' of her daughter. Sometimes people do this by asking her why she takes her daughter out everywhere:

> I have no shame that my daughter cannot talk so I will leave her at home and go (*amar kono lojja nei, amar meye bolte parena bole ami ghore phele rekhe jabo*). I don't have that. I take her everywhere. After all she is my child. What is there to be ashamed about (*lojja ta kisher?*)? Won't she have feelings that I want to go with mother and father (*oro to asha hoi, aami ma babar shonghe jabo, hoina?*)? If we ourselves don't love her who will?

The commitment of the parents to challenge any societal pressures to feel ashamed was evident in the efforts they made to take their children to different environments and provide them the support to negotiate these environments.

The Basus take Debayan everywhere. They are not only proud of how comfortable he is in these places but the relationships that he has built with people in the community. One place that they regularly visit is the hair-cutting salon close to their place. According to Mrs Basu, the barbers there like Debayan very much and call him respectfully and affectionately as *bhai* (brother), a term generally used for young men of his age:

> Sometimes when shaving he may get cut if he moves, so they tell him '*Dada* (big brother), sit quietly nothing will happen. I will cut it very nicely for you'. They will say 'See *bhai* (brother), we are putting powder so you are comfortable'. If he does not go for a few days they will ask 'Where is *dada*? Why did he not come?'

The strong sense of family identity provided a powerful anchor of support for both the child and the family. However, the family's use of the family policy to protect their child from discrediting identities was also deeply anchored to their perception of the humanness of their child.

'Can understand but cannot counter back': The child as an individual

As far as the families were concerned their children had a specific difficulty in 'expression'; having difficulties in expression did not necessarily connote that their children lacked feelings or the ability to understand. The families viewed their children as individuals who had the ability to think and feel. They believed that the minds of their children had a constant inner speech. Mrs Banerjee feels sad that people often failed to recognize this humanness in Arnob:

> One day when Arnob was small, a neighbour got all the children ice-cream. He came and told me, 'They gave me a stick but all of them had a cup'. I tried to console him, 'OK, they gave you a stick so what? You can suck on it for a long time and it will last much longer. The cup is useless'. But the hurt remained in his mind. He knows who likes him and who does not but he does not have the ability to express (*bakto korte parena*).

Families not only talked about the ability of the children to have feelings for issues that concerned them but also their ability to feel empathy for somebody else's feelings.

Debayan's mother takes a lot of pride in his attachment to his brother. From a younger age, Debayan acted like a protective older brother:

> Since Tarun was still a baby I could not get down from the rickshaw holding the baby. The rickshaw man took the baby in his hands. Debayan ran and held the rickshaw man's hand tightly. He thought he was taking the baby and going away. I liked that a lot, that he had these feelings and reacted so normally (*khub normally react korlo*).

Families not only recognized that their children had feelings but they also felt that their children were smart. Not being able to express did not mean that their children were not bright. It was just that they expressed their brightness in ways not limited to speech. Mrs Dutta believes very strongly that Joi should not be deceived about anything. In her opinion, most people deceive or mislead children who cannot speak. Mrs Dutta treats her son as a person who is fully capable of understanding whatever is explained to him:

> Sometimes it happens, not intentionally but his father might say, 'Today it is raining we will not take him to his uncle's place' but before that we would have told him we are taking him to his uncle's place. Now we suddenly change the programme. Our reason for not taking him was because he may get wet and sick. But sometime later it slips out that my husband did go to his uncle's place. Then I see that Joi gets silent. Now we don't do that. We tell him immediately. We don't lie to him. I find that is very effective. He accepts that (*oh setake mene nai*).

Since they felt that their children were smart, the mothers considered it the responsibility of family members to figure out what the child was trying to communicate.

'Putting the hand on the rolling pin': Taking the commitment to understand and support the person with disabilities.

Mrs Banerjee gets exasperated with her husband at times. She feels that instead of appreciating the tremendous strides that Arnob has made and the various good qualities that he has, her husband keeps focusing on what he does not have. Mrs Banerjee argues that it is not Arnob who has the problem but her husband who has not taken the challenge to understand Arnob. She compares this skill of understanding Arnob to a skill like rolling absolutely round *rutis* (tortillas) which one can develop only if one is committed to learn it. If her husband is not even ready to put his hand on the rolling pin, how could he ever hope to even make a *ruti*, leave alone a round *ruti*? Similarly, if he is not even willing to view the world from his son's perspective, how could he ever understand his son?

> My husband would ask, 'Why cannot he do this or that?' I would say, 'You know what all this is?' It is a kind of technique just like making a ruti (*eitao ekta kaida dharun jemon ruti belata*). When I go to roll the

ruti, the ruti keeps turning by itself becoming absolutely round. But when you try, you are not able to do at all. You are not able to get the technique at all (*kichu tei kaida hocchena*). If you want to learn the technique you have to put your hand on the roller (*belontar opore hathta rakhte hobe*).

The families felt that support and encouragement were crucial in order to help their children express themselves. When Joi tries to express something through words, Mrs Dutta never makes him feel that the problem is his speech. Instead, she makes it appear like the problem is with herself and her inability to understand. She says, 'I never told him he could not speak. I used to tell him, "See mother cannot do it, mother is foolish because she cannot understand".'

Having a disability did not mean that the child remained stagnant in their growth. The mothers perceived their child as continually growing, and evolving. For Mrs Haldar, some of these changes are significant. Paroma used to be afraid of meeting new people but now she can not only interact with people but also grasp the complexities of some of the social interactions:

Previously before she said a world she would be quiet and very scared. Like supposing someone new has come, she would not talk to them. She would feel scared but now she has none of that. She knows what to do now, who to call what and how to give respect (*kake kirokhom sonman dite hoi*).

The families in this study made use of an age old system which already existed. The structure of family identity had two sides: one of shame, the other a protection from discrediting identities. In this study, the families used the group identity to preserve the identity of their child as a family member. The strong sense of family identity helped develop a cohesive front which questioned prevalent attitudes towards disability and protected the child from pejorative labels. The perception of the child as a person focused on the humanness of the child. Instead of blaming the child for the disability, the parents considered it the responsibility of family members to understand the child and lend support.

DISCUSSION

Findings from this study reveal how some Bengali families of children with disabilities construct their children's identities and the ways in which they draw on local epistemologies to resist potentially pejorative constructions of their children. The mothers categorically rejected local deficit-oriented constructions of their children as well as those emerging from the medical model. They relentlessly drew attention to the critical role that the family policy in particular and the family in general played in presenting a positive construction of each member of the family to the external community. They also emphasized the importance of recognizing the unique attributes of their child rather than defining their child by disability alone. The families strategically drew on the epistemologies anchored in collectivist orientations to resist deficit-based constructions of their child. Some insights ore lessons that emerge are as follows:

First, the findings challenge potentially global deficit-based narratives of families of children with disabilities in the Global South that highlight how families are susceptible to feeling ashamed of their children and thus tend to isolate their children or exclude their children from family- or community-based activities. The findings indicate that while the pressure to experience shame exists, not all families succumb to it. In addition, while the very collectivist orientation of family and community could set the stage for feeling ashamed, the very same collectivist orientation also has strengths to resist this pressure. Data indicate that families use collectivist orientations along with creative approaches to push the community to think about human differences in complex ways. The epistemologies anchored in these collectivist orientations have the potential to protect family members from pejorative identities and to preserve the cohesiveness of the family.

Second, the findings also present a cautionary note for continuing efforts to export Northern ideologies of disability and inclusivity without understanding existing local understandings of human differences. The unwavering and determined efforts of these mothers to ensure their child's inclusion provide insights into the power of untapped local epistemologies of inclusion especially within the context of the current efforts to export prescriptive templates of disability (see Campbell 2011, 2015). The mothers draw on the innate sense of interdependence and reciprocal nature of relationships within the family: an approach that is distinctively different from the Western emphasis on independence and self-advocacy. These local epistemologies are crucial in terms of uncovering indigenous approaches that are powerful, effective and already in use. The findings resonate with the commentary of other scholars who have drawn attention to the need to tap into local social, cultural and historical epistemologies of disability (Anand 2015; Grech 2011, 2015; Kalyanpur and Rao 2015).

Finally, the findings also draw attention to the complex, hybrid and fluid constructions of human differences and identity in the Global South. They challenge the hegemonic concept of disability and the assumption that there is a universal template to define the term. They draw attention to the heterogeneity in the constructions of human differences in the Global South and the ways in which they resist the imposition of universal templates. They provide insights on constructions of identity that are hybrid and challenge the simple binaries of ability/disability and the concomitant notions of identity that are typically visible in the understandings of disability originating in the Global North. They also challenge the often simplistic renditions of the interpretations of disability in the Global South and call for an approach that is complex and nuanced.

REFERENCES

Addlakha, R. 2013. *Introduction*. In *Disability Studies in India: Global Discourses and Local Realities*, edited by R. Addlakha, 1–31. New Delhi: Routledge.

Appleby, S. D. 1983. 'A Study of the Attitudes and Responses of Parents in New Delhi, India Towards Their Mentally Retarded Child.' Master's thesis, University of California, Berkeley.

Anand, S. 2015. 'Corporeality and Culture: Theorizing Difference in the South Asian Context.' In *South Asia and Disability Studies: Redefining Boundaries and Extending Horizons*, edited by S. Rao and M. Kalyanpur, 154–70. New York, NY: Peter Lang.

Ananth, J. 1981. 'Is Western Training Relevant to Indian Psychiatry?' *Indian Journal of Psychiatry* 23 (2): 120–27.

Annapurna, M. 1997. *Mentally Handicapped Children and Family Stress*. New Delhi: Discovery Publishing House.

Balachandran, R. 1985. 'The Role of a Family in the Promotion of Mental Health of One of Its Members: A Case Study.' *Indian Journal of Social Work* 45 (4): 403–13.
Biklen, D. 1992. *Parents, Educators, and Inclusive Education*. Philadelphia, PA: Temple University Press.
Biklen, D., D. Ferguson, and A. Ford. 1989. *Schooling and Disability*. Chicago, IL: NSSE.
Bogdan, R., and S. Biklen. 2006. *Qualitative Research for Education: Introduction to Theories and Methods*. Boston, MA: Allyn & Bacon.
Campbell, F. K. 2011. 'Geodisability Knowledge Production and International Norms: A Sri Lankan Case Study.' *Third World Quarterly* 32 (8): 1455–74.
———. 2015. 'The Terrain of Disability Law in Sri Lanka: Obstacles and Possibilities for Change.' In *South Asia and Disability Studies: Redefining Boundaries and Extending Horizons*, edited by S. Rao and M. Kalyanpur, 73–98. New York, NY: Peter Lang.
Devkumari, R. N. P. 1986. 'An Involvement on the Parental Anxieties for the Future of Their Handicapped Children.' Thesis for Diploma in Special Education, Spastics Society of India, Bombay.
Ferguson, P. M., D. L. Ferguson, and D. Jones. 1988. 'Generations of Hope: Parental Perspectives on the Transitions of Their Children with Severe Retardation from School to Adult Life.' *The Journal of the Association for Persons with Severe Handicaps* 13 (3): 177–87.
Fetterman, D. 1988. 'Ethnographic Educational Evaluation.' In *Qualitative Approaches to Evaluation in Education: The Silent Scientific Revolution*, edited by D. Fetterman, 45–67. New York, NY: Praeger.
Flick, U. 2002. *An Introduction to Qualitative Research*. Thousand Oaks, CA: SAGE.
Gandotra, V. S. 1985. 'Management Problems and Practices of Homemakers with a Disabled Member in the Family.' *The Indian Journal of Social Work* 45 (4): 484–90.
Giel, R., M. V. D. de Arango, A. Hafeiz Babikir, et al. 1983. 'The Burden of Mental Illness on the Family.' *Acta Psychiatrica Scandinavica* 68 (3): 186–201.
Glaser, B., and A. L. Strauss. 1967. *The Discovery of Grounded Theory: Strategies for Qualitative Research*. Chicago, IL: Aldine.
Grech, S. 2011. 'Recolonising Debates or Perpetuated Coloniality? Decentring the Spaces of Disability, Development and Community in the Global South.' *International Journal of Inclusive Education* 15 (1): 87–100.
———. 2015. *Disability and Poverty in the Global South: Renegotiating Development in Guatemala*. New York, NY: Palgrave Macmillan.
Gupta, A., and N. Singhal. 2005. 'Psychosocial Support for Families of Children with Autism.' *Asia Pacific Disability Rehabilitation Journal* 16 (2): 62–83.
Gurung, C. 2015. 'Gender Sensitivity in Disability Initiatives: Perspectives on South Asia.' In *South Asia and Disability Studies: Redefining Boundaries and Extending Horizons*, edited by S. Rao and M. Kalyanpur, 99–124. New York, NY: Peter Lang.

Hammad, T., and N. Singal. 2015. 'Disability, Gender and Education: Exploring the Impact of Education on the Lives of Women with Disabilities in Pakistan.' In *South Asia and Disability Studies: Redefining Boundaries and Extending Horizons*, edited by S. Rao and M. Kalyanpur, 197–223. New York, NY: Peter Lang.

Harry, B. 1992. *Cultural Diversity, Families and the Special Education System: Communication and Empowerment*. New York, NY: Teachers College Press.

Hodkinson, A., and C. Devarakonda, C. 2009. 'Conceptions of Inclusion and Inclusive Education: A Critical Examination of the Perspectives and Practices of Teachers in India.' *Research in Education* 82 (1): 85–99.

Kalyanpur, M. 1994. *Culture, Empowerment and Low-income Families of Children with Disabilities in India*. Doctoral dissertation, Division of Special Education and Rehabilitation, Syracuse University, Syracuse, New York.

———. 2014. 'Distortions and Dichotomies in Inclusive Education for Children with Disabilities in Cambodia in the Context of Globalization and International Development.' *International Journal of Disability, Development and Education* 61 (1): 80–94.

———. 2015. 'Mind the Gap: Special Education Policy and Practice in India in the Context of Globalization.' In *South Asia and Disability Studies: Redefining Boundaries and Extending Horizons*, edited by S. Rao and M. Kalyanpur, 49–72. New York, NY: Peter Lang.

Kalyanpur, M., and B. Harry. 2012. *Cultural Reciprocity in Special Education: Building Family–Professional Relationships*. Baltimore: Paul H. Brookes.

Kalyanpur, M., and S. Rao. 2015. 'Conclusion.' In *South Asia and Disability Studies: Redefining Boundaries and Extending Horizons*, edited by S. Rao and M. Kalyanpur, 289–303. New York, NY: Peter Lang.

King, J. A., and M. J. King. 2014. 'The Lived Experiences of Families Living with Spinal Cord Disability in North East Thailand.' In *The Global Politics of Impairment and Disability: Processes and Embodiments*, edited by K. Soldatic and H. Meekosha, 107. New York, NY: Routledge.

Maudslay, L. 2014. 'Inclusive Education in Nepal: Assumptions and Reality.' *Childhood* 21 (3): 418–24.

Miles, M. 1986. 'Misplanning for Disabilities in Asia.' In *Childhood Disability in Developing Countries*, edited by K. Marfo and M. J. Thorburn, 101–28. New York, NY: Praeger Publishers.

Muthukrishna, N., and H. Ebrahim. 2014. 'Motherhood and the Disabled Child in the Contexts of Early Education and Care.' *Childhood* 21 (3): 369–84.

Peshawria, R., D. K. Menon, R. Ganguly, S. Roy, P. R. S. Rajam Pillay, and S. Gupta. 1998. 'A Study of Facilitators and Inhibitors that Affect Coping in Parents of Children with Mental Retardation in India.' *Asia Pacific Disability Rehabilitation Journal* 9 (1): 1–9.

Raka, P. 1989. 'Problems Faced by Parents of Physically Handicapped Children in the Slums of Bombay.' Unpublished dissertation for the diploma in the education of the physically handicapped, Spastics Society of India, Bombay, India.

Rao, S. 2000. 'Perspectives of a Low-income, African-American Mother on Parent–professional Relationships in Special Education.' *Mental Retardation* 36 (6): 475–88.

———. 2001. 'A Little Inconvenience: Perspectives of Bengali Families of Children with Disabilities on Labeling and Inclusion.' *Disability and Society* 16 (4): 531–48.

———. 2006. 'Parameters of Normality and Cultural Constructions of "Mental retardation": Perspectives of Bengali Families.' *Disability and Society* 21 (2): 159–78.

———. 2015a. 'Colloquial Language and Disability: Local Contexts and Implications for Inclusion.' In *South Asia and Disability Studies: Redefining Boundaries and Extending Horizons*, edited by S. Rao and M. Kalyanpur, 171–93. New York, NY: Peter Lang.

———. 2015b. '"Just a Member of the Neighborhood": Bengali Mothers' Efforts to Facilitate Inclusion for Their Children with Disabilities Within Local Communities.' In *South Asia and Disability Studies: Redefining Boundaries and Extending Horizons*, edited by S. Rao and M. Kalyanpur, 224–43. New York, NY: Peter Lang.

Richard, B. O. 2014. 'Families, Well-being, and Inclusion: Rethinking Priorities for Children with Cognitive Disabilities in Ladakh, India.' *Childhood* 21 (3): 308–23.

Ross, A. D. 1961. *The Hindu Family in Its Urban Setting*. Toronto: University of Toronto Press.

Saraswathi, T. S., and R. Dutta. 1988. *Invisible Boundaries: Grooming for Adults Roles*. New Delhi: Northern Book Center.

Shanmugavelayutham, K. 1999. *Mentally Retarded Children and Their Families: Challenges Ahead*. New Delhi: Mittal Publications.

Singal, N. 2006. 'Inclusive Education in India: International Concept, National Interpretation.' *International Journal of Disability, Development, and Education* 53 (3): 351–69.

Sinha, D. 1984–1985. 'Some Recent Changes in the Indian Family and Their Implications for Socialization.' *Indian Journal of Social Work* 45 (3): 271–86.

Srinivasan, B., G. R. Karlan. 1997. 'Culturally Responsive Early Intervention Programs: Issues in India.' *International Journal of Disability, Development and Education* 44 (4): 367–85.

Titchkosky, T., and K. Aubrecht. 2016. 'WHO's MIND, Whose Future? Mental Health Projects as Colonial Logics.' In *Disability and Colonialism: (Dis)encounters and Anxious Intersectionalities*, edited by K. Soldatic and S. Grech. New York, NY: Routledge.

Tuli, M. 2012. 'Beliefs on Parenting and Childhood in India.' *Journal of Comparative Family Studies* 43 (1): 81–91.

Turnbull, H. R., and A. P. Turnbull. 1986. *Parents Speak Out: Then and Now*. Columbus, OH: Merrill.

Chapter 19

Inclusive Education in India
Concept, Practice and the Way Forward

Ankur Madan

As a country, India has been resolute in its commitment towards creating an equitable society based on the ideals of social justice and human rights, and education is widely recognized as a means of achieving this goal. Yet, even to a cursory observer, the near-complete absence of children with disabilities in regular classrooms across schools in India is starkly evident. It is important to examine this confounding reality in order to understand why children with disabilities are excluded from this national agenda. I explore the issue of the education of children with disabilities from the standpoint of inclusive education, an elusive concept that occupies only a peripheral position in the education discourse in India and remains largely misunderstood and misinterpreted by academics and practitioners alike.

This chapter is divided into three sections. In the first section, I examine the concept of inclusive education, tracing its origins and analysing its complex nature in the Indian context. In the second section of the chapter, sources of knowledge that inform inclusive education and the nature of research in the field are explicated. The final section of the chapter deals with inclusive practice. Issues in inclusive practice are discussed, and some broad submissions are made for realizing inclusive education in the context of schools in India. For the purpose of this chapter, I make a deliberate distinction between the concept of inclusive education and its implementation, recognizing the tension that exists between the theoretical concept of inclusion and the pragmatic considerations of realizing it in practice.

THE NATURE OF INCLUSIVE EDUCATION

Education is widely viewed as an endeavour that contributes to human flourishing and attaining social justice. Drawing interlinkages between education, law and rights, Rioux (2014, 132–47) laments about how little attention has been paid to putting a human rights lens on education despite its obvious importance in ensuring equitable access. Invoking Sen (2000), Rioux (2014) points out that there is a need for social action in removing deprivation, gender inequality, illiteracy and barriers to schooling. With specific reference to education of children with disability, Rioux makes several pointed observations about the extent to which children with disabilities are denied access to school in developing countries and about the impact that such a missed opportunity has on their access to resources throughout their life cycle. The rise of inclusive education in the late 1980s and early 1990s was the result of a powerful emerging critique of several such issues in education in the West.

The rationale for inclusive education is broadly based on the belief that segregation of children with disabilities at the school level leads to social isolation and vulnerability and deprives them of their social, cultural and economic rights. According to Armstrong, Armstrong and Spandagou (2010, 26–36), parents, teachers and advocates of students with disabilities promoted inclusion as a way of challenging the restrictions to 'access' and 'participation' imposed by existing models of integration and mainstreaming. The development of the social definitions of disability influenced the critique of the role of education, and special education in particular, in the oppression and exclusion of the disabled. Criticizing special education for creating a separate subsystem of education, Barton (1995, 157) maintained that there cannot be any justification for special education in a perspective that promotes social justice and equal participation. The origins of inclusive education therefore may be traced to a movement against the existing education reforms and the paradigmatic shift in thinking about disability from the functional limitations about an individual with impairment onto the problems caused by disabling environments, barriers and cultures—the development of the social model of disability. Its origins also lie in efforts towards 'normalization' and deinstitutionalization in the West, and a strong resistance to the special education discourse. At a theoretical level, it is broadly agreed that inclusive education is concerned with 'all' children. It is seen as a transformative process to increase access (or presence) of all children into school systems, enhance acceptance of all children (not just those belonging to marginalized categories), maximize students' participation in all domains of activity and increase the achievement levels of all children (Artiles et al. 2006, 65–108).

Several important legislative markers in the international arena provided impetus to the inclusion movement. Among them, the ratification of the UNCRPD and the Salamanca statement are most significant. The Salamanca statement, an outcome of the UNESCO Conference held in Salamanca, Spain, in 1994 reaffirmed the uniqueness and diversity of all children for whom educational systems should be designed, and states that 'regular schools with an inclusive orientation are the most effective means of combating discriminatory practices, creating welcoming communities, building an inclusive society and achieving education for all' (Chowdhury 2011, 10). The Salamanca statement is considered to be the most important document to have appeared in special education so far.

INCLUSIVE EDUCATION IN INDIA

Referring to the complex origins of inclusion, Armstrong, Armstrong and Spandagou (2010) wrote, 'it is a common adage that *inclusion means different things to different people*' (p. 29). Perhaps the adage aptly sums up the nature of inclusive education in the Indian context as well. Tracing the origins of inclusive education in India is an onerous task as several scholars have noted that inclusive education as a concept in India is fraught with multiple interpretations and has not been adequately engaged with. Singal (2006, 351–69) contends that the term has been simply borrowed from the West without any serious deliberation on what it implies for us. Alur (2007, 91–106) refers to this 'West is best' kind of sloganeering as a form of neocolonialism wherein the romanticized, child-centred notion associated with inclusive education (Sharma 2010, 125–49) has led to its widespread usage and rhetorical references without any critical engagement with the concept per se.

Lack of engagement with the concept is starkly evident in the way inclusive education finds representation in the different policy provisions and Government of India programmes. While inclusive education was mentioned in several important policies and programme initiatives since the early 1990s (such as the DPEP, PIED, PWD (1995), SSA, etc.), it is apparent that there was no real clarity of its purpose or concept even when the term was incorporated in these policy documents. For instance, in her comprehensive review of inclusive education literature in India, Singal (2005, 331–50) found that the terms 'integration' and 'inclusion' often occurred interchangeably in several official documents as well as in commentaries by disability experts. While India was a signatory to both the UNCRPD and the Salamanca statements, Indian policy provisions and programme documents that brought inclusive education into prominence had several discrepancies and incongruities. The *Sarva Shiksha Abhiyaan* (SSA), for instance, prescribed several measures to accommodate children with different abilities into the mainstream. However, it continued to encourage establishment and funding of special schools for children who could not be integrated into the mainstream. Likewise, it adopted a 'zero rejection policy' and suggested multiple levels of intervention such as the Education Guarantee Scheme, Alternative and Innovation Education and home-based education as available alternatives to achieve the 'education for all' goal (SSA 2000). Hence, without any conceptual clarity and a sense of the larger purpose of what inclusive education was meant to achieve, it became just one among several other initiatives of the government to achieve the education for all goal. More recently, Bhattacharya (2010, 18–23) expresses some measured optimism following the Right to Education Act (RTE 2009), hoping that a careful deliberation of the RTE Act can provide a legal framework for implementation of inclusive education for children with disabilities in the country. He suggests several measures that can be taken at the level of inclusive practice to ensure access and meaningful participation for children in the regular education system. Rose (2017, 5–22) too sees the RTE as an important platform for achieving inclusion but warns against adopting a factionist approach to addressing the issue of exclusion. According to him, viewing inclusive education only from a disability perspective and excluding other equally disadvantaged groups, such as scheduled castes/tribes, girls and other minority groups as fellow travellers on the road to inclusion, will never achieve the 'education for all' goal. Gabel and Danforth (2008, 1–13) make a similar appeal in the context of all developing countries.

In concurrence with the above views, I contend that for developing an understanding of inclusive education in India, it is important that we engage with the broader context and the complex issues that are unique to the situation of children with disabilities in India. While presenting an overview of these issues is beyond the purview of this chapter, I briefly mention a few. Wolbring and Ghai (2015, 667–85) point towards the marginalization that disabled children in India face based on their caste, class, ethnicity, gender and the rural/urban divide, depriving them of a voice, space, power and any semblance of identity. The authors refer to this form of oppression as social and cultural apartheid. Problems with arriving at accurate numbers instead of rough estimates of children with disabilities, lack of consensus on acceptable definitions of different disabilities that are concomitant with cultural beliefs and religious philosophy of the society (and are not simply borrowed categories from the West) and the shame and stigma attached to disability that prevents its disclosure are some other issues that exacerbate the challenges that children with disabilities in India face (Gabel and Chander 2008, 70–80).

Specifically, in the context of education, it is important to keep in mind the vastness and complex nature of the elementary education system in India, the paucity of resources, the diversity and the problems of access and engagement that children from all marginalized sections of the society face in seeking quality education in the country. Besides, while the rationale for inclusive education in the developed world historically rested on the widely prevalent practice of segregation, India as a society has always traditionally accommodated people with disabilities into schools and communities (Rao 2011, 531–48). Hence, an understanding of inclusive education in the Indian context needs to evolve such that the rationale on which it is based is rooted in the contexts and constraints that exemplify the situation of children with disabilities in our country and is not simply borrowed from the developed world.

As is clear from the above discussion, inclusive education in India is imbued with multiple interpretations and lack of conceptual clarity. It is perhaps important then to examine the sources of knowledge that have contributed to building these ambiguous perceptions. Before discussing the implications of this on realizing the goals of inclusion in practice, I turn to a brief examination of the epistemological challenge of building scholarship in the domain of inclusive education in India, the emerging discipline of disability studies in education (DSE) and the possibilities it holds for the field of inclusive education in India.

SOURCES OF KNOWLEDGE IN INCLUSIVE EDUCATION

Noting that the literature in India on inclusive education is both scant and not so easily accessible, Singal (2006, 351–69) laments about the quality of educational research in the country. In her comprehensive review of inclusive education literature, she observes that most of the literature available for review is in the form of personal commentaries of individuals working in the field, with only a few claims supported by empirical research. Rose (2017, 5–22) identifies a lack of empirical research base in India as the major challenge in understanding the conditions that support or inhibit the progress of inclusive education practices in the country. In his literature review, Rose found only two dominant themes in which empirical work is available in the Indian context. One, a consideration of teachers concerns, attitudes and readiness for the promotion of inclusive schools, and two, enrolment of children who have been traditionally marginalized within the education system. The need to expand the scope of research that can inform inclusive practice is strongly expressed by other authors as well (Lindsay 2007, 1–35).

As an instructor of a course in inclusive education in a Masters' in Education programme in a university in India, I have continually struggled to find resources to share with my students that can provide an indigenous, situated understanding of inclusion as a concept and practice. With hardly any children with disabilities to observe in regular classrooms in India and notions about childhood still situated in a singular, universalized idea of the 'normal' child, inclusive education becomes a hard concept to promote in a mainstream education programme. Besides, most empirical studies tend to borrow Western connotations of the concept, applying them to contexts that are markedly different from the ones from which they have been extrapolated, providing little insight into the challenges of inclusion in the Indian context.

Armstrong, Armstrong and Spandagou (2010, 26–36) point out that in general, conducting research in inclusive education has several methodological and ethical concerns. Lately, the dominance of the positivistic framework in inclusive education research too has come under severe criticism as has special education being used as a 'default box' for dumping all research on disability-related issues (Conner et al. 2008, 441–57). Referring to the positivistic framework as insular and one-dimensional, the authors observe that special education has failed to recognize the emergence of any alternative forms of inquiry and forms of scholarship, and has remained grounded in the positivistic discourse. Thomas (2009, 13–23) makes a similar appeal to inclusive education practitioners to forsake the traditional knowledge base of special education and educational psychology as sources of knowledge to construct an epistemology of inclusive education.

Since the discourse on inclusive education is still evolving in India and its sources of knowledge are only just taking shape, it is germane that we too take cognizance of the rising unrest and discomfort with the traditional sources of knowledge and look towards fresher, contemporary approaches to view research in the field and to construct an epistemology of inclusive education that is rooted in our cultural contexts or what might be referred to as 'local knowledge' (Geertz 1985 as cited in Gabel and Danforth 2008, 1–13).

A sense of direction in this regard is perhaps provided by the tenets of the field of inquiry referred to as the DSE Disability Studies in Education) (Connors et al. 2008, 441–57). The DSE evolved as a result of a disenchantment with the traditionalism of special education and the limitations of the positivistic framework in the West. Still in its fledgling stage as a discipline though, the primary mission of the DSE is 'to promote understandings of disability from a social model perspective drawing on social, cultural, historical, discursive, philosophical, literary, aesthetic, artistic and other traditions to challenge medical, scientific and psychological models of disability as they relate to education' (Connors et al. 2008, 447). The DSE proposes an approach to research that welcomes scholars with disabilities and without disabilities to work together, recognizes and privileges knowledge derived from lived experiences of people with disabilities, encourages interdisciplinary approaches to disability and challenges methodologies that objectify and oppress people with disabilities (Connors et al. 2008). The authors view DSE to be one of the most important developments in the field of inclusive education, 'a discipline in which we can "talk back" to forces in education that undermine inclusive values' (p. 455). According to Moore and Slee (2012, 225–39), the DSE holds the potential to ensure that inclusive education becomes a platform for disabled people in changing educational structures, practices and cultures. Perhaps a similar conceptualization of inclusion and inclusive education could be envisaged for India by adopting the epistemological tools of DSE.

At another level, it is also important to 'free', so to speak, the sources of knowledge in inclusive education from the silos of academia. In other words, it is pertinent to ask the question, who participates in the generation of knowledge and whose contribution counts? Thomas (2014, 268–79) privileges the role of practitioners and tacit knowledge of teachers over scientific methods, and suggests that the participants in research should include practitioners of inclusion-teachers in regular classrooms, resource room teachers, parents, administrators and children, as they can all contribute to creating valuable knowledge by capturing and reflecting upon real classroom experiences of inclusive practices. In another article, Thomas (2009, 13–23) recommends that teachers take on the role of scholar practitioners and pick up the tools of critical inquiry: Making a similar appeal, Rose (2017, 5–22) says that in India it is absolutely essential that teachers are seen as partners in research in order to understand fully processes that support inclusion in schools. In doing so, the author believes that teachers also carry the additional responsibility of sharing their innovative practices with other practitioners leading to their professional development and growth. The author further recommends use of local languages, taking into account local contexts and evolving innovative means of disseminating research as important measures for ensuring that the knowledge is freely available and accessible to all stakeholders.

Some specific areas of critical inquiry that can contribute to understanding inclusion and inclusive practices in the Indian context could be, but not limited to, studying the nature and characteristics of programmes where inclusion has been implemented, understanding the ideology and philosophy that guide implementation, issues of governance, collaboration and preparation that schools undertake, the curriculum and pedagogic considerations which guide inclusive practices in the classrooms, the barriers and beliefs that enable and impede processes of inclusion, the learning opportunities created within the schools for teachers to develop skills for working with children and efficacy studies to understand inclusion outcomes. Involving teachers, school administrators, peers and parents as partners in generating this knowledge is of utmost importance.

As can be evinced from the above discussion, building scholarship in inclusive education in India requires that the approaches and methodologies adopted to examine it are rooted in its diverse social, cultural and historical contexts. It is also essential that inclusive practice is informed by the lived realities of those who experience it every day, and that knowledge generated in the area does not remain confined within the insular walls of the academia alone.

I now turn to the important questions of 'what constitutes inclusive practice and how can it be realized'. I address the two questions by first explicating some important issues in inclusive practice, followed by a description of an inclusive education programme in a school that I have observed. I conclude by listing the key factors in creating inclusive schools.

REALIZING INCLUSION

As mentioned at the beginning of this chapter, inclusive education is best understood by separating the theoretical concept from the pragmatic considerations of realizing it in practice. However, the dilemma for practice is that unless there is a consensual understanding of the concept, the question of what might be construed as desirable practice cannot be debated! Defining inclusion is an arduous task, as has been discussed in the previous sections of the chapter, and as Armstrong, Armstrong and Spandagou (2010, 26–36) explain that inclusion is better known by what it is not, rather than what it is, and in this proliferation of so many multiple understandings, it ends up meaning everything or nothing at all. According to the authors, while in the origins of inclusive education lay the premise of the potential role of schooling in creating inclusive and democratic societies, in practice, this insight has been largely diluted. What remains is a rhetoric of convenience which embraces the 'feel good' aspects of the inclusive discourse without any serious engagement with the real issues. While this is an important observation, I believe that in conceptualizing inclusive practice, it is important to distinguish the desirable from the pragmatic. Practice must be viewed with due consideration of the systemic constraints of educational systems and challenges that prevail in implementing inclusive practices in schools. One such consideration could be related to who gets included and whose voice counts in such decisions? Although 'inclusion for all' is a powerful slogan, it is important to realize that the experience of inclusion can mean different things to different people and that the outcomes of inclusion may be different for different groups. In fact, a powerful critique of inclusion rests on the argument that inclusion may not be suitable for all and that there are indeed limits to it. The example of the deaf community's resistance to being included in regular schools is a case in point. A similar case has also been made for children with autism. Hence, while 'inclusion for all' is an important message, decisions about whether or not it is suitable for all should be with due consideration of the heterogeneity that exists within disability itself, readiness of the setting to provide an enabling environment to all and, most importantly, the agency of those who are included.

On the other hand is the question of the basis on which decisions about who gets included are taken. According to Armstrong, Armstrong and Spandagou (2010, 31), '…the right to participation is given to some groups with the proviso that the rights of other groups (and especially of the "majority") are not affected'. Further, the right to participation has 'clauses of conditionality' such that children with disabilities are included only when they cause no harm to the rights of the majority within the mainstream. Corroborating the above view and ascribing it to 'bell curve thinking', Florian (2014, 14) says that 'schools are organized based on a utilitarian principle of the greatest good for the greatest number' such that the right to participation is seen as conditional, and the agency to establish it is assigned to others. Such thinking originates from deterministic beliefs about children's abilities wherein it is held that the 'special needs' of children with disabilities are markedly different from the learning needs of other children and require drastic adaptations to classroom processes. Hence, disturbing the status quo, so to speak, is considered to be detrimental to the interest of a larger majority of the non-disabled children. Likewise, it is also widely held that classroom practices adopted for children with disabilities in regular classrooms are beneficial only for them, and hence, adopting such practices compromises the learning of other children in the class.

What constitutes inclusive practice then is a question with conceptual as well as pragmatic underpinnings. In a context like India where the education system is faced with a multitude of systemic challenges and constraints imposed by scarcity of resources, social and cultural diversity, lack of political will and no clear vision of inclusion as reflected in policy, the challenge of realizing inclusion is an arduous one. Hence, who gets included? Is 'inclusion for all' a realistic goal? To what extent can schools make accommodations such that their 'status quo' is not disturbed? What is the degree of readiness and preparedness that schools undergo to ensure that children who are included have a meaningful academic and social engagement in the settings in which they are included? are all important questions for consideration.

For the purpose of this chapter and based on my conviction, I focus on inclusive practice in the context of and from the perspective of school as a dynamic organization responsible for implementing inclusive practices within its settings. My conviction is based on several documented and undocumented examples of inclusive practice that show that inclusive practices in a school are most effective when driven by a clear vision, ideology, a strong leadership committed to creating an inclusive environment and the will of all participating members. Hence, the envisioning of an inclusive setting begins at the school itself and need not depend entirely on extraneous factors such as unyielding policy measures imposed by external agencies (Madan 2002, 2016, 8–11; Madan and Sharma 2013, 1–13). My conviction is supported by Kinsella and Senior (2008) according to whom,

> Inclusion cannot be effectively created simply at the insistence of national, regional or school administrators. Teachers in schools have to construct the meaning of inclusion for themselves as part of an overall cultural transformation of their schools.... Schools will have to learn as organizations to embrace, implement and manage change, and this will involve not only structural and procedural change but also possible changes in the ethos, values and cultures of the schools. (p. 660)

To illustrate my point, I describe below the inclusive practices in a school that I have observed in Bengaluru (a metropolitan city in South India) which embraced inclusion almost three decades ago, long before any policy provisions or programmes were in place to support inclusion in schools in India.

AN INCLUSIVE SCHOOL

The school, which I will refer to as SJ for the purpose of this chapter, is a low fee paying, aided school run by a Hindu religious organization in a middle-class suburb of Bengaluru. At SJ, on a typical day, I observed the following scenes:

Shreya, a seven-year-old deaf girl, was laughing hysterically seated on a crude wooden bench in a really small-sized classroom that accommodated at least six other children. Shreya had accidently spilt water on the bench from her water bottle that had wet her friend's pants. The friend, also seven- or eight-year-old deaf girl, made exaggerated gestures with her hands to express her displeasure. This made Shreya erupt in laughter. Soon all the children as well as the teacher realized what had happened and joined in. Both Shreya and her friend use hearing aids.

In another VI grade classroom with about 25 children, a teacher is teaching math. At least five children in that classroom have disabilities, mostly deafness. I pay attention to a girl almost in the last row intently watching the teacher's gestures (not sign language) and copying everything in her notebook that the teacher is writing on the blackboard. The teacher is using the board extensively, and I see her making gestures with her hands in order to explain fractions, the topic for the day. There is nothing extraordinary about the way the teacher is conducting the class. It is a typical, traditional classroom where the teacher uses mostly didactic methods of teaching. When the teacher pauses, the girl turns towards her hearing friends for a quick conversation (mostly through sign language). I observe that the girl is at ease in her surroundings. I also find she is receiving support from her peers. From time to time, her friend goes through her notebook, perhaps to check if she is copying correctly.

I describe the above episodes from a typical day at the SJ School in order to illustrate how an ordinary school with very limited resources is able to practice inclusion in some form by involving members of the community effectively. Every year the school admits at least 10 to 15 children with disabilities in the age group of 4 to 7 years and places them in segregated classrooms for a year or so in order to 'prepare' them, mostly through literacy and speech training for inclusion. Subsequently, all the children are included in regular classes with the non-disabled children. Altogether, the school has about 200 children on its rolls. A few teachers work separately with the disabled children after school hours. Some of these teachers have undergone training in special education, while others have picked up skills in working with the disabled children along the way and now are referred to as special educators. Regular teachers in the classrooms provide support by using gestures, repeating instructions, speaking slowly or using the blackboard extensively. However, not all classroom practices seem inclusive and supportive. For instance, one does not see any extensive use of teaching aids or visual material that deaf children may find useful.

There are no blind children in the school, but several of them are deaf, physically or mentally challenged and autistic. There is an emphasis on speech training over sign language for the deaf children.

Once included, the children are not segregated for any curricular or co-curricular activities. The peer group is extremely sensitive towards the children and at no point does one feel that the children with disabilities are excluded or isolated. The support staff go about their daily chores extending a helping hand wherever needed, with sensitivity and humour. No special treatment is accorded to any child. No major curriculum adaptations are made for any of the children except the exemptions granted to deaf children by the school boards for learning additional languages. The school has witnessed several success stories of their students pursuing higher education and taking up mainstream jobs across different sectors.

The head of the institution is a middle-aged woman who has been with the school for three decades and has been a witness to several phases of the journey towards inclusion. She is a certified special educator by training. She remembers the time when the earlier school head faced strong resistance from parents and teachers alike when the idea of inclusion was first discussed. She says that the journey has not been easy but for the cooperation from a dedicated staff. She shared that building capabilities of teachers, preparing the peer group and the support staff were important elements of the process, but were relatively easier to achieve. At the SJ, learning from experience is given importance over formal training of teachers. The principal did not think that formal training was necessary for her teachers. In fact, she believed that a certificate of formal training does not help teachers overcome attitudinal barriers that working with children on a daily basis does. Nothing mattered more than a sensitive approach and learning from one's own day-to-day experiences, picking up skills along the way.

In my interactions with the SJ School, I realized the following. One, a school need not have access to unlimited resources in order to implement inclusion. Two, ordinary schools can become inclusive with their own convictions, without much support from external agencies. Three, a visionary leader can create a community of practice that can overcome attitudinal barriers of fellow co-workers. Four, inclusion need not be seen as an end, but a process. While an ideal situation would be wherein children with disabilities are completely supported in their learning by classroom teachers and curricular and pedagogic adaptations are made to meet their individual needs, until that happens, any kind of support, in whatever form, that can be extended to scaffold children's learning, making their educational experience a meaningful one, is important. Five, an institution, where one sees happy children all around, must be doing some things right.

PREPARING SCHOOLS FOR INCLUSION

I list below three important components of inclusive practice that may be considered essential for developing inclusive schools. It is important that the suggested practices are not viewed as prescriptive in any way. A school may interpret these practices in view of their unique situations and adapt them to suit their individual needs. Likewise, it is not my intention to provide a list of the range of disabilities that could be considered for inclusion and those that cannot be. Such decisions are best left for institutions to make, based entirely on their level of preparedness and access to resources. As long as there is commitment to inclusion in principle, inclusive practice may be considered as a process and not an end that all institutions strive to achieve in due course.

Readiness

A strong belief in providing meaningful educational experiences to all children in the school should be the vision that drives an institution to create an inclusive environment in its setting. This vision may be translated by making elaborate infrastructural adaptations if resources permit or by making small changes to the existing structures such that all children attending the school have a barrier-free access to all available facilities in the school. However, infrastructural adaptations, though of utmost importance, are not the only way schools need to prepare themselves for inclusion. Preparation also requires schools to judge the readiness of all stakeholders and to prepare them adequately to overcome the attitudinal barrier or lack of acceptance and insensitivity towards having children with different learning needs in the school. In order to do so, school administration needs to work with teachers, parents, the peer group and the support staff in a sustained and sensitive manner. It is important that a whole school approach is adopted, and each and every member of the school is involved at every stage of the preparation.

Provide Teachers with Skills

Providing adequate pedagogic skills to teachers to work with children with different learning needs in the regular classrooms is essential for the success of a programme. Several competencies and skills have been identified that teachers must develop in order to work effectively in inclusive classrooms. A few of these are peer tutoring, cooperative learning, differentiated instruction, activity-based learning, classroom management skills, culturally responsive teaching and use of assistive technology (Das, Sharma and Singh 2012, 1–15). In addition to this, and perhaps of utmost importance, is helping teachers overcome their negative attitudes towards including children with disabilities in their classrooms. A lot of the resistance that teachers show comes from their poor psychological and sociological understanding of disability, their perception about their lack of preparedness and skills/knowledge to work with different types of disabilities and poor availability of resources such as appropriate teaching and learning materials that can be used and adapted according to individual learning needs of children. In order to provide these capabilities to teachers, a collaborative and cooperative environment of support must be facilitated in the school.

Cooperation and Communication

Cooperation and communication among different stakeholders is the key to the success of an inclusive programme. At least three different levels of collaboration are desirable: One, among regular teachers, school administration and special educators/therapists/psychologists (if any) who all must work together to find the most conducive classroom practices and resources to provide all the children in the school with meaningful learning experiences; two, between teachers and parents such that they work as partners complementing the efforts of one another; and three, between the school and the community such that there is cooperation and sensitivity in identifying, admitting and retaining children with disabilities in school. It is imperative that schools

CONCLUDING REMARKS

Inclusive education in India is an evolving concept. Several incongruities become apparent in arriving at a critical understanding of its nature and implementation. Resolution of these requires a concerted effort at multiple levels. Academic scholars, practitioners and policymakers must join hands to develop scholarship in the area which is indigenous and informed by the state of the economy, societal beliefs, cultural practices and the situation of children with disabilities in this country. At the same time, schools, both private and public, irrespective of their challenges and constraints, must realize that participation in the inclusion agenda for them is no longer a matter of choice. By creating communities of learning, sharing best practices and participating in knowledge creation, administrators, teachers and parents must come together wholeheartedly to participate in this agenda, such that every child in this country can have a meaningful, enriching and empowering educational experience.

REFERENCES

Alur, Mithu. 2007. 'The Lethargy of a Nation: Inclusive Education in India.' In *Policy, Experience and Change: Cross-cultural Reflections on Inclusive Education*, edited by Lee Barton and Felicity Armstrong, 91–106. Dordrchet: Springer.

Armstrong, Ann Cheryl, Derrick Armstrong, and Ilektra Spandagou. 2010. *Inclusive Education: International Policy and Perspective*, 26–36. London: SAGE.

Artiles, Alfredo J., Elizabeth B. Kozleski, Sherman Dorn, and Carol Christensen. 2006. 'Learning in Inclusive Education Research: Re-mediating Theory and Methods with a Transformative Agenda.' *Review of Research in Education* 30 (*Special Issue on Rethinking Learning: What Counts as Learning and What Learning Counts*): 65–108.

Barton, Lee. 1995. 'The Politics of Education for All.' *Support for Learning* 10 (4): 156–60.

Bhattacharya, Tanmoy. 2010. 'Re-examining Issues of Inclusion in Education.' *Economic and Political Weekly* 45 (16): 18–23.

Chowdhury, Payal R. 2011. 'The Right to Inclusive Education of Persons with Disabilities: The Policy and Practice Implications.' *Asia Pacific Journal of Human Rights and the Law* 12 (2): 1–35.

Connor, David J., Susan L. Gabel, Deborah J. Gallagher, and Missy Morton. 2008. 'Disability Studies and Inclusive Education—Implications for Theory, Research, and Practice.' *International Journal of Inclusive Education* 12 (5–6): 441–57.

Das, Ajay K., Sushama Sharma, and Vinay K Singh. 2012. 'Inclusive Education in India: A Paradigm Shift in Roles, Responsibilities and Competencies of Regular School Teachers.' *Journal of Indian Education* 37 (4): 1–15.

Florian, Lani. 2014. 'Reimagining Special Education: Why New Approaches are Needed.' In *The SAGE Handbook of Special Education*, edited by Lani Florian, 9–22. Vol. 1. London: SAGE.

Gabel, Susan L., and Jagdish Chander. 2008. *Inclusion in Indian Education, Disability and the Politics of Education: An International Reader*. New York, NY: Peter Lang.

Gabel, Susan L., and Scot Danforth. 2008. *Disability and the Politics of Education: An International Reader*. New York, NY: Peter Lang.

Kinsella, William, and Joyce Senior. 2008. 'Developing Inclusive Schools: A Systemic Approach.' *International Journal of Inclusive Education* 12 (5–6): 651–65.

Lindsay, Katharine G. 2007. *Inclusive Education in India: Interpretation, Implementation and Issues*, 1–35. Create Pathways to Access No.15. Brighton: University of Sussex.

Madan, Ankur. 2014. 'Inclusion Is the Way Forward.' In *Learning Curve*, 2–5. Bangalore: Azim Premji University.

———. 2016. 'Meeting the Inclusion Agenda: Taking the Matter into Our Own Hands.' *The New Leam* 2 (12): 8–11.

Madan, Ankur, and Neerja Sharma. 2013. 'Inclusive Education for Children with Disabilities: Preparing Schools to Meet the Challenge.' *Electronic Journal of Inclusive Education* 3 (1): 1–23.

Ministry of Human Resource Development, Government of India. 2009. *Right of Children to Free and Compulsory Education (RTE) Act*. Available at: http://mhrd.gov.in/rte (accessed May 9, 2018).

———. 2000. *Sarva Shiksha Abhiyaan: Programme for Universal Elementary Education in India*. New Delhi: Government of India.

Moore, Michele, and Roger Slee. 2012. 'Disability Studies, Inclusive Education and Exclusion.' In *Routledge Handbook of Disability Studies*, edited by Nick Watson, Alan Roulstone and Carol Thomas, 225–39. London: Routledge.

Rao, Shridevi. 2001. 'A Little Inconvenience: Perspectives of Bengali Families of Children with Disabilities on Labelling and Inclusion.' *Disability & Society* 16 (4): 531–48.

Rioux, Marcia. 2014. 'Disability Rights in Education.' In *The SAGE Handbook of Special Education*, edited by Lani Florian, 132–47. Vol. 1. London: SAGE.

Rose, Richard. 2017. 'Seeking Practice Informed Policy for Inclusive Education in India.' *Asian Journal of Inclusive Education* 5 (1): 5–22.

Sen, Amartya K. 2000. *Development as Freedom*. New York, NY: Anchor Books.

Singal, Nidhi. 2005. 'Mapping the Field of Inclusive Education: A Review of the Indian Literature.' *International Journal of Inclusive Education* 9 (4): 331–50. doi:10.1080/13603110500138277.

———. 2006. 'Inclusive Education in India: International Concept, National Interpretation.' *International Journal of Disability, Development and Education* 53 (3): 351–69.

Sharma, Neerja. 2010. 'Education for Children with Disability: Reflections on Best Practices to Assimilate Children in the Mainstream.' In *The Social Ecology of Disability*, edited by N. Sharma, 125–49. Technical Series 3. Delhi: Lady Irwin College.

Thomas, Gary. 2009. 'An Epistemology for Inclusion.' In *Psychology for Inclusive Education: New Directions in Theory and Practice*, edited by Peter Hick, Ruth Kershner and Peter T. Farrell, 13–23. Abingdon: Routledge.

———. 2014. 'Epistemology and Special Education.' In *The SAGE Handbook of Special Education*, edited by Lani Florian, 268–79. Vol. 1. London: SAGE.

Wolbring, Gregor, and Anita Ghai. 2015. 'Interrogating the Impact of Scientific and Technological Development on Disabled Children in India and Beyond.' *Disability and the Global South* 2 (2): 667–85.

Chapter 20

The Emancipatory Potential of a Structural Understanding of Disability
A Response to Linda Ware

Suchaita Tenneti

INTRODUCTION

In her essay 'Many Possible Futures, Many Different Directions: Merging Critical Special Education and Disability Studies' (2005), Linda Ware explores the contributions that disability studies could make to critical special education. She observes that the regressive history of special education with its focus on behaviourist and positivist approaches and the preponderance of the medical model of disability have limited the success of critical special education studies. This is primarily because of the persistence of the term 'special education' even in critical appropriations of this body of knowledge. But disability studies, she says, can revitalize critical special education by providing an epistemological frame of reference within which fundamental conceptions and assumptions about disability can be questioned. Disability studies carry the potential of transforming disability from a minority discourse to a universal one, thereby countering the reification of disability that takes place within special education.

While Ware's arguments for the establishment of linkages between critical special education and disability studies are immensely useful in foregrounding disability as a political category, it is worrisome that she emphasizes a 'humanities-based disability studies' (p. 103) over social science approaches. It could well be observed, as Ware does, that positivist and functionalist orientations have dominated the study of disability and have thereby segregated and marginalized people with disabilities. But the social sciences cannot be reduced to positivism or functionalism. Instead, the social sciences could help in the understanding of disability as an axis of 'structural' inequality, which has significant bearings on the field of education and on efforts to increase teachers' awareness about disability.

This chapter commences with a mention of the ways in which Ware herself acknowledges the role of the social sciences in constructing a disability praxis, especially given the interdisciplinary nature of disability studies. It proceeds to an exploration of three implications of the structural nature of disability for awareness efforts for teachers. Firstly, there is a thrust on the need for teachers to situate disability within its structural matrix beyond the domain of education and to shift their attention from the study of difference to the study of ableism and normalcy (see Fiona Kumari Campbell in this volume). Secondly, teachers need to be able to locate disability alongside other structural categories such as caste, class and gender in order to develop a holistic understanding of the construction and ramifications of structural inequality. Thirdly, the limits of attitudinal changes alone in challenging inequality need to be acknowledged and clearly outlined. This can be achieved by analysing phenomena within the education system at large that restrict teacher agency and by enabling teachers to understand the tenacity of structures of ableism over their own consciousness.

WARE'S NOTIONS ABOUT THE INTERDISCIPLINARY NATURE OF DISABILITY STUDIES

Ware (2005) describes disability studies as an '*interdisciplinary* [emphasis added] critical genre [that] draws from scholarship in history, literature, philosophy, anthropology, religion, medical history, and rhetoric to re-create a developed portrait of disabled people across histories and cultures' (p. 103). Although Ware emphasizes the humanities within the category of 'the interdisciplinary', she makes important uses of social science approaches and 'the social' throughout the essay. She identifies as critical Roger Slee's claim that 'being disabled is a relational concept within a sociological discourse' (p. 104). She later refers to Lous Heshusius's hope of special education abandoning its behaviourist history in favour of a 'social/political/cultural' understanding of disability (p. 107). The significance of 'the social' and the sociological in these arguments is critical because it foregrounds the interdisciplinary nature of disability studies with the social intermingling with other kinds of analytical categories.

Furthermore, the 'relational' is an instance of a concept that is relevant to both the humanities and the social sciences. There are other such instances where Ware's concerns are relevant to the social sciences. She observes, '…disability studies offers a plot that differs from that of special education, one that speaks to the humanity that we share rather than the one that estranges and others our differences' (p. 103). The expression 'humanity that we share' could refer to the philosophical/existentialist question, 'What does it mean to be human?' which is central to disability epistemology. But it could also be interpreted in terms of establishing structural solidarities with other marginalized groups. Such an approach would help locate disability within broader networks of structural oppression and help develop a more holistic foundation for praxis—a point that shall be discussed in the second section.

It is also significant to compare Ware's earlier observations of the interdisciplinary nature of disability studies with a conception that she offers later in the essay where she says:

> [G]iven the field's interdisciplinary origins in the social sciences, humanities and rehabilitation science efforts have just begun to bridge these fairly complex boundaries in pursuit of integrative approaches to develop a coherent field of inquiry. Disciplinary distinctions, divisions, subdivisions, and departments characterize the existing structure of higher education and simultaneously pose the greatest obstacles to responsive teaching in the twenty-first century. (p. 109)

Ware's observation in this quote precisely describes the risk of arbitrarily segregating disciplines. Therefore, despite the historical dominance of 'social science methods' over all other modes of enquiry referred to earlier, the truly emancipatory potential of disability studies lies in its embrace and critical recuperation of multiple domains of enquiry. This sentiment is reflected by other scholars of disability studies. In his research 'Debating Disability', Tom Shakespeare (2008) foregrounds the importance of medical sociology and medical ethics in disability studies despite the role of medicine in the pathologization of disability. Shakespeare makes a further important point about methodology that could be analysed in relation to Ware's observation about social science methods. He says,

> I believe that while academics should be engaged with contemporary political issues, they should also aspire to the best possible standards of data collection and analysis. If they allow their moral, emotional or political preconceptions or affiliations to contaminate their research, then they will produce shallow data or misleading arguments which will be incapable of serving broader political objectives. (p. 12)

Although Shakespeare's allusions to the 'disinterestedness' of the researcher could be debated, his statement could be used to argue in favour of the selection of 'appropriate' methods in accordance with the questions being raised rather than resort to any kind of a priori dismissal of methods on political grounds. Thus, social science methods continue to be relevant to disability studies, although they might be subject to constant interrogation with epistemological and methodological dialogues emerging from other disciplines (and post-disciplines).

Thus, it could be inferred that Ware makes significant positive use of the social sciences in her essay, although her confidence in the emancipatory potential of the social sciences is uncertain. This offers an interesting comment on disability studies: no discipline or field of enquiry can be dismissed in terms of its relevance to the study of disability despite the historical relationship that that particular discipline or mode of enquiry has had with disability rights and politics.

THE STRUCTURAL MATRIX OF DISABILITY AND TEACHER AWARENESS ABOUT DISABILITY

During her research project with secondary and post-secondary teachers on helping them understand disability 'as a concept and a constituency' (p. 110), Ware uses texts that could be said to fall into the domain of the humanities. Her narrations of the teachers' journey through the process of conscientization are extremely persuasive and encouraging. The teachers became conscious of the presence of stigma at the level of unconscious thought, the universality of experiences such as shame and the construction of difference. The task of enabling teachers to think of disability beyond the challenges that it poses to schools, as Ware notes, is indeed successful. But it is equally critical for teachers to specifically reflect on disability as an axis of structural inequality. At a broad level, this implies an understanding of how social, economic, political and other resources are distributed based on notions of one's ability/disability. Iris Young (2005) would call structural inequality 'the politics of positional difference' as opposed to 'the politics of cultural difference', which would validate the distinctive identity of people with disabilities.

Young defines the politics of positional difference as follows:

> This approach theorizes social groups as constituted through interactions that make categorical distinctions among people in hierarchies of status or privilege. The production and reproduction of 'durable inequality', as Charles Tilly calls it, involves processes where people produce and maintain advantages for themselves and disadvantages for others, in terms of access to resources, power, autonomy, honor, or receiving service and deference by means of application of rules and customs that assume such categorical distinctions.... (p. 6)

She consistently defines this kind of difference as having a certain prevalence over varying cultural contexts, thereby constituting a structural inequality or a generalized form of inequality. Young acknowledges the value of cultural difference in assisting in the attainment of freedom by providing specific insights into the manifestations and implications of axes of structural inequalities across diverse contexts. But Ware's focus seems to be largely on the latter. She seems to be emphasizing the need for teachers to reflect on the differences in the construction of disability across cultures and within their own specific culture as opposed to thinking of disability as a social category.

Shridevi Rao's work on Bengali families with children with disabilities demonstrates how variations in the use of terminology of disability reflect differential attitudes regarding the stigma associated with disability. In her work 'A Little Inconvenience': Perspectives of Bengali Families of Children with Disabilities on Labelling and Inclusion' (2001), Rao observes how families use the term 'inconvenience' to describe the challenges their children face and to persuade others to enable the inclusion of their children. The term 'inconvenience' could be read as a euphemism for disability, but it could also be seen as a significant attempt to de-stigmatize disability.

Teachers could use Rao's work to reflect on the ways in which cultural resources could help develop a healthy vocabulary about disability. At the same time, a structural understanding of disability would serve as a reminder to teachers that despite the use of potentially emancipatory terminology, disability remains a 'marked' category within the cultural contexts that Rao writes about. Thus, a structural understanding of disability precludes risks of cultural relativism while allowing scope for the specific understanding of disability across varying contexts.

The structural understanding of disability plays a further role in helping teachers understand the construction of disability beyond the school which, as mentioned earlier, is one of Ware's aims. Consider work on neoliberalism and employment in the context of disability in India. In their work 'Trapped between Ableism and Neoliberalism: Critical Reflections on Disability and Employment in India', Arun Kumar, Deepa Sonpal and Vanmala Hiranandani (2012) analyse the exploitation of people with disabilities as workers and the manner in which this exploitation is concealed and even rewarded on the grounds of the 'independence' that employment provides people with disabilities. A study of works such as these would help teachers reflect on the relationship between education and employment, the meaning of emancipation and independence and subtle forms of discrimination across various domains of social existence.

Focusing on the role of structural phenomena in shaping disability would help shift teachers' attention away from people with disabilities themselves and on to the ways in which normalcy and ableism are constructed and then used as forces of marginalization. Lennard Davis (2006) emphasizes this shift from disability to normalcy and ableism:

> [A]s with recent scholarship on race, which has turned its attention to whiteness, I would like to focus not so much on the construction of disability as on the construction of normalcy. I do this because the 'problem' is not the person with disabilities; the problem is the way that normalcy is constructed to create the 'problem' of the normal person. (p. 3)

Davis traces the history of the 'bell curve' mode of thinking to understand the construction of ableism and normalcy including the role of industrialization in developing eugenics and the idea of 'the average'. This historical and sociological analysis could be used as a point of discussion among the teachers and pave the way for ethical discussions about what their ideas are of a life that is worth living. But it could also be used to help them critically engage with the centrality of the average in thinking about the aims of education itself and other related concepts such as merit, assessments and standardization. Analysing these concepts alongside critiques of neoliberalism would prove to be an enlightening exercise for teachers in the context of understanding disability as an axis of structural inequality.

There is a possible pessimism within this structural understanding of disability because there is nothing that teachers can immediately 'do' with it. Nevertheless, it is vital for teachers to grasp the full import of the tenacity of structures on thought and action.

CRITICAL INTERSECTIONALITY

Analysing disability as an axis of structural inequality creates possibilities for teachers to think about how it fares alongside caste, class, gender and other social categories. This would, in turn, create scope for discussing the very construction of disability. For instance, Gobinda Pal (2010) analyses the intersection between caste and disability where he writes about chronic illnesses and malnutrition among people from lower castes besides other impairments. This raises the question about whether chronic illness or malnutrition should be understood as disabilities and the significance of this question for the meaning of disability. Pal also observes that many families belonging to lower castes do not send their disabled children to school because of economic challenges or the absence of suitable schools and not because of stigma associated with disability unlike upper caste families who tend to conceal their disabled children out of a sense of shame. Thus, analysing the intersection of caste and disability reveals the differences in stigma, accessibility, education and other concerns across caste boundaries. It further offers scope to explore the possibilities of the experiences of disabled people from upper caste communities dominating disability studies.

THE LIMITATIONS OF TEACHER AGENCY

Ware acknowledges the limits to teachers' understanding of disability owing to institutional restrictions:

> The tensions in schools of education specific to disability and 'inclusive education' parallel those in K-12 settings where educators are constrained by institutional structures that insure exclusion and where cultural barriers obscure alternative understandings of disability. (p. 105)

Besides training institutions, the ability of teachers to exercise any agency in their places of work, schools or universities, with respect to constructing a disability praxis, is limited. McNeil's criticism of Henry Giroux's idea of teachers as change agents is relevant in this context. McNeil is sceptical of teachers' ability to escape the 'technocratic rationality pervasive in schools' (1981, 207). She cautions that an overemphasis of teachers' agency 'ignores the extent to which much teacher practice is an accommodation to institutional realities, including those realities which embody the very societal inequalities teachers are supposed to enable their students to question' (p. 207). Institutional structures as constraining forces are essential to take into account while assessing the aims and outcomes of programmes for disability awareness. Given the institutionalization of ableism, teacher educators could realistically reflect and enable collective reflection among teachers about realistic ways in which a disability praxis could be achieved and what its possible manifestations could be.

But a structural understanding of disability reveals another set of limits on teacher agency, which could be explained through Bourdieu's

(1972) concept of the habitus. The habitus refers to the set of durable dispositions that individuals possess through various social structures that shapes their worldview. The habitus is so deeply embodied that it functions as a kind of tacit knowledge that orients actions without the explicit awareness of the social actors. Nevertheless, the habitus does not entirely determine one's actions—it strongly orients actions—and leaves scope for agency. Of course, social structures restrict the scope of this agency but it is also important to recognize that these structures are also *enabling* of agency. Thus, the restrictive and enabling features of social structures need acknowledgment. In the context of disability, this would entail facilitating reflection among teachers about the manner in which their potential to bring about a disability praxis is restricted both by institutional structures and their own deeply internalized belief systems. These belief systems are so deeply ingrained owing to their constant reiteration and reinforcement by various social institutions that their tenacity should not be underestimated: hence, the need for constant debate and critical self-reflection.

CONCLUSION

In conclusion, Ware's acknowledgement of the interdisciplinary nature of disability studies and her attempts to introduce a disability studies perspective into critical special education are extremely relevant and well argued. However, there is a need to foreground a structural understanding of disability through an inclusion of social science perspectives within disability studies that could, in turn, enrich efforts to create awareness about disability among teachers. Ware draws on social science perspectives and accepts their relevance while maintaining a scepticism of them. However, despite the negative histories of positivist and functionalist approaches in disability studies, the social sciences cannot be reduced to either of these approaches. Instead, a structural understanding of disability could help teachers understand the manner in which disability affects various aspects of life through disparities in the distribution of resources within and beyond education. It helps shift their attention from disability as difference to the construction of normalcy and enables an understanding of the intersectional nature of disability. Finally, it creates a sense of critical self-reflection and vigilance in teachers by foregrounding the tenacity of structural forces and making teachers aware of the limits of their agency. Thus, although a structural understanding of disability might appear pessimistic and does not directly provide a heuristics of praxis, it is a critical component of conscientization (and arguably praxis, as well) and the project of 'de-reifying' disability by transforming disability from a narrow domain concerning people with impairments to an epistemological lens through which fundamental questions about society and existence could be posed.

REFERENCES

Bourdieu, P. 1972. *Outline of a Theory of Practice*. Cambridge: Cambridge University Press.

Davis, L. J. 2006. 'Constructing Normalcy: The Bell Curve, the Novel, and the Invention of the Disabled Body in the Nineteenth Century.' In *The Disability Studies Reader*, edited by L. J. Davis, 3–16. New York: Routledge.

Kumar, A., D. Sonpal, and V. Hiranandani. 2012. Trapped Between Ableism and Neoliberalism: Critical Reflections on Disability and Employment in India.' *Disability Studies Quarterly* 32 (3). Available at: http://dsq-sds.org/article/view/3235/3109 (accessed 22 May 2018).

McNeil, L. 1981. 'On the Possibility of Teachers as the Source of an Emancipatory Pedagogy: A Response to Henry Giroux.' *Curriculum Enquiry* 11 (3): 205–10.

Pal, G. 2010. *Dalits with Disabilities: The Neglected Dimension of Social Exclusion*. Working Paper Series, 4 (3). New Delhi: Indian Institute of Dalit Studies.

Rao, S. 2001. 'A Little Inconvenience: Perspectives of Bengali Families of Children with Disabilities on Labelling and Inclusion.' *Disability and Society* 16 (4): 531–48.

Shakespeare, T. 2008. 'Debating Disability.' *Journal of Medical Ethics* 34 (1): 11–14.

Ware, L. 2005. 'Many Possible Futures, Many Different Directions: Merging Critical Special Education and Disability Studies (Chapter 7).' In *Disability Studies in Education: Readings in Theory and Method*, edited by S. Gabel, 103–24. New York: Peter Lang.

Young, I. M. 2005, May 22. 'Structural Injustice and the Politics of Difference.' Paper for AHRC Centre for Law, Gender, and Sexuality Intersectionality Workshop, Keele University, UK, 1–46.

Chapter 21

Disability at Work? Media Representations, CSR and Diversity

Arun Kumar and Nivedita Kothiyal

In this chapter, we map and problematize representations in the mainstream media of practices enhancing the employment of persons with disabilities within the private sector in India. Commonly understood as corporate social responsibility (CSR) and/or diversity management, such practices include, for example, targeted employment schemes, scholarships to individuals working in the private sector for pursuing higher education and livelihood training and skill upgradation programmes for persons with disabilities. They have gained their legitimacy through incentives and promotion by the State; extensive coverage by mainstream media promoting wider adoption and awards and recognitions offered variously and jointly by governments, industrial associations and disability-related organizations.

Drawing on a corpus of print and online news items published in the English language in leading national and regional dailies and widely read news websites online, we problematize the text, probe the subtext and map the absences in the representations of disability and persons with disabilities. Beyond the favourable representation of such corporate practices, we argue that they mask the denial of reasonable accommodation to persons with disabilities in private-sector employment, persist with the ableist constructions of disability and perpetuate the cult of the 'supercrip' (Clogston 1994). The (able-bodied) employer and (disabled) employee relationship continues to be characterized through tropes of dependence and gratitude.

DISABILITY AND EMPLOYMENT

With the rise of industrialization and global capitalism, transformations in the material relationships of production, reconfiguration and reorganization of work, establishment of control and surveillance, and shifts in the ideas of care resulted in reformulation of disability (Oliver 1990; Oliver and Barnes 2012; Ryan and Thomas 1980). Discussing the impact of industrialization on persons with disabilities, Ryan and Thomas (1980, 101) have noted that:

> The speed of factory work, the enforced discipline, the time-keeping and production norms—all these were a highly unfavourable change from the slower, more self-determined and flexible methods of work into which many handicapped people had been integrated.

As a result of the increasing standardization and normalization of machines, work processes, standards and time, persons with disabilities rapidly moved to the bottom and outside of the labour market (Oliver 1990). They were seen as deviants, individual workers who slowed down the pace of the mechanized assembly line and therefore needed to be separated out. With the rise of institutionalized control or controlling institutions, including the workhouses, persons with disabilities were separated as those who 'could not' work from those who 'would not' work. While in the past, the primary responsibility of taking care and providing for those who could not work essentially resided within the family and the community, it changed with the coming of capitalism. Persons with disabilities who had withdrawn from the wider (economically productive) society were then institutionalized under the care of the State (Oliver 1990).

While the rise of industrial capitalism excluded persons with disabilities from work and workplaces, it also reconstituted them as individuals.

Discussing the rise of individualism and disability, Oliver and Barnes (2012, 82) argue that:

> Under industrial capitalism... disability became individual pathology; people with impairments could not meet the demands of wage labour and so became controlled through exclusion. Wage labour became the distinction between the able and less able poor crucially important.

With this, the able-bodied norm came into being while persons with disabilities became deviants or abnormal, which resulted in their further exclusion. The able-bodied norm has since been institutionalized extensively. According to Wolbring (2008, 252–53), ableism refers to

> a particular understanding of oneself, one's body and one's relationship with others of humanity, other species and the environment, and includes how one is judged by others... Ableism reflects the sentiment of certain social groups and social structures that value and promote certain abilities, for example, productivity and competitiveness, over others....

It produces a preference for certain sets of abilities, while those deficient in or deviating from this preferred set, whether perceived to be or for real, are considered to be lesser, thus resulting in their discrimination and subjection (Wolbring 2006, 2008). For persons with disabilities, the ableist constructions of disableism force them to strive to either become able themselves or distance themselves from the able-bodied (Griffin, Peters and Smith 2007). Discussing the ableist conceptions of disableism within the world of work, Kumar, Sonpal and Hiranandani (2012) have argued that it continues to be the pivotal conception around which job design and employment for persons with disabilities are organized. With their disabilities 'cast [aside] as a diminished state of being human' (Campbell 2001, 44), employers and related employment exchanges focus exclusively on the 'ability' of persons with disabilities. Jobs are designed according to the abilities of the employees and not redesigned according to their disabilities. This obsession with ability has severely compromised the many related rights of persons with disabilities as workers. Persons with disabilities are never encouraged and often openly discouraged from speaking about their disabilities.

The enforced demand on persons with disabilities to become 'normal' or prove their abilities has led to the emergence of the 'supercrip' (Clogston 1994), or the 'superhero' or the 'disabled hero' (Wendell 1997). According to this, persons with disabilities are often represented as individuals who have had to overcome their disabilities and have managed to become like the able-bodied. Persons with disabilities are glorified into 'heroes' who must recover from their despondency, stop focussing on their 'inabilities', work hard to benefit from and continue to acknowledge the role of the able-bodied 'other' who provided them with the opportunity to work in the first place, thus re-emphasizing the narrative of the 'disabled hero'. This perpetuates a 'hierarchy of disability' (Crawford and Ostrove 2003) by showcasing these individuals as exemplars to be emulated by others suffering from similar afflictions or benchmarks against which other persons with disabilities are assessed and deemed as failures if they do not fit the mould (McDougall 2006).

REPRESENTING DISABILITY

Media plays an important role in how we 'make disability' (Higgins 1992). This is achieved through both (a) agenda setting, which refers to ways by which frequent and prominent coverage is used to make an issue more or less significant for the public (Coleman et al. 2009);, and (b) framing, that is the presentation of 'some aspects of a perceived reality and make them more salient… to promote a particular problem definition, causal interpretation, moral evaluation, and/or treatment recommendation' (Entman 1993, 52). In the case of disability, media content, stereotypes and absences have framed the mainstream discourse on it (Haller 2000; Stadler 2006).

Informed by the social construction of disability (discussed previously) and the critical role of mainstream media in making disability, we focus on media coverage of CSR and/or diversity management practices aimed at promoting employment of persons with disabilities in the private sector in India. We do so by analysing articles published in the English language in leading national and regional dailies and widely read news websites online, over the last 15 years. A total of 220 articles were archived, of which 102 articles were selected for further analysis and 118 were rejected as they contained reference to disability in passing as part of one or more vulnerable social groups in the country. For the purpose of analysis, an inductive analytic approach was adopted where 'the patterns, themes and categories emerge(d) out of the data rather than being imposed on them prior to data collection and analysis' (Patton 1980). Following our analysis, six key themes emerged from the media coverage. These related to nature of work, workers, merit and dis/ability, reasonable accommodation, supercrips and superheroes, and textual authorship. These are discussed in greater detail next.

Nature of Work

The workforce participation rates of persons with disabilities are significantly lower than those for the overall population (Bhalla 2015; Mitra and Sambamoorthi 2006). This workforce participation rate falls further and drastically when it comes to employment in the organized private sector, especially in leading corporations and businesses (DEOC 2009; NCPEDP 1999; Somvanshi 2015). From among those working in private-sector organizations, persons with disabilities are often assigned to stereotypical jobs within the old economy, such as junior clerks and stenographers, receptionists, telephone operators, typists, machine operators, polishing watch cases and putting head straps, jewellery making, tailoring, wood carving and so forth (Bhadra 2010; Mishra 2004; *The Financial Express* 2005). Or in the case of new economy, persons with disabilities find employment in retail fast-food industry, in lower-end, low-skilled jobs as housemasters or brewmasters, or in the burgeoning outsourcing BPO and IT/ITeS industry (Golikeri 2012; Kela 2012; Raja and Chandramouly 2005; Rangan 2011; Srikanth 2005; *The Hindu* 2011). Such jobs are concentrated in back-end service provision categories such as quality control, telemarketing, e-mail processing and support, transaction processing, voice and accent training with some promises of future possible openings in administration, training and human resource departments, or similar support functions in any typical organization (Katakam 2011). Most of the jobs are entry-level and involve low-level skills (Raghavendra and Vasi 2006; Raja and Chandramouly 2005). Commonly understood as

'Mcjobs' and 'iMcJobs' in the new economy, persons with disabilities are not only poorly rewarded (Ribeiro 2009), such jobs are often highly stressful, physically exhausting, emotionally exacting, unstable and devoid of autonomy and discretion.

Relatively fewer jobs are available to persons with disabilities as professionals, senior managers and other positions of power despite being qualified and capable of it (Fernades 2010; Kurup 2007). The stories of difficulties that persons with disabilities face when seeking employment commensurate with their experience and are narrated in only six of the articles collected by us (*Deccan Herald* 2012; Kelekar 2008; Kurup 2007; Sharma 2007; Venugopal 2010). Each of these stories recounts the individual initiative and effort from the employee in proving their competence for a specific job or having to overtrain themselves just to get their first job. There are only a handful who have managed to breach the glass ceiling and have risen within the managerial jobs (*The Financial Express* 2005). Persons with disabilities, therefore, become 'token' employees in high-skilled, remunerative jobs. As representative icons, persons with disabilities in such jobs are subject to undue workplace pressures on two counts: (a) they have to constantly struggle to prove themselves, be as good as or even better than all the other employees just to fit in and be accepted; and (b) when differences are highly visible, token employees feel the fate of people like them resting on their shoulders, and therefore they cannot afford to make mistakes or fail (Agócs and Burr 1996). For example, Basu (2017) writes:

> 'It is a fantastic thing that organisations are focusing on creating an inclusive culture,' said BS Nagesh, founder of Trust for Retailers and Retail Associates of India (TRRAIN) that runs Pankh, an initiative to train PWDs to make them part of inclusive growth in the retail sector. 'We have seen the impact this has at the lowest level. At management levels, when students from institutes such as the IIMs go on to become managers, not only does the effect percolate down, they also become brand ambassadors of inclusiveness in the organisation,' Nagesh said.

This uneven distribution—over-representation in low-skilled employment and under-representation in managerial/professional positions—has remained unacknowledged, by and large, in mainstream media's portrayal of employment of persons with disabilities.

Loyal and Hardworking Employees

Although prior research has shown that persons with disabilities are frequently portrayed negatively by mainstream media coverage (Mike 1996; Philips 2012b), our analysis suggests otherwise. Mainstream media's coverage of employment of persons with disabilities was often celebratory and heart-warming in tone and content, extolling other corporate organizations and associations to do the same (Katakam 2011; *The Hindu* 2011); or lauding individual employees (Ramanathan 2011; Subramani 2006). Even collectively, persons with disabilities are showcased as loyal employees who were unlikely to leave the organization once they have been trained by it (e.g., *Business Line* 2010; Deshpande 2011; Kably and Rajadhyaksha 2012; Katakam 2011; Menon 2006; Raja and Chandramouly 2005; Subramani 2006; *The Indian Express* 2012; *The Times of India* 2011).

In comparison with others, persons with disabilities were described as follows: 'these employees are stable and do not leave for a better salary' (Srikanth 2005); '[t]hey are more sensitive towards others (leading to better team work) and are also more disciplined, sincere, organized and loyal' (Kably and Rajadhyaksha 2012); '[n]ot only are these people hardworking as you or me, but their shortcomings give them an unnatural sense of humour and zest for life; they take that to their jobs, thus also creating a friendly environment all around where they work' (Bhadra 2010). Their attitude and behaviour towards work and at workplaces, respectively, were frequently noted (Bhatia 2008; Charan 2005a). As was the benefit they offered corporations in attaining competitive advantage through diversity management (Cox and Blake 2001). Bhattacharjee (2011), for example, surmised the business case as follows.

> From the organizations' point of view, working with PwDs has a positive impact on its customer base. As the employees already have the experience of interacting with PwDs, it reflects on their dealings with such customers as and when required. The PwDs bring a diverse

culture to the organization. Other employees also become accustomed to aspects like sign language, which in the long run can be beneficial to the organization.

Merit and Dis/ability

The stronghold of ableism is further reinforced when merit and abilities are projected as the only basis of selection for persons with disabilities. For example, media coverage analysed by us emphasized that the selection of persons with disabilities is only on the basis of their individual 'merit' (Fernandes 2010; Kelekar 2008; Naidu 2008; Roy 2012). As part of which, private-sector organizations frequently reiterated their commitment to 'become equal opportunity employer without compromising on merit' (Deshpande 2011). Instructive to note here is that merit is framed, as if, in contradiction to the ideals and ideas of providing equal opportunity to persons with disabilities.

In locating merit, private companies frequently used the services of recruitment consultants and voluntary organizations in mapping jobs (Charan 2005b) and to 'help [them] understand specific jobs that suit a person with a certain disability' (Pal 2008). As part of which, principles and practices from mainstream industrial/organizational psychology such as 'person-job' fit are used extensively (Reddy 2012). For example:

> [i]t is just about following the HR principle of having the right person in the right job. Just like qualifications and work experience, the type of disability should be an assessment criterion instead of blanket rejection. (Pal 2008)

As a result of which, BPO jobs are found to be most suitable as these are:

> primarily desk-oriented, which are conducive for physically challenged people, many of the processes are non-voice and transaction based that are suitable for persons with hearing disabilities. (*The Economic Times* 2006)

And elsewhere:

[t]asks with low levels of body risk, the least physical movement and minimum verbal communication were identified and categorised ability-wise. The physically impaired were engaged to polish watchcases and assemble components and the hearing impaired to strap watch heads, while the visually impaired found a place in the [Titan's] packaging and despatch division. (*The Financial Express* 2005)

Thus, persons with disabilities are left with little control or say over the kind of jobs and nature of work being offered to them (Duff and Ferguson 2011), and how and with whom they should work. For example, the call centre EuroAble which employs only persons with disabilities (Ghosh 2011) invokes the trope of community to highlight the comfort of persons with disabilities in working with those who are like them. Similarly invoking community, Ramanathan (2011) noted that from the fast-food industry that the:

challenge [to assemble the order in under a minute] was soon overcome, as is evident to anyone visiting the KFC outlet in Newmarket, Kolkata-the outlet is almost entirely staffed by the differently-abled. After extensive training for six months, they work in groups to have the comfort of being in the same community.

Merit and productivity, therefore, are presented as sacrosanct norms, without recognizing how such 'merit' is defined or 'productivity' norms are set by others to meet the 'needs of the enterprise' (Annamalai 2012; Dick and Nadin 2006; Ghosh 2011). This is evident from the quote by a senior manager in a call centre employing persons with disabilities:

'Productivity was also an issue in some cases. When we started off, we had 50-60% productivity. Now, it has improved to 75%. We will soon reach even 110%! These people have a point to prove. They want to show they can be as good as anybody else. (Ramanathan 2011)

By converting the disability of a person into ability, which can then be exploited by the employing organization (Kabli 2012; Kably and Rajadhyaksha 2012; Sardesai 2012; Subramani 2005b), the real needs for reasonable accommodation are conveniently rejected (Raja and Chandramouly 2005).

Reasonable Accommodation

As we have argued that the employment of persons with disabilities is frequently framed as part of voluntary CSR and/or diversity management, the provision of reasonable accommodation is cited as evidence of social contributions of private-sector companies in the news coverage (Bhatia 2008; Bhattacharjee 2011; *Business Line* 2010; Ghosh 2011; Naidu 2008; Raja and Chandramouly 2005; *The Financial Express* 2005; *The Times of India* 2011; Venugopal 2010). Such reports further emphasize that the provision of reasonable accommodation for persons with disabilities has not, in any way, compromised the financial imperatives of private-sector organizations (Bhadra 2010; Ghosh 2011; Golikeri 2012; Katakam 2011; Kela 2012; *Mint* 2010; Raja and Chandramouly 2005; Rangan 2011). Instead, they suggest that such initiatives have created a 'win-win' situation for employers and the employees.

However, a more detailed analysis suggests that more often than not, employers provide reasonable accommodation only when it benefits them. For example, news reports suggest that owing to the expenses involved, assistive technologies are procured only when they offer economies of scale. The BPOs, for example, tend to provide assistive technologies only when persons with disabilities are recruited in sufficient numbers. There is little mention of private-sector organizations offering financial support to its employees with disabilities for any individualized technologies or aids, including those relevant to their daily living. This is the case despite the recognition that persons with disabilities expend additional time and effort in routine activities of everyday living and on account of which Barnes and Mercer (2005) have called for reformulating our conception of work itself.

Expectedly so, there is little modification of work/labour processes as any change in these would require, according to Wilton (2004, 423):

> the employers to adjust how, when and where essential work tasks are performed to meet the needs of a disabled employee. In this sense, reasonable accommodation constitutes a challenge to the logic of contemporary capitalist economies, where flexibility is first and foremost a privilege of capital.

The physical remodelling of office work spaces is considered enough, at best, to 'normalize' work conditions for persons with disabilities; and subsequently, workers are expected to cope with the usual pressures of work (Ghosh 2011; *Mint* 2010; Naidu 2008). The private-sector organizations take pride in the fact that following selection (with minor modifications in selection procedures for reasonable accommodation), persons with disabilities are not given any preferential treatment in promotions, career advancement and compensation (Raghavendra and Vasi 2006; Raja and Chandramouly 2005; Thanuja 2007). This is contested by persons with disabilities, as the following testimony suggests 'It's great that companies are willing to remodel offices to accommodate us, but that's not enough', says Jagdale, 22.

> A little leeway, in terms of targets, deadlines and office timings, or even a small adjustment to make a chair more comfortable, shows us the company cares. But we will always be the minority in most organisations, so they are reluctant to make any big changes for us.

Supercrips and Yet

Given the typical absorption of persons with disabilities in low-skilled, back-end jobs within private-sector organizations, and a near dogmatic emphasis on merit, there are only a few who manage to move into senior managerial positions. Those who do are represented as heroic individuals who have managed to overcome the odds and have worked harder than others to prove their merit (*Deccan Herald* 2012; Nagrath 2010; Nayak 2012; *The Indian Express* 2007). For example, it was reported that:

> Ashwin Karthik S.N., a software engineer at Mphasis, and Chidambar Vishnu Joshi, senior delivery manager at IBM India, have something in common. Both are heroes in their own right. Twenty-four year old Karthik is the first BE graduate in India who has a condition of Celebral Palsy–Quadriplegic, the severest form that affects all four limbs. Joshi, 38 who is unable to use his left leg due to polio, received the National Award for Life Time Professional Achievement in 2006. (Pal 2008)

Such celebratory accounts of successes of persons with disabilities have been understood as the making of the 'supercrip' (Clogston 1994). They focus on portraying particular senses and skills of persons with disabilities to superhuman levels, in overcoming their disabilities, material conditions and social backgrounds.

Related to this is a less frequent descriptor in mainstream media's coverage of employment of persons with disabilities that relates to their formulation as victims, disadvantaged and in need of a supportive hand to overcome their destitution and poverty (Bhatia 2008; Ghosh 2011; Handique 2009; Katakam 2011; Rangan 2011). Not unexpectedly, such a portrayal conveniently sidesteps substantive discussion on reasons behind it. Instead, persons with disabilities and their families are portrayed as grateful (Fernandes 2010; Subramani 2005a). For example, Deshpande (2011) has reported the following testimonies from persons with disabilities and their families:

> I run a lemon juice stall at Ghatkopar. I want to soar high in life. I knew I could do nothing sitting on an iron rod, selling lemon juice. I thank Eureka Forbes for selecting us. We will soar higher now.

And:

> There is nothing we cannot do if given the right opportunity. Till now, people only looked at our drawbacks, not our strengths. You (employers) recognised our strength. We will never let you down.

And further still:

> I am grateful that these people recognised their abilities and gave our children the opportunity to work.

Thus, the representations of persons with disabilities as employees in the private sector in the country vacillate between their formulation as superheroes who overcome their disabilities, poverty and social backgrounds or as victims in need of (able-bodied and corporate) support. In either case, such representations conveniently ignore the pasts and presents of persons with disabilities.

Authorship of the Text: Who Speaks? On Whose Behalf?

The experiences of persons with disabilities as workers are all too frequently, and we argue deliberately, silenced in the mainstream media's coverage. Instead, far greater attention is provided to the employer, the manager or the industrialist who is portrayed as a 'silent contributor' to relevant social causes (Katakam 2011). One news report, for example, noted the following: 'It is part of our strategy to promote the spirit of "I can" as opposed to "I cannot"', says a senior industrialist. (*Business Standard* 2008).

As a result of which, persons with disabilities, their employment and experiences of it are largely presented through the voice of the Other: the able-bodied employer, benefactor, business leader or the reporting journalist.

Among the news reports carrying quotes, only 18% of the quotes came from persons with disabilities themselves. Mainstream media coverage, therefore, mirrors the recurrent experience of persons with disabilities of being overlooked and deliberately silenced, as the able-bodied managers, business leaders and colleagues assume that persons with disabilities cannot speak for themselves. For example, Bagchi (2015) reports:

> Ghousiya Nishat is a project coordinator with EMC's Professional Services department, and her colleague Gayathri Shenoy, a project manager in the same department, is helping her settle in. Ghousiya has muscular dystrophy and is tetraplegic—she has full-body paralysis. She also has low vision. 'Initially, I gave her smaller targets. But she finished in a few days the work I'd planned to assign to her over three months. Now the challenge for me is to find more challenging work for her', says Shenoy.

This form of speaking for and over tends to universalize the opinion of the able-bodied and their experience of employment of persons with disabilities as a seemingly neutral and transparent record of reality. In effect, it works to ignore the opaqueness of power and the privilege associated with it.

CONCLUSION

Following the reformulation of disability with the onset of industrialization and capitalism (Oliver 1990; Oliver and Barnes 2012; Ryan and Thomas 1980), characterized by the pathologization, segregation and institutionalization of disability, how might we understand contemporary practices of employment of persons with disabilities in the private sector in India? Although employing persons with disabilities, their disabilities are secreted away behind the tropes of ableism, merit, community, supercrip and so forth.

The private-sector's response to disability, we would argue therefore, can be problematized by way of neoliberalization of global capitalism. In a race to cut costs among global corporations, outsourcing, subcontracting and subsidiarization of economic activity have grown extensively. Persons with disabilities are being employed increasingly in such jobs, commonly understood as McJobs and iMcjobs. Despite the high rates of attrition in such industries, persons with disabilities are seen as loyal and diligent employees. But this is a part of the story.

Following the renowned political scientist, Brown (2005, 38), we understand neoliberalism as a political rationality that 'both organises these (referring to economic and social) policies and reaches beyond the market'. This carries a social analysis that, when deployed as a form of governmentality, reaches from the soul of the citizen-subject to education policy to practices of empire (Brown 2005, 39).

It reconceptualizes and reconstitutes the individual as rational and calculating whose 'moral autonomy is measured by their capacity for 'self-care'—the ability to provide for their own needs and service their own ambitions' (Brown 2005, 42). As part of which, individuals no longer make demands of the State and the market, instead they must take responsibility for their own lives.

The employment practices and experiences of persons with disabilities in the private sector, we would argue, are undergirded by neoliberalism's core principle of self-care. Instead of demanding employment as a right from the State, or its regulation of the market, private companies are expected to manage diversity voluntarily and regulate themselves, thus making their employment of persons with disabilities evidence of their CSR (Subeliani and Tsogas 2005). At the same time, persons with disabilities are expected to assume responsibilities for their employment, experience and lives. In this, the focus is not on their disabilities, but on their abilities. Ableism not only helps private corporations to reconfigure person-job fits but also circumvents demands for reasonable accommodation. On top of which, merit becomes a frequently deployed trope to assess ability and performance, while disability remains secreted away. The rights of persons with disabilities are, therefore, reformulated as privileges to be earned in exchange of performance of key responsibilities, the most significantly through economic contribution. The supercrip, therefore, becomes an icon that other persons with disabilities aspire to. This conflation between ableism and neoliberalism is now reconfiguring disability in deeply problematic ways (Kumar, Sonpal and Hiranandani 2012).

REFERENCES

Agocs, C., and C. Burr. 1996. 'Employment Equity, Affirmative Action and Managing Diversity: Assessing the Differences.' *International Journal of Manpower* 17 (4/5): 30–45.

Annamalai, S. 2012, June 1. 'Efficiency, Hallmark of BPO Run by Visually Challenged Persons.' *The Hindu*. Available at: http://www.thehindu.com/news/national/tamil-nadu/efficiency-hallmark-of-bpo-run-by-visually-challenged-persons/article3477469.ece (accessed May 9, 2018).

Bagchi, S. 2015, March 15. 'IT Firm EMC Shows the Way, Hires Profoundly Disabled.' *The Economic Times*. Available at: http://economictimes.indiatimes.com/tech/ites/IT-firm-EMC-shows-the-way-hires-profoundly-disabled/articleshow/46581918.cms (accessed May 9, 2018).

Barnes, Colin, and Geof Mercer. 2005. 'Disability, Work, and Welfare: Challenging the Social Exclusion of Disabled People.' *Work, Employment and Society* 19 (3): 527–45.

Basu, S. 2017, April 11. 'India Inc Opens Doors Wide for Differently-abled IIM Graduates'. *The Economic Times*. Available at: http://m.economictimes.com/news/company/corporate-trends/india-inc-opens-doors-wide-for-differently-abled-iim-graduates/articleshow/58037371.cms (accessed May 9, 2018).

Bhadra, V. 2010, April 13. 'Honing the Skills of the Differently-abled.' *The Economic Times*. Available at: http://economictimes.indiatimes.com/news/company/corporate-trends/honing-the-skills-of-the-differently-abled/articleshow/5790048.cms (accessed May 9, 2018).

Bhalla, J. S. 2015, March 22. '5 Lakh Differently-abled to be Skill-ready by '18.' *The Pioneer*. Available at: http://www.dailypioneer.com/sunday-edition/sunday-pioneer/landmark/5-lakh-differently-abled-to-be-skill-ready-by-18.html (accessed May 9, 2018).

Bhatia, M. 2008, December 8. 'IT Firms Give a Leg-up to the Differently-abled.' *The Economic Times*. Available at: http://economictimes.indiatimes.com/liveitup/it-firms-give-a-leg-up-to-the-differently-abled/articleshow/3806539.cms (accessed May 9, 2018).

Bhattacharjee, S. 2011, June 7. 'PWDs, an Untapped Talent Pool.' *The Times of India-Ascent*. Available at: http://www.timesascent.com/career-advice/PWDs-an-untapped-talent-pool/21195 (accessed May 9, 2018).

Brown, W. 2005. *Edgework: Critical Essays on Knowledge and Politics*. Princeton, NJ: Princeton University Press.

Business Line. 2010, December 3. 'Companies that Make a Difference.' *Business Line*. Available at: http://www.thehindubusinessline.com.

Business Standard. 2008, February 26. 'We Want to Promote the "I can" Spirit Among People.' *Business Standard*. Available at: http://www.rediff.com/money/2008/feb/26inter.htm?print=true (accessed May 9, 2018).

Campbell, F. A. K. 2001. 'Inciting Legal Fictions: Disability Date with Ontology and the Ableist Body of the Law.' *Griffith Law Review* 10 (1): 42–62.

Charan, S. 2005a, June 19. 'Training Them for a Better Future.' *The Hindu*. Available at: http://www.thehindu.com/2005/06/19/stories/2005061917140300.htm (accessed May 9, 2018).

———. 2005b, July 28. 'Their Special Abilities Are Tapped Here.' *The Hindu*. Available at: http://www.thehindu.com/2005/07/28/stories/2005072818080400.htm (accessed May 9, 2018).

Clogston, J. S. 1994. 'Disability Coverage in American Newspapers.' In *The Disabled, The Media, and the Information Age*, edited by J. A. Nelson, 45–57. Westport, CT: Greenwood Publishing Group.

Coleman, R., M. McCombs, D. Shaw, and D. Weaver. 2009. 'Agenda Setting.' In *The Handbook of Journalism Studies*, edited by K. Wahl-Jorgensen and T. Hanitzsch, 147–60. New York: Routledge.

Cox, T. H., and S. Blake. 1991. 'Managing Cultural Diversity: Implications for Organizational Competitiveness.' *The Executive* 5 (3): 45–56.

Crawford, D., and J. M. Ostrove. 2003. 'Representations of Disability and the Interpersonal Relationships of Women with Disabilities.' *Women & Therapy* 26 (3–4): 179–94.

Deccan Herald. His employers banked on his abilities and they came in handy. (2012, December 3). *Deccan Herald*. Available at: http://www.deccanherald.com/content/296177/his-employers-banked-his-abilities.html (accessed May 9, 2018).

DEOC. 2009. *Employment of Disabled People in India: Baseline Report*. Delhi: National Centre for Promotion of Employment for Disabled People (NCPEDP).

Deshpande, V. 2011, April 1. 'A Job Centre to Call Their Own.' *The Hindu*. Available at: http://www.thehindu.com/todays-paper/tp-national/A-job-centre-to-call-their-own/article14666496.ece (accessed May 9, 2010).

Dick, P., and S. Nadin. 2006. 'Reproducing Gender Inequalities? A Critique of Realist Assumptions Underpinning Personnel Selection Research and Practice.' *Journal of Occupational and Organizational Psychology* 79 (3): 481–98.

Duff, A., and J. Ferguson. 2011. 'Disability and the Professional Accountant: Insights from Oral Histories. *Accounting, Auditing & Accountability Journal* 25 (1): 71–101.

Entman, R. M. 1993. 'Framing: Toward Clarification of a Fractured Paradigm.' *Journal of Communication* 43 (4): 51–58.

Fernandes, J. R. 2010, May 23. 'Can and Able.' *The Times of India*. Available at: timesofindia.indiatimes.com.

Ghosh, L. 2011, April 5. 'Companies Unwittingly Discriminate Against Differently Abled.' *The Economic Times*. Available at: http://economictimes.indiatimes.com/jobs/companies-unwittingly-discriminate-against-differently-abled/articleshow/7870126.cms (accessed May 9, 2018).

Golikeri, P. 2012, March 29. 'BPO for Differently Abled Has Sound Future.' *DNA*. Available at: http://www.dnaindia.com/money/report-bpo-for-differently-abled-has-sound-future-1668674 (accessed May 9, 2018).

Griffin, P., M. L. Peters, and R. M. Smith. 2007. 'Ableism Curriculum Design.' In *Teaching for Diversity and Social Justice*, edited by M. Adams, M. A. Bell and P. Griffin, 335–58. New York: Routledge.

Haller, B. 2000. 'How the News Frames Disability: Print Media Coverage of the Americans with Disabilities Act.' In *Expanding the Scope of Social Science Research on Disability*, edited by B. M. Altman and S. N. Barnartt, 55–83. Oxford: JAI Press.

Handique, M. 2009, October 5. 'Conspiracy of Silence Obscures Numbers.' *Mint*. Available at: http://www.livemint.com/Home-Page/ZJFv59tIC8RcmrnLH0hpZP/Conspiracy-of-silence-obscures-numbers.html (accessed May 9, 2018).

Higgins, Paul C. 1992. *Making Disability: Exploring the Social Transformation of Human Variation*. Springfield: Charles C Thomas.

Kably, L. 2012, September 5. Sops can Boost jobs for Disabled Persons. *The Times of India*. Available at: http://timesofindia.indiatimes.com/city/mumbai/Sops-can-boost-jobs-for-disabled-persons/articleshow/16256672.cms (accessed May 9, 2018).

Kably, L., and M. Rajadhyaksha. 2012, December 1. 'Can and Able.' *The Times of India Crest Edition*. Available at: http://www.youth4jobs.org/pdf/can-and-able-society-times-crest.pdf (accessed May 9, 2018).

Katakam, A. 2011. 'Miracle Workers.' *Frontline* 28 (3). Available at: http://www.frontline.in/static/html/fl2803/stories/20110211280308500.htm (accessed 12 May 2018).

Kela, A. 2012, April 30. 'The Disabled as an Economic Resource.' *The Financial Express*. Available at: http://www.financialexpress.com/archive/the-disabled-as-an-economic-resource/943345/ (accessed 9 May 2018).

Kelekar, A. 2008, November 17. 'Upwardly Immobile.' *The Computer Express*.

Kumar, A., V. Hiranandani, and D. Sonpal. 2012. 'Trapped Between Ableism and Neoliberalism: Critical Reflections on Disability and Employment in India.' *Disability Studies Quarterly* 32 (3). Available at: http://dsq-sds.org/article/view/3235/3109 (accessed May 9, 2018).

Kurup, D. 2007, December 24. 'Private Sector Reluctant to Hire Disabled.' Available at: http://www.thehindu.com/todays-paper/tp-national/tp-karnataka/Private-sector-reluctant-to-hire-disabled/article14900779.ece (accessed May 9, 2018).

McDougall, K. 2006. '"Ag Shame" and Superheroes: Stereotype and the Signification of Disability.' In *Disability and Social Change: A South African Agenda*, edited by B. Watermeyer, L. Swartz, T. Lorenzo, M. Schneider and M. Priestley, 387–400. Pretoria: Human Sciences Research Council.

Menon, S. 2006, December 3. 'Cos Need to Enable Equal Options.' *The Economics Times*. http://economictimes.indiatimes.com/news/company/corporate-trends/cos-need-to-enable-equal-options/articleshow/690624.cms (accessed May 9, 2018).

Mick, Kristin Anne. 1996. 'Framing Disability: A Content Analysis of Disability-related Newspaper Coverage from 1986 to 1994.' Master's Thesis submitted to San Jose State University. Available at: http://scholarworks.sjsu.edu/etd_theses/1245 (accessed 10 December 2012).

Mint. 2010, December 6. 'Society Has to Come to Terms with Pwd.' *Mint*. Available at: http://www.livemint.com/Leisure/UrQZsS9nXLLC1UFNrzzM7K/8216Society-has-to-come-to-terms-with-PwD8217.html (accessed May 9, 2018).

Mishra, R. 2004, January 5. 'Celebrating Ability.' *Business Line*. Available at: http://www.thehindubusinessline.com/life/2004/01/05/stories/2004010500020200.htm (accessed May 9, 2018).

Mitra, S., and U. Sambamoorthi. 2006. 'Employment of Persons with Disabilities: Evidence from the National Sample Survey.' *Economic and Political Weekly* 41 (3): 4026–29.

Nagrath, S. 2010, July 28. 'Definitely Abled.' *The Business world*. Available at: http://www.businessworld.in/index.php/After-Hours/DefinitelyAbled.html (accessed May 9, 2018).

Naidu, V. 2008, March 12. 'The Miracle Worker.' *The Times of India-Ascent*.

Nayak, M. 2012, July 7. 'Not a Smooth Ride.' *Business World*. Available at: http://businessworld.in/article/Not-A-Smooth-Ride/08-11-2014-64666 (accessed May 9, 2018).

NCPEDP. 1999. *Employment Practices of the Corporate Sector*. Delhi: NCPEDP. Available at: http://www.ncpedp.org/employ/em-resrch.htm (accessed February 12, 2012).

Oliver, M. 1990. *The Politics of Disablement*. London: Macmillan.
Oliver, M., and C. Barnes. 2012. *The New Politics of Disablement*. Basingstoke: Palgrave Macmillan.
Pal, A. 2008, October 8. 'Making a Difference.' *Outlook Money*. Available at: https://www.outlookindia.com/outlookmoney/archive/making-a-difference-91054 (accessed May 9, 2018).
Patton, M. Q. 1980. *Qualitative Evaluation Methods*. Beverly Hills, CA: SAGE.
Phillips, Sarah. 2012. *Women with Disabilities in the Europe and Eurasia Region*. Washington, D.C: USAID. Available at: http://socialtransitions.kdid.org/sites/socialtransitions/files/resource/files/Women%20with%20Disabilities_formatted_12AUG20_final.pdf (accessed 15 December 2012).
Raghavendra, R., and N. Vasi. 2006, April 26. 'Desi BPOs Lend a Hand to Disabled.' *The Times of India*. Available at: http://timesofindia.indiatimes.com/business/india-business/Desi-BPOs-lend-a-hand-to-disabled/articleshow/1506570.cms (accessed May 9, 2018).
Raja, S. T. E., and A. Chandramouly. 2005, February 4. 'Calls for Special Skills.' *Business Line*. Available at: http://www.thehindubusinessline.com/todays-paper/tp-life/calls-for-special-skills/article2204785.ece (accessed May 9, 2018).
Ramanathan, A. 2011, June 11. 'Level Playing Field.' *Outlook Business*. Available at: http://archive.outlookbusiness.com/article_v3.aspx?artid=272169 (accessed May 9, 2018).
Rangan, P. S. 2011, October 17. 'More PWDs in Today's Workforce.' *The Hindu*. Available at: http://www.thehindu.com/news/cities/Hyderabad/more-pwds-in-todays-workforce/article2539958.ece (accessed May 9, 2018).
Reddy, M. 2012, March 19. 'Being Mutually Inclusive at the Workplace. *The Times of India-Ascent*. Available at: http://www.timesascent.com/hr-zone/Being-mutually-inclusive-at-the-workplace/77208 (accessed May 9, 2018).
Ribeiro, J. 2009, March 24. 'In Bangalore, a BPO With a Heart.' *PC World*. Available at: http://www.pcworld.com/article/161878/article.html (accessed May 9, 2018).
Roy, S. 2012, July 5. 'Taking a Different Approach to Business.' *Business Line*. Available at: http://www.thehindubusinessline.com/news/variety/taking-a-different-approach-to-business/article3602643.ece (accessed May 9, 2018).
Ryan, J., and F. Thomas. 1980. *The Politics of Mental Handicap*. Harmondsworth: Penguin.
Sardesai, C. 2012, May 22. 'Making Disabilities Work.' *Mumbai Mirror*. Available at: http://timesofindia.indiatimes.com/life-style/relationships/work/Making-disabilities-work/articleshow/12004205.cms (accessed May 9, 2018).
Sharma, R. 2007, December 25. 'Tapping the Disabled Workforce.' *Mint*. Available at: http://www.livemint.com/Industry/orr9ozreNMwzb6PXrPanII/Tapping-the-disabled-workforce.html (accessed May 9, 2018).
Somvanshi, K. K. 2015, December 3. 'India Inc Still a Challenge for Disabled, 10 cos Employ 90% of Disabled Employees Working in Nifty 50 Firms.' *The Economic Times*. Available at: http://economictimes.indiatimes.com/

jobs/india-inc-still-a-challenge-for-disabled-10-cos-employ-90-of-disabled-employees-working-in-nifty50-firms/articleshow/50019057.cms (accessed May 9, 2018).
Srikanth, B. R. 2005, May 29. 'BPOs Spot Stability—Industry Starts to Hire Physically Challenged.' *The Telegraph*. Available at: https://www.telegraphindia.com/1050530/asp/frontpage/story_4804069.asp (accessed May 9, 2018).
Stadler, J. 2006. 'Media and Disability.' In *Disability and Social Change: A South African Agenda*, edited by B. Watermeyer, L. Swartz, T. Lorenzo, M. Schneider snd M. Priestley, 373–86. Pretoria: Human Sciences Research Council.
Subeliani, D., and G. Tsogas. 2005. 'Managing Diversity in the Netherlands: A Case Study of Rabobank.' *The International Journal of Human Resource Management* 16 (5): 831–51.
Subramani, L. 2006, January 6. 'Brewing Sound Sense.' *Deccan Herald*. Available at: http://archive.deccanherald.com/Deccanherald/jan62006/Metro134540200615.asp (accessed April 28, 2012).
———. 2005a, July 5. 'Better Jobs, Better Future. *Deccan Herald*. Available at: http://archive.deccanherald.com/Deccanherald/jul52005/spectrum112225200574.asp (accessed December 30, 2011).
———. 2005b, September 15. 'Special People Come with Special Skills.' *Deccan Herald*. Available at: http://archive.deccanherald.com/deccanherald/sep152005/state1834242005914.asp (accessed December 23, 2011).
Thanuja, B. M. 2007, December 5. 'A Leg-up for Disabled.' *The Economic Times*. Available at: http://economictimes.indiatimes.com/liveitup/a-leg-up-for-disabled/articleshow/2596268.cms (accessed May 9, 2018).
The Economic Times. 2006, June 12. 'BPOs Eye Differently-abled Pros. *The Economic Times*. Available at: http://economictimes.indiatimes.com (accessed May 9, 2018).
The Hindu. 2011, January 11. 'IT Companies Urged to Employ Persons with Disabilities.' *The Hindu*. Available at: http://www.thehindu.com/todays-paper/tp-national/tp-karnataka/IT-companies-urged-to-employ-persons-with-disabilities/article15515121.ece (accessed May 9, 2018).
———. 2011, February 1. 'They're Ready to Take on Life Now.' *The Hindu*. Available at: http://www.thehindu.com/todays-paper/tp-national/tp-karnataka/article1144491.ece (accessed May 9, 2010).
The Financial Express. 2005, September 11. 'When the Differently Abled Come into Their Own.' *The Financial Express*. Available at: http://www.financialexpress.com/archive/when-the-differently-abled-come-into-their-own/144570/ (accessed May 9, 2018).
The Indian Express. 2007, December 4. 'Specially-abled Persons Should be Treated Equal.' *The Indian Express*. Available at: Indianexpress.com.
———. 2012, August 19. 'Training and Recruitment Programme for Educated Disabled Persons.' *The Indian Express*. Available at: http://archive.indianexpress.com/news/training-and-recruitment-programme-for-educated-disabled-persons/990239/ (accessed May 9, 2018).

The Times of India. 2011, July 30. 'Disabled as Good as Regular Employees.' *The Times of India.* Available at: http://timesofindia.indiatimes.com/city/gurgaon/Disabled-as-good-as-regular-employees/articleshow/9416284.cms (accessed May 9, 2018).

Venugopal, V. 2010, December 13. 'Left Out in the Workplace.' *The Hindu.* Available at: http://www.thehindu.com.

Wendell, Susan. 1997. 'Toward a Feminist Theory of Disability.' In *The Disability Studies Reader,* edited by Lennard J. Davis, 260–78. London: Routledge.

Wilton, R. D. 2004. 'From Flexibility to Accommodation? Disabled People and the Reinvention of Paid Work.' *Transactions of the Institute of British Geographers* 29 (4): 420–32.

Wolbring, G. 2006. 'Ableism and NBICS.' Available at: http://www.innovationwatch.com/choiceisyours/choiceisyours.2006.08.15.htm (accessed 11 January 2012).

———. 2008. 'The Politics of Ableism.' *Development* 51 (2): 252–58.

PART 6

Legal Discourses of Disability in India

Chapter 22

A Disability Studies Reading of the Law for Persons with Disabilities in India

Amita Dhanda

Before evaluating lawmaking from a disability studies perspective, it is necessary to examine how lawmaking is commonly understood. Even as customs and judicial decisions are accorded the status of law, such status is more evolutionary than created. In comparison to custom and judicial decisions, enacting legislation is a direct act of lawmaking. The law in legislation continues to grow through judicial interpretation, but interpretation is ordinarily perceived as refining or embellishing a finished product. In more recent times, courts have written judgements which are seen less as judicial decisions and more as judicial legislations. Insofar as such lawmaking is occasional and not seen as primary role of the courts, this article shall not concern itself with it. Instead the focus of the chapter shall be on the making of law by enacting legislations.

In formalist understanding, the power of enacting the law resides with the State. Since India is a federal polity, this power is divided between the Union and the states according to subjects specified in Lists I and II of the Seventh Schedule, respectively. According to this schedule, disability as a subject resides with the states. However, since the power to make law to enforce international obligations resides with the Union and legislative intervention in the field of disability has been prompted to fulfil such obligation, the Union has emerged as the primary lawmaker in the field. India has opted for a parliamentary form of government, which means that the party which enjoys majority in the house forms the government. And whilst the enactment of legislation is undertaken by the Union or state legislature, the executive which is constituted by the party in power is generally expected to initiate the process of enactment.

For this enactment to clear the test of legality, it would need to pass the test of jurisdiction, that is, the body making the law should have the power to make it. The enactment is undertaken according to prescribed procedure, which includes matters such as the house in which it is introduced or the number of readings, the examination by parliamentary select committees and so on. The legislation should not breach fundamental rights, which means that the State should exercise its powers whilst respecting the rights of the people. Any crossing of the permissible limits could render the legislation unconstitutional. Since this consequence ensues only after a judicial pronouncement, till such pronouncement is made, the enactment is presumed to be constitutional. This rule itself brings home how despite allowing the people to question state power, the legislators continue to wield power and dictate meaning till the people are able to convince the courts that their interpretation of the fundamental rights should trump the enunciation from the State. A far from easy task for anyone, but especially onerous for persons with disabilities as the attributions of independence, reason and autonomy, which post-enlightenment were presumed to be possessed by all humans (or rather all men), was routinely denied to them (Davies 2017).

This denial emanated from dominant perceptions of disability as deficit—an inadequacy which needed to be fixed by significant others such as educators, trainers and medical or rehabilitation professionals. The same deficiency was cited as the reason behind denying autonomy to persons with disabilities (Mackelprang and Salsgiver 2016). Depending upon the nature and severity of impairment, the authority to decide for persons with disabilities was conferred on others be it family, guardian, a designated trust or other such like individuals and authorities (Arstein-Kerslake 2017). In consequence of the non-recognition of legal personhood, the exclusionary properties of laws relating to persons with disabilities were firstly questioned by the non-disabled, who also constructed the charter of socioeconomic entitlements for persons with disabilities. These non-disabled perspectives still largely occupy the spaces of lawmaking on disability. In this chapter, it is this legal regime on disabilities put in place from non-disabled perspectives that shall be used as the comparator to the disability studies approach to lawmaking.

Unlike the non-disabled perspectives on lawmaking, the Disability Studies Approach accords primacy to the voice of persons with disabilities. The approach challenges the primacy accorded to the allegedly objective knowledge possessed by professionals of the human mind and body. Such claims of objectivity are made because the process of peer review, whereby this professional power is accorded exclusive authority to determine knowledge, is an unquestioned but invisible process. This power denies the experiential understanding possessed by persons with disabilities, the status of knowledge. Disability studies demonstrate how the processes of formulating rules to recognize authentic knowledge were discriminatory as they were made without the participation of persons with disabilities and oblivious of the disability perspective. Thus, the recognition or non-recognition of a body of knowledge greatly depends upon the connection between power and knowledge. This power is possessed by professionals operating in the field of disability and denied to persons with disabilities.

This insight also informed negotiations on the Convention on the Rights of Persons with Disabilities (hereinafter CRPD). The CRPD, unlike the other instruments of the United Nations on disability has been drafted, adopted and is being enforced with active participation of persons with disabilities. Nothing about us without us, the ruling slogan during the CRPD negotiations, epitomized the resistance of persons with disabilities at several critical junctures. Disabled people drew upon the slogan to push back retrograde provisions and to incorporate text which they perceived to be more in accord with their rights and aspirations. To illustrate, the CRPD does not have a provision which permits the use of forced treatment; guardianship has not been expressly endorsed; and even as all other United Nations instruments prior to the CRPD find explicit mention in the preamble, the MI principles of 1991, which allowed compulsory treatment and guardianship, were not included due to the active resistance of the World Network of Users and Survivors of Psychiatry. Further unlike the other United Nations instruments on disability, which primarily concentrated on socioeconomic rights, the CRPD has addressed both civil–political and socioeconomic rights.

In this chapter, I contend that the recognition of the voice of persons with disabilities in the CRPD has made it possible to undertake lawmaking from a disability studies perspective. The chapter therefore firstly elaborates on how the absence of this perspective has impacted upon the making of disability laws in the country and next dwells on what a disability studies compliant approach would require from lawmaking in India. I initiate this inquiry by firstly examining the disability-centric legislations subsisting on the statute book before the CRPD. I next examine the processes by which lawmaking on disability was undertaken after the CRPD and how despite wide ranging consultations the laws were not made in accord with the demands of the sector. Since a disability studies approach would not brook such a consequence, I conclude the chapter by enunciating what procedures would be needed to be adopted for lawmaking to be informed by the insights of disability studies.

LAWMAKING ON DISABILITY BEFORE THE CRPD

The traditional approach towards making laws for persons with disabilities can be tracked through the four disability legislations which were inducted into the Indian Statute Book from 1987 to 1999. The four legislations are the Rehabilitation Council of India Act (RCIA) of 1992, Persons with Disabilities Act (PWDA) of 1995, the National Trusts Act (NTA) of 1999 and the Mental Health Act (MHA) of 1987. The inclusion of the last named legislation in this list could be questioned as the disability status of persons with mental illness has often been questioned in India. A challenge which became sharper as the MHA excluded persons with intellectual disability from its purview. I have included it here because the statute provided the statutory justification for denying persons with mental illness of their liberty. It also put in place procedures by which persons with mental illness could lose their freedom to make decisions, and guardians of person and managers of property could be appointed to act for them. The inclusion of the MHA could be further justified by the fact that mental illness was included in the definition of disability in the PWDA. Nevertheless in recognition of its grey status, though the MHA is the earliest entrant in this pantheon, I have it bring up the rear instead of leading the way.

In what follows, I especially highlight those aspects of the aforesaid legislations that are antithetical to a disability studies-informed lawmaking. The description aims to highlight how persons with disabilities lose when laws are not made from a disability studies approach.

The RCI Act

The RCIA was enacted to usher in the process of licensing for rehabilitation professionals. This move was prompted by the belief that quality assurance necessity necessitated that rehabilitation services should be provided by licensed professionals This belief was promoted in a factual scenario where rehabilitation services were being provided through civil society initiatives, a number of which were started by parents who were attempting to educate and train their wards (Chauhan 1994). In the first instance by the enactment of the law, all these pioneering enterprises were rendered illegal by a legislative sleight of hand.

Subsequently, through the medium of bridge courses and other such procedures, the derecognized were brought back into the fold. And thus slowly the protest which had erupted on the enactment of the Act dissipated and died down. The RCIA displaced the self-taught culture of rehabilitation, whereby a community fought for its own inclusion by demonstrating that all kinds of minds and bodies were capable of education and learning provided opportunity was given and the right kinds of skills were employed. An evangelical zeal coupled with a high level of self-belief drove those programmes. This experiential knowledge (though not of persons with disabilities) was subsumed within the model of professionalism where an expert is only one who has been educated and trained to so operate and possesses certification, which states so. The RCIA was enacted with the aim to weed out the charlatans. However, the strategy it adopted to do so mixed the wolves and the sheep. And then in order to save the sheep from undeserved slaughter, its bridge courses opened possibilities of re-inducting the very wolves it was aiming to destroy.

A disability studies approach would not have privileged the academically trained professionals who adopted a deficit approach towards disability. Instead, it would have advantaged evidence-based knowledge whether acquired by academic study or by hands-on experience. Moreover, the manner in which any body of knowledge addressed the dignity concerns of persons with disabilities would be a relevant factor in its evaluation. The RCIA privileged the expert model of knowledge creation wherein persons with disabilities were only passive partakers of knowledge. If power provides the leverage to pronounce upon the authenticity and status of knowledge, then knowledge allows entry to the portals of power (Foucault 1980; Stehr and Ericson 1992). The RCIA model blocked this entry to the experiential knowledge possessed by persons with disabilities. Such knowledge could at best be smuggled in, if persons with disabilities acquired the recognized professional qualifications.

PWDA, 1995

Two features of the PWDA, 1995, are of special significance for the analysis being undertaken in this chapter. The first is the definition of disability, and the second is the total silence on the matter of civil-political rights of persons with disabilities. The statute provided an exhaustive list of impairments which were to be considered disability for the purposes of the statute. For the particular impairment to make the mark, it was important that the impairment should be of the degree specified in the statute. According to the PWDA, an individual was recognized as a person with disability only when the impairment made the severity cut-off of 40%. The fact that the individual due to socio-economic circumstances may have experienced more exclusion with lesser impairment or that a person with higher impairment may be able to do more due to technological or social support was accorded no significance. The attribution of disability due to association or perception was not even in the realm of contemplation.

A major consequence of the medical model of defining disability was that it objectified the human body and mind and trumped lived reality with medical diagnosis. The reason for this preference could be attributed to the fact that the definition of disability in the statute had been constructed to prioritize amongst disabilities to determine which persons with disabilities were deserving of the special entitlements of positive discrimination such as reservations in education and employment, rehabilitation and unemployment allowance, land and housing at reduced rates, employees insurance and so on. The medical measurements it was believed would identify the deserving more accurately and hence had to be relied upon for undertaking the selection process. That this so-called objectivity in not taking note of the social obstacles often ousted those who despite lower severity of impairment were more in need of affirmative action measures was not considered. Further, this exclusive focus on the severity of the impairment kept persons with disabilities entrapped in the stranglehold of severity where capabilities had to be diminished in order to obtain much-needed support. The demands of dignity were compromised. From a statist perspective, it was important to ensure that there were no wrongful inclusions, and the dignity losses such procedures may ensue got dismissed as necessary evils. From a disability perspective, wrongful exclusion and the manner in which an entitlement was distributed were equally important. The travails surrounding the disability card provide a useful example. Persons with disabilities sought a permanent card which was valid across the country. Even when the demand was conceded, caveats on time and place of validity were continually added.

The PWDA may have adopted a more holistic definition of persons with disability if the statute was not only limited to socioeconomic rights but also extended to civil-political rights and also took on board the need to address questions of discrimination and prejudicial exclusion. Once human rights are accepted as indivisible, the demands of dignity and choice are automatically factored into the calculation. This delicate balance gets lost when enunciation of rights is restricted to any one manifestation. Since socioeconomic rights are progressively realizable and limited by economic capacity, dignity is routinely compromised in making provision for them. The struggles surrounding reasonable accommodation are a case in point.

In comparison to socioeconomic rights, civil-political rights are articulated in more non-negotiable terms. Both their immediate availability and their justiciability contribute to this perception. This non-negotiability causes civil-political rights to be more routinely asserted without embarrassment or shame (Shue 1996). There was no mention of civil-political rights in the PWDA, and this looming absence, in my view, greatly contributed to the denial of autonomy, agency and voice to persons with disabilities. The PWDA allowed for persons with disabilities to be beneficiaries, and this dominant identity infantilized them and failed to advance their claims of citizenship.

NTA 2000

In comparison to the other two statutes, this legislation was envisioned as a special law for persons with autism, cerebral palsy, mental retardation and multiple disabilities. The enactment (which remains on the statute book) was enacted to answer the perennially expressed concern of parents, of what would happen to their wards after them. The original idea was that the Trust would be a pubic kitty for persons with the specified disabilities, and the beneficiaries would obtain benefits or services commensurate to the contribution made by their parents or guardians. Since such a classification would not withstand a constitutional challenge on equality, this investment-linked plan was dropped even before the legislation was introduced in the Parliament. For the rest, in the first five years of its existence, the Trust promoted guardianship as the means of providing protection to persons with specified disabilities.

Guardianship as a legal artefact may be of some benefit, if at all, to those persons with disabilities who had resources or property, and the guardian as caretaker ensured that the resources or property were not frittered away. Guardianship means nothing to people who have no resources. And guardianship systems are not self-implementing nor do they guard against the abuse of power by the guardians themselves. Except for the fact that the NTA allowed for the appointment of guardians through a highly simplified procedure, there was little proactive protection that was being provided by the Trust to persons with the named disabilities. Even as local-level committees started to be set up in nearly all the districts of the country, the process of the Committee appointing guardians only started in 2003–04 when 810 guardians were appointed by the local-level committee. As the numbers climbed and four-digit numbers were reported by the Trust in its 2007–08 Report, the highest reported number was 2,875 in 2004–05. The statutory provision and its subsequent implementation did not obtain as much traction as its welfare schemes such as *Niranmaya*. The Trust took a more empowering pathway when it launched a series of support-based schemes such as *Samartha* and *Sahyogi*.

The NTA as already stated was a statutory effort to put in place a regime which provided protection with substitution. However, the statute unlike most laws on guardianship did not make the appointment of a guardian an all or nothing game. Section 14(3) of the NTA required the local-level committee to consider whether the individual concerned needed a guardian at all, and if yes, then for what purposes? The subtext of this provision was that just the fact of the impairment did not render a person legally incompetent. This provision allowed guardianship to not be a mechanical formality, which the Trust facilitated. Instead of relying on this section and other provisions which obligated the Trust to encourage self-advocacy and autonomous living, the Trust could invest in building the competencies of persons with the specified disabilities.

From 2005 onwards, the Trusts directed its attention towards social change, and instead of seeking to have their wards adjust to the expectations of society, it moved to change social understanding of its wards and made a series of pro-active interventions. Thus, the *Badhte Kadam* campaign was an awareness-building program which travelled through the length and breadth of the country celebrating the capabilities of persons with disabilities. The campaign was operating on the insight that social acceptance was integral to the growth of capabilities. With social acceptance, the inherent capabilities would grow and develop, whereas social disbelief or rejection would cause the inherent capabilities to shrivel up and die. On a similar logic, the Trust launched ARUNIM in its own effort to encourage entrepreneurship in persons with disabilities and to market the products made by persons with disabilities in a competitive manner. There was an effort to launch a support persons scheme to facilitate independent living along with drafting persons with disabilities into leadership positions whereby they could present their point of view from a position of power. Along with these path-breaking initiatives, the Trust also undertook more traditional welfare programmes such as a health insurance scheme and group living projects.

The NTA was a legislation which had interspersed in its largely protective regime some stray provisions which expressed the aspiration for self-reliance and autonomy. In shifting its programmatic attention towards the realization of those goals of self-reliance, the Trust demonstrated that like protection, self-reliance also required time, attention and investment. Such time, attention and investment were routinely granted to the non-disabled because they were presumed capable and equally routinely denied to persons with disabilities. I have focused attention on the NTA programmatic experiment because it shows the importance of perspective. The disability-friendly approach of NTA allowed many more people with disabilities to take charge of their lives because they were presumed capable of doing so, and this happened without changing the law. The Trust or rather the then chairperson's effort to change the law and to bring the NTA in conformity with the CRPD faced a lot more opposition and ultimately (as the next section would show) could only provide food for thought and some forward-looking discourse.

After India's ratification of the CRPD, the National Trust was the first State entity to explore how universal legal capacity and support could be inducted into law. Insofar as the legislation had a nominal recognition to the fact of support, the first round of reform effort attempted to expand the list of beneficiaries to also include persons with mental illness. This move met with great resistance from the representatives of the existing beneficiaries as they believed they would be stigmatized by association. It was next proposed that let the support needs of all persons with disabilities be addressed by the National Trust. In order to obtain traction for the support model, in one of the many amendment proposals, it was next suggested that let the NTA incorporate a provision whereby a National Support Mission could be established. This mission was to promote alliancing between all vulnerable groups whether disabled or non-disabled.

All these proposals generated a lot of fire and heat. They also promoted a more progressive discourse around universal legal capacity and support. However, the resistance to the proposal showed the double consciousness subsisting within the disability community which caused them to simultaneously seek acceptance for themselves from the non-disabled world and refuse entry to others with less glamorous impairments. This resistance ultimately resulted in the NTA not being amended in any manner due to the CRPD. As failed efforts also carry their own lessons, the NTA amendments provide live illustrations on what lawmaking for all from a disability rights perspective could be made to do.

MHA

The MHA replaced the Indian Lunacy Act of 1912. The statute was ostensibly enacted to replace the unscientific outmoded lunacy law, which it did by abandoning the pejorative language of the Lunacy law with more therapeutic terminology. The metaphor of illness and cure was employed to veil the custodial objectives of the law (Dhanda 2000). Thus, the practice of compulsory care was continued only in this legislative manifestation in which therapeutic reasons were added to the social control motivations of the repealed Lunacy law. The practice of appointing guardians of person and property was also continued. And significantly, whilst the powers of medical practitioners, especially of the psychiatric kind, were upgraded, the person with mental illness was further demoted. The Lunacy Act allowed a person who had voluntarily sought treatment to also seek discharge, and the hospital was obligated to release the voluntary patient within a period of 24 hours. In comparison, the MHA introduced a provision whereby even a voluntary patient could be retained in the psychiatric hospital provided a medical board opined that such retention was in the interest of health and safety. Incompetence, dangerousness to self and others, and the stereotypical perceptions in relation to persons with mental illness were present in full measure in the MHA. This statute in more ways than one reinforced stereotype of the dangerous incompetent person with disability for persons with mental illness.

The MHA can be perceived as the ideational counterpoint to the disability studies approach as it treats persons with mental illness as objects that have to be fixed, and being objects, their will and preference had little meaning. A protest was permissible, but primarily for persons who were misdiagnosed. A person with mental illness who was correctly diagnosed was not seen as a bearer of rights. The same fear of wrongful denial of autonomy and choice informed the chapter providing for the appointment of guardians of person and mangers of property. Once the threshold condition of mental illness was established, the other grounds of dangerousness and incompetence were virtually presumed. The law thus sealed the subsisting social prejudice against persons with mental illness.

LAWMAKING AFTER THE CRPD

As already mentioned, both the text of the CRPD and the process of making it privileged the voice of persons with disabilities. Article 4(3) of the CRPD specifically obligated states to not make laws or policies concerning persons with disabilities including children with disabilities without consulting with them through their organizations.

In the lawmaking process, which was launched in the country after India ratified the CRPD, this obligation was surely observed in the letter. The question that I wish to raise is that whether it was observed in spirit? And if it was not observed in spirit, then can it be seen as fulfilment of the mandate of the CRPD or more importantly for this chapter: would a nominal participation of persons with disabilities in the lawmaking process be viewed as lawmaking stemming from a disabilities studies perspective.

In what follows, I outline the process, which preceded the enactment of the Persons with Disabilities Act, 2016, and the Mental Health

Care Act of 2017. The process of preparing the law was started by both the ministries of social justice and empowerment (hereinafter MSJE) and the ministry of health (hereinafter MOH) setting up committees to prepare draft legislations. Whilst the MSJE set up a high-powered committee, which provided representation to central and state governments, non-governmental organizations and persons with disabilities, it addressed the issue of technical expertise by having a disability communications specialist, who was also parent to a young man with cerebral palsy, head the Committee and appointed the Centre for Disability Studies of a law school as a legal consultant to the Committee. The MOH opted for a technocratic team of a psychiatrist and a law professor to formulate the draft. The drafts of both legislations were opened for consultations, though the extent of the consultation was far from the same. The MHCA was deliberated upon in a couple of meetings called by the MOH in Delhi and Bangalore. The PWDA draft was translated in every major language of the Union, and the Committee travelled with it to the capital of every major state in the country. Significantly, the Committee invited suggestions from the people at every state capital it visited. A number of these suggestions were incorporated with due acknowledgement in the final Bill submitted by the Committee to the government.

The drafts put out by the MHCA Committee operated on the principle that psychiatric treatment was beneficial for persons with psychiatric illness, and the law should facilitate access to such treatment. This insight was incorporated in the legislation by making ambulance services available, making available essential mental health services in each district, creating an essential drugs list and making the drugs available free of cost at all community health centres and above all, providing insurance for mental illness on an equal basis with physical illness and making government reimburse the expenses incurred if any essential medication was found to be unavailable. The therapeutic tilt of the statute can also be deduced from the manner in which it addressed matters of autonomy, consent and choice. Thus, the statute prohibits the use of certain parameters for determining mental illness, along with laying down competencies a person with mental illness should possess to make treatment decisions. The use of support did not negate the presence of legal capacity. A provision is made for advance directives and nominated representatives. The latter entity could come into operation by force of law, even if the person with disability has not nominated anyone and the advance directives may not be followed if the treating doctors think otherwise. Both quasi-judicial and judicial reviews are available to a person aggrieved with an order, but the disagreement of the person receiving treatment is at no place accepted as a reason not to administer treatment. The CRPD requires support to be constituted in accordance with the will and preference of the person with disability. The MHCA makes the matter of will and preference a contest between legal and medical professionals. The will and preference of a person with disability would be respected provided a medical or legal authority agrees with it. These core features of the MHCA were in place from the very first draft put out by the expert committee. Subsequent drafts saw greater sophistication of language and sequencing of legal provisions, but the substance of the law did not dramatically change. It is true that the MHCA was subjected to lower public participation than the PWDA. Disabled people and their organizations asked for a reconsideration of the manner in which questions of will and preference were addressed; however, the legislation reached the Standing Committee of Parliament without any amendments being introduced in the law. Some changes were introduced in the MHCA as finally enacted, but these changes primarily came on the suggestion of the Standing Committee who heeding to the representations of the people asked the government to change a few of the ancillary provisions of the Act, and the core legislation except for semantic modifications remained intact.

The PWDA was exposed to a trajectory opposite to that of the MHCA. The original preparation was undertaken with the active involvement of all stakeholders. There was governmental representation, but evidently the Committee was perceived as a civil society venture, hence the governmental members preferred to observe a strategic silence. The silence was broken when the PWDA Committee draft began to be considered in government circles. Every draft issued out by the government diluted an additional feature of the Committee draft. This process of undermining the Committee's draft came to such a pass that the ministry planned to introduce the PWD Bill, 2013, in the Parliament without making its content public. The text of the Bill got leaked, and the resulting furore caused the government to step back. As a result, the legislation was reworked, and a hurriedly upgraded PWD Bill, 2014, was instead of being enacted only introduced in the Rajya Sabha. The Bill was subsequently sent to the parliamentary standing committee on welfare, which yet again undertook a process of consultation and submitted its report. The Committee noted the dissatisfaction of civil society with the continuance of the guardianship provisions and asked the government to address the matter. The recommendation was noted but no more happened.

THE ROLE OF DISABLED PEOPLE AND THEIR ORGANIZATIONS IN LAWMAKING

There is a need to ask this question on the role of the Disabled People's Organisation's (DPO) because at the end of the day, after six years of consultation, the new act enhanced the number of impairments covered by the law, but restricted the beneficiaries of affirmative action measures. Thus, reservations in education and employment, social security and other concessional measures are only being extended to persons with benchmark disability. Civil-political rights were accorded a notional mention. The recognition of legal capacity was confused, and guardianship was retained. Each of these choices is contrary to the consensus reached during the wide-ranging consultations undertaken through the length and breadth of the country. Ultimately, the law whilst tipping its hat at the CRPD primarily inducted what the State was willing to concede.

The question this chapter is raising is not whether what the government did was better or worse? The central question of this chapter is that if the State can go ahead and enact exactly what it would have enacted without the consultation, then what is the purpose of the consultation? Is the mandate of Article 4(3) of the CRPD fulfilled just by holding a consultation? If one looks at the text of the article, such a contention can be made. However, if the purpose for including the obligation in the Convention is examined, then the answer has to be in the negative. The purpose of placing this obligation was to give room for the voice of persons with disabilities to be heard. Consultation is about dialogue about reciprocity. Charade consultations cannot be seen to fulfil that requirement.

If the aforesaid conclusion is correct, then it is important to ask what next? Does the holding of a charade consultation nullify the law made subsequent to it? If this query is answered in the negative, then why would governments follow such like directives? And would an affirmative answer be an invitation to chaos?

Being not consulted or being roped into charade consultations is not unique to persons with disabilities. Such like procedures are also practised on the non-disabled and other vulnerable groups. Would I allow for such a consequence to ensue when they are subjected to similar non-consultative lawmaking? Or is this consequence only limited to persons with disabilities? I would answer this question by firstly distinguishing between the non-disabled and other vulnerable groups. The other vulnerable groups are in a position similar to persons with disabilities, and non-consultation with them should yield similar consequences, especially if their presence in governance structures is as sparse as that of persons with disabilities. This is of special relevance to persons with disabilities, as they are both the victims of wrongful attribution and unfair exclusion. Consultation is a way of filling knowledge gaps and offsetting prejudice subsisting against vulnerable groups. The consequences should be inversely proportional to the absence experienced by the particular constituency. The greater is the exclusion, the stronger is the consequence. Thus, the invalidation of the law could be the strongest consequence, which could be followed by mandatory involvement of the constituency in the rule-making process. Directions to induct the concerns of the vulnerable group whilst implementing the law or an obligation to provide a reasoned response to the representations of the people could be other ways of addressing governmental recalcitrance.

This DS approach to lawmaking could be used by all citizens to challenge State monopoly in lawmaking. Such monopoly, I think, needs to be questioned as I agree with Aristotle when he holds that good citizens need to be both rulers and ruled, and there can be no training in playing rulers if citizens are only passive recipients of legal products made by the State. Just an enhancement of the consultation-linked obligations in the law cannot on its own usher change. If the existence of legal provisions could ensure compliance, then there would be no need to introduce the aforesaid sanctions on sham or no consultation. As the sanctions again are legal provisions, how would their induction improve matters? A deeply felt obligation to act according to the law is integral to any rule of law society. The fact that they are acting according to the law and not on whim and caprice is a claim which substantially contributes to the legitimacy of power wielders. The desire of lawmakers to be seen to act in accordance with the law is the resource on which citizens need to draw to obtain conformity from State authorities. The existence of this desire makes it worthwhile to induct citizen-friendly practices such as informed consultation in the law.

CONCLUSION

Consultation alone may not make the voice of the people heard, but consultation is the vital first step. It opens the doors for conversation and demonstrates how lawmaking is continuous and evolving and not one time and fixed. The act of creating legal meaning should be inclusive of all people and not excluding of any. The disability studies approach could allow for such democratization of lawmaking, the benefit of which could extend beyond disability. However in the first instance, persons with disabilities could use the CRPD banner to press for lawmaking which is in active engagement with the disability studies approach even if not in strict conformity with it. The analysis in this chapter showed how the present spate of lawmaking in disability made short shrift of the demands of the disability studies approach and primarily relied upon statist perspectives to enact the laws. This sidelining needs to be challenged and course correction demanded, if the voices of persons with disabilities are not to be yet again muffled and silenced. As it stands, the statist and disability studies approach have been so conflated that the hard-won right of participation stands compromised. There is need to devise strategies of recovery, some of which have been suggested in this chapter.

REFERENCES

Arstein-Kerslake, Anna. 2017. *Restoring Voice to People with Cognitive Disabilities.* Cambridge: Cambridge University Press.

Chauhan, R. S. 1994. The Triumph of the Spirit: The Pioneers of Education and Rehabilitation Services for the Visually Handicapped in India. New Delhi: Konark Publisher.

Davies, Margaret. 2017. *Law Unlimited.* Melbourne: Taylor & Francis.

Dhanda, Amita. 2000. *Legal Order and Mental Disorder.* New Delhi: SAGE Publications.

Foucault, Michel. 1980. *Power/Knowledge: Selected Interviews and Other Writings 1972–77.* New York: Pantheon Books.

Mackelprang, Romel W., and Richard Salsgiver. 2016. *Disability: A Diversity Model Approach in Human Service Practice.* Oxford: Oxford University Press.

Shue, Henry. 1996. *Basic Rights: Subsistence, Affluence, and U.S. Foreign Policy.* Princeton: Princeton University Press.

Chapter 23

Reimagining Kinship in Disability-specific Domesticity
Legal Understanding of Care and Companionship

Rukmini Sen

According to the Rights of Persons with Disabilities Act, 2016, a caregiver has been defined as 'any person including parents and other family members who with or without payment provide care, support or assistance to a person with disability'. In contrast, the caregiver in the Mental Healthcare Bill, 2016, is 'a person who resides with a person with mental illness and is responsible for providing care to that person and includes a relative or any other person who performs this function, either free or with remuneration'. The most important difference in these two legal definitions of caregiver, which itself is an absolutely new idea in the Indian legislative framework, is that of the residential requirement. In the latter, the caregiver needs to reside with the person with mental illness, which is not the case in the former law. This chapter will be an attempt to understand and conceptualize care in the context of disability—to trace backwards into the disability movement as well as judgements on persons with disabilities in India to unearth how care has come into the legal landscape for persons with disabilities. Clearly, there has been a shift from the 'naturalness' of care, to be provided usually by women of the family within the domesticity to 'skilled' care to be also offered by women inside the familial space. The economy of care has undoubtedly brought into the fold a legal need to recognize the caregiver, mainly because the function of caring is shifting hands from the 'familial' to the 'professional'.

Similar to the concept of care entering the disability legislation, family and its responsibility towards the child/adult with disability also have found space in the 2016 Act. This chapter will also explore the trajectory shift from the independent living movement of the US disability legislation dominating the Indian framework as well, in the early 1990s, towards a discourse on locating the disabled person within the family and community while implying interdependence and not just dependence through it. The right of the disabled child to be with the family and the entitlement of an adult disabled person to form a family are both ensured through this legislation.

Through this chapter, this parallel, yet interconnected, thread of care and companionship (within the family), which is now part of the Indian legal landscape for persons with disabilities, will be assessed. It is necessary to map as well as argue that these entitlements have not entered our legislation merely because the 2007 United Nations Conventions of the Rights of Persons with Disabilities had these provisions. Rather, it is necessary to inscribe that parents' associations as well as women's movement activists had played an important role in shaping the movement discourse on disability in India. There is thus an inherent connect that the disability movement has with many other social movements in India, and the present legislation, which is markedly different from the 1995 one, owes its existence to this intersecting manner in which disability has emerged as an issue. It is therefore important to locate disability and disability-specific domesticities within the kinship matrix. Personal zencounters with age-related disability in the immediate family and an academic interest in new kinds of kinships emergent in the neoliberal care economy are the primary reasons to explore the politico-legal landscape of care and kin/kin-like companionship keeping persons with disabilities at the centre of this enquiry.

This chapter around the (legal) meanings of care is at one elementary level, a difference drawn between the noun care and the verb care. Care as provision and care as a feeling of affection show an important distinction marked in legal discourses around illness and disability. In fact, one of the ways to map disability legislations in India is a shift from the absence of care provisions to the acknowledgement of right to care of the person with disability. However, the latter is couched within the right to health framework, more within care as health care provision, rather than care as affection. A 2014 report on Right to Health of Persons with Disabilities in India only focuses on health care services—questions of access to and discrimination experienced, post access of these services by persons with disabilities. In a context where right to health and health care services did not find any mention in the Persons with Disabilities Act (1995), it is important to ascertain how in the recent 2016 Act, care has been addressed, albeit within the health discourse. It may be worth interrogating the care jurisprudence around disability in India, which is what this chapter intends to discuss by interpreting provisions of the different laws.

CARE IN A RIGHTS-BASED LEGISLATION

According to the Rights of Persons with Disabilities Act, 2016, caregiver has been defined as 'any person including parents and other family members who with or without payment provide care, support or assistance to a person with disability'. Similarly, an institution is defined as one for the reception, 'care', protection, education, training, rehabilitation and any other activities for persons with disabilities. In the section on home and family, there is a concern expressed in the law about a condition in which when the parents are incapable to take 'care' of a child with disability, then the competent court needs to ensure care from near relations or from community-based familial setting or from a government- or non-government-run shelter home. Within the section on social security, health, rehabilitation and recreation, health 'care services' and prenatal, perinatal and postnatal 'care' of mother and child have been included. In a section on human resource development, there is a provision to 'initiate capacity building programmes including training in independent living and community relationships for families, members of community and other stakeholders and *care providers* on *care giving* and support'. Let us try to assess conceptually the different meanings in which care finds place in the 2016 legislation as distinct from the 1995 one and of course as a post United Nations Convention on the Rights of Persons with Disabilities (UNCRPD) law. Firstly, with respect to institutional care, there is an understanding of the service provision of care. This service necessarily includes availability and attendance of doctors and nurses, and other kinds of treatment-related support that the person with disability requires. This provision is mostly about the need to locate care within health care services and the right to health framework of Constitutional obligations. This notion of care compliments the pre- and postnatal care of the mother and the child, another health care service that has become important and necessary service within the mother and child schemes as well as reproductive rights of the pregnant woman. Secondly, the kind of care that is expected to be extended to a child with disability is another provision of the legislation. This comes as a clear response to the concern that children with disability are either hidden from the family and kinship networks or are uncared for. Similar kind of provision exists since 1999 through the National Trust for Welfare of Persons with Autism, Cerebral Palsy, Mental Retardation and Multiple Disabilities Act which has in its objectives the need to promote measures for the care and protection of persons with disability in the event of death of their parent or guardian. What is important to note is that the legal ideas on care were present and imagined for people with specific kinds of disability, and post their legal age for adulthood, when they legally required a guardian. This legislation was contained within the 1990s human rights framework of independent living but in close connection and support from within the family and community. However, what is necessary to foreground is that the notion of welfare, support and care was all thought only with respect to those kinds of disabilities which were assumed to cause 'more' dependence and required a legal recourse to get support by the parent/guardian and care after the death of the parent/guardian. It is quite clear that the life of the parent/guardian was construed in relation to the child with autism or cerebral palsy or other forms of disability as separate from those identified in the Persons with Disabilities Act of 1995. The most important paradigmatic shift that has taken place in the 2016 legislation is the right of any child with disability towards parental care, in the absence of it care from family/community. If that also seems not possible to be found, then care through shelter homes is an option. Thirdly, a context in which care is identified in this legislation is that of the caregiver/care provider. An Indian legislation specifically mentioning a caregiver in the context of disability clearly indicates the manner in which a care economy has been recognized. More importantly, the care giver could be one who is paid or not—this itself means that care is a service and not merely labour that is meted out primarily by women domestic/professional caregivers or women of the family extending support and care towards family members with disability. Through the former, that activity which has constantly been naturalized as a role that women perform now gets a legal acknowledgement, in the category/language of the caregiver. The latter reinforces the care industry reality and thereby the need for capacity building of the care providers. This also indicates that caring is a function that can be learnt or at least the skills of it can be improved. Not only is there a formalization of the care roles, there is also an expectation about a set of people being present in order to take charge of the care functions. This comes through this argument that 'this continuous responsibility, in the absence of any formal support networks, has many negative consequences for caregivers, including the suppression of feelings such as not wanting to do it anymore' (Chakravarti 2008, 354). Another important difference that is needed to be remembered in this context is that between the paid caregiver (usually women) and the unpaid caregiver (usually women of the domestic space)—while for the former, care is work, for the latter, care is a duty or a role tied around the effect of love, from which there cannot be any respite. 'Love, in this context, often becomes fractured or distorted by feelings of obligation, burden and frustration. But the prevailing ethos of family based care suggests that normal tasks are being performed, that roles enacted are straightforward, expected and unproblematic' (Chakravarti 2008, 360). In most care scholarship, what has been the focus is the paid care worker/giver. The context of the care work however can vary along two continuums: public- to market-based work, and formal to informal work, and care workers may be hired as public servants, self-employed care workers, care workers operating in informal markets, family assistants and informal family care workers (Zelnick 2017, 3). Since care has to be understood in cultural contexts, it becomes necessary to talk about the woman in the family emerging as the primary caregiver in Indian contexts as distinct from the paid woman care worker. Caring as part of housework and care work as a constituent of care industry are the binary through which care operates; and the (scholarly, legal, economic) focus being on the latter questions around work conditions, work locations, minimum wages and other kinds of social security measures becomes irrelevant in the context of care as inclusive of housework. Also, caring for others may lead to the non-existence, if not a complete denial, of physically and culturally caring for the self.

In all of these four senses in which care is present in the Rights of Persons with Disabilities Act, 2016, there is a continuous attempt to create the functional/service-oriented aspect of care. Care as feeling is assumed and naturalized even in this legislative framework. In other words, care in the affection/affective sense cannot be spoken about or imagined in a legislative discourse. Does this mean that the legislation promotes altruism of a certain kind to be continued within the familial relations? Unless any discussion happens within the disability movement spaces around rearrangement of domestic responsibilities or equal sharing towards caring for the disabled child or (disabled) elderly, a legal recognition of care services in itself does not suffice for the complexities around the question of care. Moreover, an assumption that members of a family will be caring towards each other, however, may not perform the services of caring, and therefore, the need for the law to emphasize on the familial responsibility towards caring for the disabled child (only) is a limited understanding of caring for and caring about the disabled.

CONSTRUCTION OF FAMILY IN LEGISLATION FOR PERSONS WITH DISABILITY

Is there a specific need in the recent legislation on disability to have a section on family? Is family defined, constructed or its roles expected in most legislations in India? If the answer to the first question is yes and the 'second no, then there is a need to specifically talk about what makes it vital for a family to find place within a legislation whose chief objective is to' ensure that persons with disabilities enjoy the right to equality, life with dignity and respect for his or her integrity equally with others. It is at the same time relevant to foreground that a legislation, which claims to have been influenced by and came into existence due to the ratification of the UNCRPD, 2006, the meaning and the responsibilities attached to the family or from the family, is limited in the domestic legislation enacted ten years after the international convention. The UNCRPD Article 23 on respect for home and family has the primary objective of taking appropriate measures to eliminate discrimination against persons with disabilities in all matters relating to marriage, family, parenthood and relationships, on an equal basis with others. Within this broad intention, an important provision which exists taking into consideration the material denial or non-consideration around marriage of the disabled person (more specifically the woman) is that of the right of all persons with disabilities who are of marriageable age to marry and to find a family on the basis of free and full consent of the intending spouses is recognized. The Indian legislation does not include this provision in its section on home and family. Rather, it talks about the right to information that persons with disability need to have regarding reproductive and family planning. Moreover, no person with disability shall be subject to any medical procedure which leads to infertility without his or her free and informed consent. The other essential provision within home and family is about the already discussed care of the disabled child. The domestic context which leads to the emphasizing on the second provision on infertility creation could be the Pune hysterectomy case (for details, check Rajan 2003). However, what is to be thought about is the complete legal non-recognition that there exists both discrimination and marginalization about consideration and possibilities of persons with disabilities creating their own adult relationships, marrying or parenting like any other person without some form of disability. At the same time, it is important to admit that in the chapter on Duties and Responsibilities of appropriate Governments, within a section on awareness campaigns, one such responsibility noted has been to foster respect for the decisions made by persons with disabilities on all matters related to family life, relationships, bearing and raising children. It is noteworthy to mark the absence of marriage in the Indian legislation. It is equally worth mentioning this difference between talking about issues related to making relationships, families and children within the (limited) framework of awareness campaign (2016 Act) as opposed to non-discrimination (2006 Convention). Is it enough to raise awareness or is it only through awareness raising that discrimination practised around consenting to and creation of relationships by persons with disability that will lead to the reduction of discrimination around the social denial of lack of accessing these intimate relationships? The Convention suggests that the family is the natural and fundamental group unit of society and is thereby entitled to protection by society and the State. Within this context, it is mandatory that persons with disabilities and their family members receive the necessary protection and assistance to enable these families to contribute towards the full and equal enjoyment of the rights of persons with disabilities. The role of the State in assisting the family with persons with disability is enshrined in the Convention 2006, but is not the case with respect to the 2016 Act. Rather, the latter is more interested in the function that the family/members need to perform—that of care, rather than what the State needs to ensure so that these caring functions can be effectively performed with support from the State. In India, where family is accepted to be the essential institution towards maintaining the social fabric, the irony however is that the State absolves itself from the responsibility of complimenting the familial role of care, by constructing more spaces of institutional care or providing any financial assistance towards families caring for person with disability. This dual character of naturalization and altruistic nature of care from the family only leads to the lack of intervention or responsibility of the state and its institutions towards extending support to families with disability.

TOWARDS INTERDEPENDENCE

Is there a way to talk within disability movements about care companionship and interdependence? One method of doing this is to remember what Morris (2001, 13) argued, that the disabled people's movement can redefine the meaning of independence to indicate having choice and control over the assistance required by the person with disability rather than doing everything by oneself. The other matter to take into consideration in a move from an independence to interdependence is the feminist ethic of care, which is based on a recognition of interdependence, relationships and responsibilities, and which criticizes notions of autonomy, independence and individual rights as being too much based on a masculine view of people as separate from each other. When disabled people in Britain first started to come together to challenge the prejudice they experienced in 1981, they drew on the following human rights perspective:

> All human beings have an equal right to live, to eat adequately, to housing, to clean water, to a basic standard of health and hygiene, to privacy, to education, to work, to marry (or not), have children (or not), to determine their own sexuality, to state an opinion, to participate in decisions which affect their lives, to share fully in the social life of their community and to contribute to the well being of others to the full extent of their capabilities. (General Recommendation, UN Convention on the Elimination of all Forms of Discrimination against Women)

It is also important to remember the tenets on ethics of care as Virginia Held proposed that

> ethics of care appreciates and values emotions and relational capabilities that enable morally concerned persons in actual interpersonal contexts to understand what would be best. In a sense, ethics of care accords primacy to sentimental reason, valuing reflexively some sentiments (such as sympathy, empathy, sensitivity, and responsiveness). (Baxi 2010, 6)

What is necessary to be challenged is this false binary between care and justice, rather the need to think of imaginative and practical coexistence between the two, returning to Baxi's (2010, 13) question 'How may a caring state ever happen' (p. 13)? Although in the year 2016 the disability legislation was passed by the Indian Parliament, many of the initial ideas around disability discrimination and entitlements for persons with disabilities have been accommodated, yet much still remains. The transformation to care dependence responsibility within a just (legal) framework is a political journey that needs to be worked upon continuously. Recognizing difference and politicizing interdependence could to be the basis of an ethic of care ensuring human rights for persons with disability.

REFERENCES

Baxi, Upendra. 2010. 'Justice and Care.' *India International Centre Quarterly* 37 (2, Autumn): 118–32.

Chakravarti, Upali. 2008. 'Burdens of Caring: Families of the Disabled in Urban India.' *Indian Journal of Gender Studies* 15 (2): 34163.

Jenny Morris. 2001. 'Impairment and Disability: Constructing an Ethics of Care That Promotes Human Rights.' *Hypatia* 16 (4, Autumn): 1–16. *Feminism and Disability*, Part 1.

Rajan, Rajeswari Sunder. 2003. 'Beyond the Hysterectomies Scandal: Women, the Institution, the Family and State in India.' In *The Scandal of the State: Women, Law and Citizenship in Postcolonial India*. New Delhi: Permanent Black.

Zelnick, J. R., S. Haviland, and J. C. Morgan. 2017. 'Caring for Care Workers.' *New Solutions* 27 (4): 1–9.

PART 7

Constructing Disability as Diversity

Chapter 24

Disability as Diversity
An Alternative Perspective

Shanti Auluck

I write this chapter from the epistemic location of a being a mother, advocate and academician. My experiences of disability are grounded in my close interactions with persons with intellectual and other disabilities, especially my forty-one-year-old son who has Down's syndrome.

DISABILITY AS A FORM OF HUMAN DIVERSITY

Thinking of disability as diversity is a relatively recent approach. For example, a person with visual or hearing impairment forms an understanding of the world which is unique in terms of the absence of visual or sound images. Similarly, a person with cognitive impairments has a world which is in some ways different because many complex abstract concepts are not part of his/her world. It is important to recognize that these are authentic experiences and world views. In the words of Allie Cannington (a young advocate and activist with locomotor difficulty), 'In order to harness the power, diversity and innovation of our society, we must realize that our bodies and minds experience the world very differently'.

My journey in life and my association with many friends and family members, including my son with Down syndrome, made me question the notions of disability. Unlike popular notions, they made me think 'Is living with disability a form of suffering?'. What creates 'suffering' is insensitivity of others and lack of opportunities as well as support systems. Whether or not disability is a form of human diversity is not a question that can be answered entirely in terms of logic and rationality but requires a stronger focus on the lived realities of disabled people.

Nature has created an amazing variety with each creation carrying its own unique place in the scheme of universe. It is true from the tiniest living cell to as complex a living being as humans. Similarly, the whole universe of plant, trees, flowers, planets, stars, galaxies, black holes, oceans, rivers, mountains, elements and molecules, to name a few, shows a wonderful variety, and at the same time intricately connected to each other's existence. Robert Paine (1966), a groundbreaking ecologist, found that removing what he called a 'keystone species' from an environment could profoundly affect the fortunes of neighbouring species. Paine demonstrated that certain species exert a disproportionate impact on their ecosystems and that their elimination—as a result of climate change, pollution or some other natural or man-made factors—can produce unexpected and far-reaching consequences for the local environment. Jo Chopra, (2005), founder of an NGO Karuna Vihar India, working with persons with disabilities and their families, has beautifully described how disability is a balancing factor in the human ecosystem.

DISABILITY IS A SOCIAL CONSTRUCT

When I look at the world from the standpoint of people with intellectual and other cognitive impairments, I am deeply reminded of the social construction of our world. The more I think about it, the more rooted I feel about the idea that disability is contextual.

As per the norms of majority, people with different sensory and cognitive world do become minority, and society overlooks their perceptions, experiences and needs.

My own understanding evolved as I understood social construction. I increasingly began to see the diversities of human world, and disability itself appeared as a part of this diversity. Each one of us is living in a make-believe world. Little do we realize that the perception of the world itself is arising from sensory and conceptual foundation as well as experiences in a given life circumstance. Our needs, feelings and aspirations give a different shape to our experiential world. Similarly, knowledge, learning and reflective thinking keep modifying our world view. A deeper look at our journey of life from infancy to old age itself would show that our perception of the world keeps changing during the whole lifespan. Thus, life is a series of social constructions. Some of them help us, whereas others create barriers. Rigid thinking, biases and prejudices are expressions of limited world views. This way of looking at people and the rest of creations in nature is a liberating thought. It enables one to become more accommodative of differences and resolve conflicts and difficulties with others. It paves way for greater harmony within and without. It certainly results in more humane approach towards everything. Recent court judgements (in last few years) have highlighted the controversy surrounding ableist and utilitarian notions with regard to disability. Ghai (2015) mentioned that on 21 July 2009, in a landmark decision, the Supreme Court of India allowed a nineteen-year-old mentally challenged orphan girl to carry on with a pregnancy that resulted from a sexual assault. Shruti Pandey, a human rights lawyer from Delhi, admits that this is a case that is 'so grey' that case is not about abortion per se. Rather, India's legal strictures recognize and protect the agency of a woman to take decisions for her life and body, especially all its nuances when the woman is a person with intellectual mental impairment. The plea was that an intellectually challenged mother will not be able to discharge the duties of a mother as she herself was an orphan living in Nari Niketan. Legal assistance along with a few NGOs contested this apprehension and took upon themselves to support and train this young woman to take care of her child. Today, the young woman is a proud mother of a teenage daughter who is studying in school. What an immense change in the life of the woman! She has somebody of her own in life, though she herself was abandoned by her parents. This is what support systems can do to a person. Some disability activists, like Jeeja Ghosh, a highly educated woman who has cerebral palsy, are not just disturbed, but actually angry with the judgement (see *Outlook* 2009). Similarly, the Bombay High Court had disallowed a mother to abort her child with

Down syndrome with 24 weeks of pregnancy. The judgement said 'children with DS are very loving and live well', so there was no reason for abortion. Research work with Ghai and Johri (2008) has raised the question of abortion with respect to a disabled foetus. Where do we draw a line indicates that consent and choice are problematic issues.

Can life ever be free of difficulties and sufferings? It is inevitable to go through ups and downs in life. My son (with Down syndrome) is constantly teaching me precious lessons of life. He lives in 'NOW', free from hankerings of the past and worry for future. He has the capacity for pure love because he is free from unnecessary biases and expectations. Small things make him happy. He is free from ego trappings. Both of us are like friends, understanding each other's feelings and needs. It is very interesting for me to visualize his world which is free from many constructs and conditionings, and it enabled me to view differences as diversities of human world and not a threat to my egoistic perception of the world. For past many years as I was learning to appreciate diverse viewpoints, the thought of him being 'NORMAL' does not occur to me. I have seen the limitations in the notion of 'normalcy', which excludes wonders and value of diversity.

As I mentioned earlier that disability is not necessarily a condition of suffering; this thought itself is an irony of utilitarian/perspective or attitude (Galton (1908)). As an extended argument, it means we should avoid or try to get rid of all situations that may bring difficulties and grief to us. To what extent one would go on in this pursuit. Tomorrow our healthy child or another family member may get interminable disease or disabling condition due to disease or injury. What will we do then? (Do not tell me 'that is different'!) It is the conditionings of our mind that limit our thinking. Life is a series of experiences, pleasant or unpleasant. Each experience teaches us if we are ready to take its lessons. Painful experiences have much greater potential to make us wiser, sensitive and compassionate.

CHALLENGING SELECTIVE ABORTION AND UTILITARIAN VIEW

A new kind of Eugenics is emerging in the society. It says that using growing knowledge, identify the disabling conditions in the growing foetus and eliminate it.

Recent discoveries in prenatal diagnosis have brought the utilitarian versus humanistic notions in sharp focus. Pragmatism persuades one to think that any form of disability is a suffering to the person and family. Therefore, allowing such foetuses/babies to be born puts them and their parents into misery, and such a situation should be avoided as foetus is only a potential human being and not yet achieved the status of complete person. It is a subtle form of insult to people with disability. Essence of being a human does not lie in crude pragmatism; it lies in finer human sensitivities and feelings. Life is a series of joys and sorrows. Successful dealing with such situations is a life-enhancing experience facilitating inner strengths and growth. There are several implications of diversity viewpoint. It opens up our mind to enable us to see strengths in people rather than only weaknesses. We are able to see the fighting human spirit which scales all obstacles to fulfil its aspirations and desires.

A condition becomes disabling when required facilities are not there. It is the obligation of the society to accommodate and provide facilities and services to everyone according to their needs. It is distressing to see how persons with disability and their families are made to feel apologetic, an attitude arising from a highly biased view. It is a lack of consideration for 'others' that I find very unfair and unjust. It has resulted in utter lack of services and infrastructure which is critical to people living with disabilities.

Every creation in nature is sacred, and life is a precious chance to experience this amazing and beautiful world. I am inspired by the courage and perseverance of so many of my friends who have struggled much harder in order to achieve and fulfil their aspirations as compared to others. Imagine for a moment the life of a person who uses wheelchair. He is denied simple pleasures like going out, visiting friends, attending educational institutions and all other public spaces. The extent to which life can be limited can be gazed by few examples. Imagine the life of a person on wheelchair. Can such a person go to friends' places, restaurants, markets and other recreational centres? Where is the accessibility even for using toilet? How does a person with visual impairment function in the absence of mobility and technology support? A hearing impaired person is deprived of so much information and knowledge because the social world is dominantly language based. A person with cognitive impairment is neglected by all growth opportunities, for example, appropriate education, employment and social and cultural life. Families having children with cognitive impairments have no place to go for guidance and support. It results in very impoverished learning environment as well as severe emotional difficulties. The list is endless.

Who is responsible for such deprivations? Clearly, it is the society who has been so self-centred that it never thought of millions of people who also need the same public spaces, physical and social, as rest of the population. Urbanization without care and sensitivity has added so many more dimensions to their problems.

Each and every public institution is responsible for this negligence. The benefit of technology and infrastructure rightfully belongs to every one of us. It is not a matter of favour! It is not a utopian idea; equality of opportunity is a fundamental right of everyone. We cannot accept the insensitivity arising out of selfish attitudes in the garb that it is not an ideal world.

NEED FOR SOCIAL SUPPORT SYSTEMS

An examination of our daily life will evidently show how dependent we are. Our lives would come to a stop if so many people were not providing us what we need, for example, food, clothing, medicines and many other essential things. We may term it as business venture, but the fact is that people depend upon such systems in the society. Irony is that when it comes to providing needed support systems to people with disabilities, it is considered to be burdensome and an issue of charity. Needless to say that people with disabilities do have some specific needs, but it cannot be an excuse for indifference and negligence. Interdependence is a key survival issue for the society at large, and ignoring the needs of minority groups is totally unjust. Accessible public spaces and public transportation, accessible information system, appropriate education, employment, safe living and family support systems are some of the important issues which need immediate attention of the government and society at large.

Is anyone immune to disability? An unfortunate accident can make one loose limbs, paralysis or brain damage. Majority people acquire disability as a result of ageing and debilitating diseases. How long we will remain insensitive and unresponsive to the needs of these citizens of our country? Though technology has eased many of our day-to-day struggles, it has also given us a false sense of self-sufficiency. In pursuit of individualistic concerns, we forget the role that our families and friends play in our lives. In early years of our life and old age, our survival hinges critically on human support. The gradual loss of family values in our society will sooner or later hit our lives negatively.

Another amusing viewpoint that some people cherish is that a person with disability also has some unique abilities. In search of such talents and abilities, one starts looking for extraordinary qualities in people with disabilities. This bias implicitly shows that people with disabilities are worthy of our recognition only when they have some qualities to boast about. Such a bias is more pronounced in case of people with visual impairment, intellectual disability and autism.

Every life is precious and valuable. Every creation in the world is amazing in terms of its complexity and wonderfully functioning systems. Each neuron, cell and tissue is a wonder; how well-orchestrated everything is. But human mind in its arrogance starts unfairly judging and discriminating. This arises from false sense of pride and deeply ingrained need for establishing self-importance. Nature has bestowed upon us the capacity for learning, discriminative intellect (*vivek*) and wisdom. This is a unique quality of every human being. It is our responsibility to use it for supporting and not destroying nature's intelligent manifestations. Box 24.1 captures the sentiments of a mother regarding her child with Down syndrome.

That is the story of majority children and adults with intellectual disability. We as teachers and parents, who have had the chance of observing their everyday challenges, often undergo inner transformations.

RIGHT TO EQUAL OPPORTUNITY

People with disabilities have been neglected too long by India. It was considered to be a family responsibility and not the State's responsibility

Box 24.1

> **Narrative of a child with Down syndrome as viewed by his mother:**
>
> I was born in this wonderful world like everyone else, but my parents did not rejoice. Rather they grieved. Why? You may ask!!! People call me 'mentally retarded'. If some error occurred when I was growing in my mother's womb, was that my fault? Does it really matter that I am not like majority of people in terms of my physique or intellect? Being different is not a crime. I too need love and recognition like all of you. I do have a right for respectful living! I do require education and training to grow up and develop! I too need to be as self-reliant as possible and work and earn like everyone else!
>
> Then why do I get only neglect, cold responses and ridicule!

to address the rights of people with disability. Charity attitude had been the dominant approach, and it has to change. Equal opportunities and required facilities alone will change the situation. Breaking myths about disability and access to growth opportunities, for example, education and employment, in an inclusive environment will dismantle the notions of incapacities and slowly substitute it with diversity approach. It does not need huge finances, it just demands changes in mindsets.

The State is duty bound to provide equal opportunities for health, education, accessibility infrastructure and employment and so on to all its citizens. Similarly, community/society owes the responsibility to dismantle unjust attitudes, for example, assumption of incapacity, disability as a curse, non-recognition of growth needs like education and employment and other basic human needs.

The World Bank (2011) report commissioned by the Ministry of Social Justice and Empowerment highlights the poor state of affairs of people with disabilities. Poor implementation of the commitments by the government continues despite creating a separate department in 2011 for the empowerment of people with disabilities. According to the report,

> India's implementation capacity is generally weak in a number of areas of service delivery which are most critical to improving the situation

of disabled people, and it is not realistic to expect that all the actions needed by many public and non-public actors can be taken all at once. It is important therefore to decide the most critical interventions and 'get the basics right' first. Obvious priorities include: (i) preventive care, both for mothers through nutritional interventions, and infants through both nutrition and basic immunization coverage; (ii) identifying people with disabilities as soon as possible after onset. The system needs major improvements in this most basic function; (iii) major improvements in early intervention, which can cost effectively transform the lives of disabled people and their families, and their communities; and (iv) expanding the under-developed efforts to improve societal attitudes to people with disabilities, relying on public-private partnerships that build on successful models already operating in India.

Education, employment, issuance of disability certificates and so on remain critical issues. The Rights of Persons with Disabilities Act has been enacted by the Parliament in December 2016. The system of implementation is yet to be in place. The Right to Education Act along with the RPD Act, 2016, gives pretty good mandate for creating opportunities for education, but it requires thoughtful systems and preparations to make it happen. There is a lack of convergence of various ministries, for example, health, education, employment and several others to bring change in the situation. Accountability systems are not there to hold the departments responsible for poor implementations.

The situation can change! It demands examining one's attitude, sensitivity and recognition of interdependence in the society. Only then it can claim to be an evolved and civilized society.

REFERENCES

Galton, F. 1908. *Memories of my Life*. Methuen and Co.
Outlook. 2009, September 14. 'A Dissenting Note.' *Outlook*.
World Bank. 2011. *World Report on Disability*. Washington, DC: World Bank.

Chapter 25

Unification of Disability in Diversity
A Different Voice

Anita Ghai

I write from a clearly marked location as a disabled woman with visible disability. Critically, I write as an academician who is in the process of designing a disability studies programme in Ambedkar University. In the volume, I have focused on diversity and its connection to disability. Many scholars have taken up diversity as an all-embracing and enticing term, as its potential is of including marginalized categories with a clear assumption that disability would inevitably be a part of the discourse on diversity. My submission is that disability to my mind has escaped critical scrutiny.

In the Indian scenario, the calls for inclusion are often met by a patronizing tokenism, which argues that though exclusion of disability is real, society and its concomitant systems are powerless to challenge its perfectionist norms. The vulnerability results from a normative mode that cannot meaningfully understand the anxieties associated with body disintegration. Theoretically, there are very strong threads common to humanity, which binds us, but in practice, exclusion is rampant. Diversity attracts an erudite liberal responsiveness, making society create a politically correct and a 'feel good' understanding about marginalized and disadvantaged categories of people.

We do recognize that complexity of diversity is to be underscored, as each diverse community represents unique issues, opportunities and approaches. Couser (2005, 96) for instance validates diversity by affirming the fact that '[d]isability is an inescapable element of human experience. Although it is rarely acknowledged as such, it is also a fundamental aspect of human diversity. It is so, first, in the sense that, world-wide, an enormous number of people are disabled'. Similarly, Davis (2015, 61) presents the following simple definition of diversity: 'that despite differences, we are all the same—that is, we are humans with equal rights and privileges'. Thus, a number of scholars celebrate diversity and argue that the formulation is candid, common and politically indisputable. Conceptually, diversity resonates with the heterogeneity of disability. However, some questions trouble me. Are we really the same? Even as a disability rights advocate, my engagement with deaf person is not easy as I am not an expert in sign language. Similarly, to respond to a Dalit person who is visually impaired is not an easy endeavour given my own identity as an upper caste person. Even if I am sensitive, I cannot assure that my inclusion in a diverse world would be without complications. Thus, any marginalized category, and in my case specifically disability, is without fail repressed and is not included under the well-known categories of caste, race, ethnicity and gender.

Notwithstanding the fact that disability has been understood as an esteemed cultural construction both factually and metaphorically, its material reality has missed its other counterparts of diversity both inside and outside the academia. So can disability justifiably be part of the diversity paradigm? The material reality of the disabled creates systemic segregation of disabled people from the core institutions of contemporary society, education employment, recreation and citizenship. If diversity celebrates empowerment, disability seems to be the reproduced disempowerment. I recall Shakespeare (1994, 298) who has argued that non-disabled people 'project their fear of death, their unease at their physicality and mortality onto disabled people, who represent all these difficult aspects of human existence'. Thus, disability as a medical and concessional category in the diversity stipulation of society and specifically academia is never recognized as knowledge.

In the earlier chapters that take up issues of higher Education for people with disabilities is aways taxing. As I have stated elsewhere (2015) 'Education has also been one area in which the discourse of "special" reigns supreme. Thus the students are routinely placed into 'standard' and non-standard populations. While diversity might be the rhetoric, the rank ordering of ability disrupts its very existence'. Thus, the binary of regular/special begins with the process of 'Othering', thereby segregating the disabled from a caring and inclusive interaction both with fellow students and teachers.

To quote William Rhodes (1995, 459), 'the metaphor of illness (e.g., diagnosis, treatment) was codified and imported directly into school system.... The imported medical metaphor of illness constructed differences in learning styles as "pathology" "handicaps" and deficiency'. As Ahmed (2012) points out, paradoxes are central to diversity work. She employs the metaphor of the brick wall, which emerges repetitively in her research to examine some of these paradoxes. I find the metaphor brick wall as a critical concept in understanding diversity. Ahmed states, 'The feeling of doing diversity work is the feeling of coming up against something that does not move, something solid and tangible. The institution becomes that which you come up against' (p. 26). In other words, paradoxes of diversity work such that those who were imaginative and excited to create uniformity in society are actively prevented from doing so. And, worse, those who point out institutional problems come to be seen as the problem. Once diversity, and particularly 'institutional diversity', is understood as routine and is that which no longer surprises us, diversity has lost its critical edge and potential to disrupt; indeed, at times, 'having a [diversity] policy becomes a substitute for action' (p. 11). I find real inclusion, and therefore diversity is a profound and deeper challenge to humanity. My contention is that diversity is used as a legitimizing tool, because the suggestion is to create a neoliberal economy for which homogeneity, predictability and stability are key. However, the rule in neoliberal economies is that the difference between the rich (read-able bodied) and the poor (read disabled) gets wider rather weakens. Diversity therefore is becoming unattainable in the profit paradigm that is predominant. It can be possible only when every human being, irrespective of the nature or degree of their marginalization, should have the right to belong to their local school, college university, office and their local community, with meaningful and appropriate support, enabling them to participate and contribute to the society. As Ahmed (2012, 163) writes,

> inclusion could be read as a technology of governance: not only as a way of bringing those who have been recognized as strangers into the nation, but also of making strangers into subjects, those who in being included are also willing to consent to the terms of inclusion.'

In this context, what worries me is the politics of identity. An affirmation of disabled identity upholds the fact that disability provides the insiders (people with disabilities) with an inimitable vantage point, which the non-disabled do not possess. Since the continuum of disability and ability is difficult to comprehend, disabled identity does set against the oppositional category of the able-bodied identity. As Mark Sherry (2008), on the other hand, points out that

> disability cannot be understood as a category shared by any minority group because disability is always a sexed, gendered, racialized, ethnicized, and classed experience [. . .] and every response to disability operates within a framework of multilayered and complex patterns of inequality and identities (p. 75).

Consequently, diversity discourse seems to be complex in simply incorporating people with disabilities. My submission therefore is that diversity does not necessarily equate to inclusion. A community has people from multiple backgrounds, but if it is not coordinated to make those individuals feel accepted and embraced, then it does not matter. Inclusion therefore needs a divergence which has a certain ethos and thinking, which initiates the process of enfolding the multiplicity.

Friedner (2017, 12), a deaf scholar in disability studies, points out that 'Disability functions as a form of non-threatening "feel good" diversity in India'. As a category, it productively constitutes and unifies the nation. Disability functions like Butler's (1993) 'constitutive outside'. My submission is that the positive part of disability can stand up to that extent when disabled people do become political and ask for citizenship right. If they can quietly assimilate themselves to the 'unity in diversity' theme, then questioning of diversity does not happen.

A concern that arises about disability as an identity category is whether everyone 'chooses' a disabled identity or not. The previous chapter underscores prenatal selection, which I posit is the most serious pointer towards the impediments in creating a diverse society. As I have stated elsewhere, 'When sex selection has evoked so much debate, the issue of selection on grounds of disability is clearly more complex' (Ghai 2015). In understanding of diversity, the questions of choice and selection are of omnipotence. As we understand mother of an unwanted daughter and that of a disabled child face tremendous difficulties. To choose to give birth to a child with disability is to challenge dominant social constructions of both motherhood and childhood. If it is possible to argue that the desire to abort a female foetus arises from the conditions of patriarchy, is a similar logic not applicable to disability selection? As one of the case in point, I am going to discuss intellectual impairment. Though very often disabilities such as mobility, visual, hearing and cerebral palsy are discussed in the discourse of diversity, intellectual impairment troubles diversity. No matter how aptly we convey to the ablest world that we must challenge the misapprehensions about intellectual disability. Michael Berube, a father and disability studies scholar, confronts the fallacy that intellectual disability undermines the value of a life, as exemplified by his son Jamie, who Berube describes as witty, inquisitive and full of a love for life. Berube (2016) asserts that like most children, when given ample amounts of love and attention, kids with Down syndrome have the best fighting chance at meeting their full potential and living a successful, happy life. Similarly, Kittay begun by describing her daughter Sesha in the negative way as she really cannot speak for her daughter Sesha. As Kittay (2001, 559–60) puts it,

> Yet this lack is a synecdoche for all that she is unable to do: feed herself, dress herself, toilet herself, walk, talk, read, write, draw, say Mama or Papa. I would have preferred to start by speaking of her capabilities: the hugs and kisses she can give, her boundless enjoyment of the sensuous

feel of water, or her abiding and profound appreciation of music. When asked about my daughter, I want to tell people that she is a beautiful, loving, joyful young woman. But then I need to tell them what she cannot be, given her profound cognitive limitations, her cerebral palsy, and her seizure disorders. When people ask how old my daughter is I always hesitate, wondering whether to give her chronological age and speak of her as a lovely and intense thirty-year-old woman [now forty-seven].

Her limitations are described only by people who do not know her. The ones who know her experience the richness and beauty of Sesha.

One instance is that of art and aesthetics in which Tobin Siebers talks about Judith Scott, a remarkable artist with an intellectual disability, a fibre artist who had Down syndrome and was severely deaf. Here, Siebers locates Scott not only for the legality of her art, but also for the drawbacks of accounting for the 'disabled mind', a term used by him (2008, 97).

Further, Siebers says,

What makes the fiber sculptures even more staggering as works of artist are the fact that Scott has no conception of the associations sparked by her object sand no knowledge of the history of art. In fact, she never visited a museum or read an art book, she did not know she was an 'artist', and never intended to make 'art' when she set to work, at least in the conventional understanding of these words.... She was warehoused at age seven in the Ohio Asylum for the Education of Idiotic and Imbecilic Youth and spent the next thirty five years of her life as a ward of the institution. (Siebers 2010, 69)

While diversity implies inclusion, can we accept Sesha as described above? Mostly people like Sesha and Jimmy are defined with 'severe cognitive impairments'. Notwithstanding the definition, they seem to be lacking personhood and excluded from discussions about diversity, as they do not figure as autonomous human beings. Diversity can reduce this violence against people with disabilities only if we change the interpretation of the society that 'fully includes' disability in a discourse on humanity. We have to question the assumption that the disabled child is constructed as economic liability and therefore a burden on family and society. In a neoliberal context, where the profit paradigm prevails, very often the justification given for preventing disabled from being born is that the state/society has to bear the cost of disability. The scarcity is often cited as a rationale for disability selection. As I state elsewhere, 'While the billions spent on wars (major source of disablement) are not lamented, the money spent on disabled people is constructed as high cost' (Ghai 2015). Monetary factors are at the root of the persistent undervaluing of disabled lives. This rationale is, however, tarnished as it is also the aspiration for the construction of a set of homogeneous, standardized persons. Somehow in the language of Divyung, disability negates the material reality of the disabled body and conceptualizes it as inspiration divine body does not get in the sociopolitical nuances. To me, diversity works as a manoeuvre in neoliberal political and economic markets that work to ratify the status quo through 'feel good' politics (see, e.g., Ahmed 2012; Vertovec 2012) My submission is that this move from disability to diversity is a difficult terrain. Siebers reminds us that disability is not just missing from a diversity consciousness, but that disability is antithetical to diversity as diversity nicely suits neoliberal capitalism. My submission is that the idea of diversity conceals the financial and cultural inequities My concern is that diversity should not take us to the historical path in which taking up a process of normalization imposes not only eradicating the difference but also entailing and signifying it as diversity. In the earlier chapter, Shanti reminds us of both utilitarianism and pragmatism, but we need to focus on not only the material bodies of the disabled, but also the reason they give to the idea of humaneness. Ngai (2007, 335) writes '… disgust is never ambivalent about its object. More specifically, it is never prone to producing the confusions between subject and object'. I think that disability, as a barely established category, would not like to dilute it with diversity. While intersections are critical, the intermingling of diversity and disability allows for the conceivable erasure between subject and object. Thus, non-disabled are contented to perceive triumphs of disabled without ignoring the role that they may play in disability oppression.

To conclude, I would want to walk the terrain of diversity cautiously. More research is needed as we work on the relationship between diversity and disability in a globalized world that can be both enabling and disabling.

REFERENCES

Ahmed, Sara. 2012. *On Being Included: Racism and Diversity in Institutional Life.* Durham, NC: Duke University Press.
Berube. 2016. 'The Value and the Virtue of Raising a Child with Down Syndrome, Point of Inquiry.' Center for Inquiry—Social Sciences. Available at: http://www.pointofinquiry.org/michael_berube_the_value_and_the_virtue_of_raising_ (accessed November 29, 2017).
Butler, Judith. 1993. *Bodies That Matter: On the Discursive Limits of 'Sex'.* New York: Routledge.
Couser, T. G. 2005. 'Disability as Diversity: A Difference with a Difference.' *Ilha do Desterro* 48: 95–113.
Davis, Lennard. 2015. 'Diversity.' In *Keywords for Disability Studies*, edited by Rachel Adams, Benjamin Reiss and David Serlin, 61–64. New York: New York University Press.
Friedner, Michele. 2017. 'How the Disabled Body Unites the National Body: Disability as "Feel Good" Diversity in Urban India.' *Contemporary South Asia.* doi:10.1080/09584935.2017.1374925.
Ghai, Anita. 2015. *Rethinking Disability in India.* Routledge: New Delhi.
Kittay, Eva Feder. 2001. 'When Caring Is Just and Justice Is Caring.' *Justice and Mental Retardation Public Culture* 13 (3): 557–80.
Ngai, Sian. 2007. *Ugly Feelings.* Cambridge: Harvard University Press.
Rhodes, W. C. 1995. 'Liberatory Pedagogy and Special Education.' *Journal of Learning Disabilities* 28: 458–62.
Shakespeare, T. W. 1994. 'Cultural Representations of Disabled People: Dustbins for Disavowal?' *Disability and Society* 9 (3): 283–99.
Sherry, M. 2008. *Disability and Diversity: A Sociological Perspective.* New York: Nova Science Publishers.
Siebers, Tobin. 2008. *Disability Theory.* Ann Arbor, MI: University Of Michigan Press.
———. 2010. *Disability Aesthetics.* Ann Arbor, MI: University of Michigan Press.
Vertovec, Steven. 2012. '"Diversity" and the Social Imaginary.' *European Journal of Sociology* 53 (3): 287–312.

About the Editor and Contributors

Editor

Anita Ghai joined as a professor in School of Human Studies, Ambedkar University Delhi, in 2015. Before this, Anita has been an associate professor in Department of Psychology in Jesus and Mary College, University of Delhi. Her interest is in disability studies and issues of sexuality, psychology and gender. As a former fellow at the Nehru Memorial Museum Library, Teen Murti Bhavan, Anita has researched on issues of care of disabled women recipients, that is, their daughters and providers of care, that is, the mothers with leanings towards feminist and disability theory. Anita has been the former President of the Indian Association for Women's Studies. She has authored *Re-thinking Disability in India*, Routledge, New Delhi (2015) and *(Dis)Embodied Form: Issues of Disabled Women* (2003), and co-authored *The Mentally Handicapped: Prediction of the Work Performance* with Anima Sen.

Contributors

Shilpaa Anand teaches in the Department of English at Maulana Azad National Urdu University (MANUU) in Hyderabad. She has an MA in English from the University of Hyderabad and a PhD in the interdisciplinary programme of disability studies from the University of Illinois at Chicago. In her doctoral work, she explored the conceptual history of disability in the Indian context. More recently, her research has focused on culturally distinct notions of corporeality and corporeal difference.

About the Editor and Contributors | 431

Shanti Auluck is the chairperson/founder member of Muskaan, an NGO working for the empowerment of persons with intellectual disability, Delhi. Muskaan (started in 1982) provides vocational training, life skill training and employment along with assisted living facility. It also provides counselling and guidance to parents/families. She as well as Muskaan has been given several awards including National Award in 2006 for best NGO working in the field of disability by the Ministry of Social Justice and Empowerment, Government of India. She taught Psychology at Lady Shri Ram College, Delhi University, from 1976 to 2005. She also published and presented papers on Psychology and Indian Philosophical Thought.

Meenu Bhambhani is a seasoned corporate social responsibility (CSR) and development sector professional with close to 20 years of experience in creating inclusive solutions for the underserved and unrepresented communities. At Mphasis, she has been leading the CSR function for over 10 years now. She has played a pivotal role in institutionalizing CSR and aligning it with the Mphasis core business and vision. Under her leadership, Mphasis CSR has received wide recognition both nationally and internationally, including recognition by the President of India as the Best Inclusive Employer for Persons with Disabilities.

Her background in the development sector is multifaceted. She is a person with disability herself, a professional in the area of human development with specialization in disability studies and social policy. Prior to joining Mphasis, Meenu spent 10 years working in diverse fields including teaching English Literature, implementing policies as Assistant Commissioner—Disabilities with Government of Rajasthan, consulting with the World Bank and advocating/spearheading policy advocacy for people with disabilities through a non-profit organization. She has been a researcher of disability studies and has published scholarly articles in renowned journals and publications. She has been widely recognized for her contribution to the field of CSR and disability inclusion. In 2008 and 2009, she was recognized by the

CEO for her outstanding contribution to CSR. In 2010, she won the President's National Award in the category of Best Individuals Promoting Employment Opportunities for Persons with Disabilities.

Meenu holds a PhD in English Literature from the University of Rajasthan. She also earned an MS in Disability and Human Development from the University of Illinois at Chicago, facilitated by a generous fellowship from the Ford Foundation.

Tanmoy Bhattacharya guides research on Syntax, Psycholinguistics, Gender, Disability, Deaf Education and Sign Linguistics, at the Centre for Advanced Studies in Linguistics (CASL), University of Delhi. He has two PhDs in linguistics, one from the University of Hyderabad, India, and the other from University College London, UK, the latter as a Commonwealth Scholar. He has published, till date, 67 journal papers and 4 books, and has delivered 174 talks at different conferences/events, out of which 80 have been invited talks. He is the Project Coordinator of Indo-Norwegian Cooperative Programme project on Syntactic Variation and Language Mixing. His most recent book is *The Sign Language(s) of India*, 2014. He has been Chief Editor of Indian Linguistics (2014–17), and his most recent writing has been a five-part essay series on 'Peopling of the Northeast of India' published since 2016. He has been a convenor member of an UGC Committee on Disability and Higher Education, member Expert Committee for Indian Sign Language, RCI, and the ex-Coordinator of the Equal Opportunity Cell, University of Delhi. Within the field of disability, he specializes in inclusive education, linguistic stereotypes and prejudices, and disability studies. He has worked on exam policy and produced blueprints for equal opportunity cells and disability studies centres at universities for the UGC.

Fiona Kumari Campbell researches with the School of Education and Social Work, University of Dundee, Scotland, and is an Adjunct Professor of Disability Studies, University of Kelaniya, Sri Lanka. Her work is concerned with the production of Disability and Abledment from within a frame of Studies in Ableism. Additionally, Campbell works around decolonized knowledge related to atypical bodies in the South Asian context.

Upali Chakravarti is with the Department of Elementary Education, Miranda House, New Delhi. Her area of work and research is disability, care work and education.

Jagdish Chander is an Associate Professor of Political Science at Hindu College, University of Delhi. He earned his PhD in Disability Studies from Syracuse University, Syracuse, New York, under which he has documented the history of disability rights movement, particularly the self-advocacy movement of the blind in India. Dr Chander has contributed several chapters in edited books published by leading international publishers and has presented papers on topics related to disability rights and disability legislations in several national and international conferences. He is currently engaged in writing the biography of the late Shri Lal Advani, who is considered to be the founding father of modern rehabilitation services for the disabled in India.

Sameer Chaturvedi graduated in Sociology (Hons), Department of Sociology, Hindu College, University of Delhi, New Delhi, post-graduated in Sociology, Department of Sociology, Delhi School of Economics, University of Delhi, New Delhi, Master of Philosophy in Sociology, Centre for the Study of Social Systems, School of Social Sciences, Jawaharlal Nehru University (JNU), New Delhi. He submitted his MPhil Dissertation entitled '"Disability" between Models: A Sociological Exploration (2015)'. He is working as a PhD Research Scholar (JRF) since January 2015 in Centre for the Study of Social Systems, School of Social Sciences, JNU, New Delhi, the title of his PhD thesis being *Disability, Desire and Relationships: A Sociological Exploration*.

Amita Dhanda is Professor of Law at NALSAR, University of Law in Hyderabad, India. Her work on the rights of persons with psychosocial disabilities contributed to the discourse on legal capacity in the UN Convention on the Rights of Persons with Disabilities. Subsequently, she has actively engaged in the law reform process in her country to bring the Indian law in conformity with the UN Convention. Professor Dhanda believes in the pluralizing of inclusion and multiplicity of voice, and her work on disability and gender is an effort in that direction. In her book *Legal Order and Mental Disorder* (SAGE, 2000) and all subsequent writings, Professor Dhanda has demonstrated how the law is both an instrument of exclusion and empowerment.

Nandini Ghosh is Assistant Professor of Sociology at Institute of Development Studies Kolkata. She has a bachelor's degree in sociology from Presidency College, Kolkata, and a master's degree from Calcutta University. She completed her PhD in social sciences from the Tata Institute of Social Sciences, Mumbai, in 2008. Her areas of interest are qualitative research methodology, sociology of gender, marginalization and social exclusion and social movements. She has published a monograph *Impaired Bodies Gendered Lives: Everyday Realities of Disabled Women* (2016). She has coedited a book titled *Pratyaha—Everyday Lifeworlds: Dilemmas, Contestations and Negotiations* (2015). She has also edited another volume *Interrogating Disability in India: Theory and Practice* (2016).

Nidhi Goyal is a disabled feminist from India. Working at the intersection of disability and gender, she is committed to changing the lives of women and girls with disabilities. Nidhi's work spans research, writing, training, campaigns, advocacy and art. She is the founder and director of Mumbai-based non-profit organization Rising Flame working for persons with disabilities with a focus on women and youth with disabilities. Nidhi has been appointed to the prestigious civil society advisory group of UN women's Executive Director, sits on the advisory board of Voice, a grant making facility by Dutch Ministry, and is the President elect of the AWID (Association for Women's Rights in Development) Board. Finally, she is India's first-ever female disabled stand-up comic artist who uses humour to challenge prevalent notions around disability, gender and sexuality.

Niluka Gunawardena is affiliated with the University of Kelaniya and the National Institute of Social Development as a visiting lecturer. She is also a secondary teacher at the Colombo International School,

Sri Lanka. Niluka is committed to developing holistic models of inclusive education based on South Asian epistemologies. She is currently involved in the 'Play for All' campaign, which is aimed at creating inclusive parks and play environments for children with all forms of abilities in Sri Lanka. She does independent research on sexual and reproductive health and rights of disabled women as well as disability in a gendered post-war context in Sri Lanka and is actively involved in promoting leadership and advocacy skills development among disabled youth. She is currently exploring modes of empowerment through the arts in collaboration with multi-disciplinary allies in her country.

Hemachandran Karah teaches English Literature at the Humanities and Social Sciences faculty, IIT Madras. He specializes in Literary Disability Studies and Medical Humanities.

Nivedita Kothiyal is currently an independent researcher and teaches part-time at the University of York. Until recently, she was an Associate Professor at Institute of Rural Management Anand (IRMA) in India. She holds a PhD in Human Resource Management and has over 15 years of experience in research, teaching, consultancy and training. Her research is interested in decent work, gender and diversity management, workforce development and skill building, and corporate social responsibility. In her research, she draws on postcolonial theory and critical management studies. Her research has been published in field-leading journals, including the *British Journal of Management* and *Indian Journal of Industrial Relations*, and edited volumes including *Undoing Boundaries* and *The SAGE Handbook of Qualitative Business and Management Research*.

Arun Kumar is a Lecturer in International Management at the University of York, United Kingdom, where he also serves as his department's Equality and Diversity Champion. He researches the history of development and management in India with a particular focus on large philanthropic organizations. His research has been supported by Economic History Society, UK, and Rockefeller Archives Centre, USA. He is currently working on a research monograph titled *Re/Imagining Modernity* about the history of Indian elites' philanthropy in the 'long' Indian 20th century. Arun holds a PhD from Lancaster

University, United Kingdom, and previously, he has worked as a development consultant and researcher on questions on social justice and inclusion, governance and accountability, and programme planning and evaluation.

Santosh Kumar is an Assistant Professor at the School of Business Studies and Social Sciences, CHRIST (deemed to be University), Bangalore. He teaches in Master Programme in English with Cultural Studies and Bachelor Programme in English Studies. He is a doctorate in Linguistics from the University of Delhi. He has taught Professional Communication, Human Values and Professional Ethics in National Institute of Technology Delhi. His areas of interest are disability studies, gender studies, sociolinguistics and paremiology. His doctoral thesis explored the representation of disability and gender in some of Hindustani proverbs.

Ankur Madan is an Associate Professor at the School of Education, Azim Premji University, Bangalore. Here, she teaches in the Masters Programme in Education. She has a masters' in Child Development and a doctorate in Child Development from the University of Delhi. She has taught in various institutions such as the University of Delhi, American University of Kuwait and Department of Psychology at CHRIST. Her areas of interest are childhood studies and inclusive education. Her doctoral work explored the scope of implementing inclusion in the regular school system in Delhi. She has coedited the book titled *Childhoods in India: Traditions, Trends and Transformations*. Her publications are mostly in the area of inclusive education and childhood studies.

Deepa Palaniappan is State Disability Consultant for Bihar Rural Livelihood Mission JEEViKA, Government of Bihar and Disability Resource Person with Odisha Livelihood Mission, Panchayati Raj and Drinking Water Department, Government of Odisha. With academic training in both political science and special education, she has engaged with disability-related fieldwork through her work and research endeavours in Bihar, Jharkhand, Madhya Pradesh, Assam, Odisha and Tamil Nadu. She has also undertaken pro bono documentation work with various grassroots disabled peoples' organizations with commitment to train community-based organizations in the disability sector to document and historicize their field-based interventions.

Janet Price is a disabled feminist based in Liverpool, UK, having links to Taranaki, New Zealand. She is an activist and writer, and has over 30 years association with India, through friendships and social justice work.

Trained as a medical doctor, Janet worked in Public Health in the UK and India, and as a researcher/academic, she was based at Liverpool School of Tropical Medicine. She retired due to disability associated with multiple sclerosis and became an honorary research fellow there, maintaining awareness of academic/health developments through membership of the LSTM's Gender Group and Liverpool University's medical humanities and sociology network. She has built connections with disability activists/organizations around sexual health/disability/gender in Africa/South Asia and globally.

Janet writes blogs, discussion and research papers and is committed to producing work with others. She is on the board of DaDaFest, a disability and deaf arts organization in Liverpool which has a growing global reach. Recently, DaDaFest has been working to develop local festival plans with disability artists/activists in India/South Asia and with African colleagues, and its work shares ideas about interdependence, support and rights through theatre, dance, visual/video art and music, presented live and online.

Shridevi Rao received her PhD in Special Education from Syracuse University, New York, in 1996. She is a Professor at the Department of Special Education, Language, and Literacy at The College of New Jersey. Her interests include cultural constructions of disability, disability and development, disability studies in education, and inclusive education. She has conducted ethnographic studies that focus on families', teachers', and teacher candidates' constructions of disability. Along with Maya Kalyanpur, she has coedited the book titled *South Asia and Disability Studies: Redefining Boundaries and Extending Horizons*. Currently, she teaches both undergraduate and graduate courses in education.

Valerian Rodrigues is currently Ambedkar Chair at Ambedkar University Delhi. He has earlier taught at Mangalore University and the JNU, and was a National Fellow of the Indian Council of Social Science Research. He has published extensively on political ideas and public institutions in India

Asha Singh had been teaching at the Department of Human Development and Childhood Studies at the Lady Irwin College for about three decades. Her doctoral work used methods of theatre to explore sociocultural contexts, teacher-taught relations and perceptions of school. She guided masters' students to develop child appropriate methods in researching with children. Her interests are early childhood care and education, arts in education, children's orientation to play and working with teachers in these areas to deepen understanding of inclusive practices in the classroom. She also has taught arts and its significance for early learning to graduate students at Azim Premji University as well as at the National School of Drama at Tripura. She also developed and guided curriculum and content for children's educational television series *Galli Galli Sim Sim* emphasizing inclusion and diversity.

Sandeep R. Singh is an Assistant Professor in Comparative Literature and Translation Studies at the School of Letters in Ambedkar University Delhi, India. His current area of research interest includes disability studies, narrative discourse and life-writing. He also teaches in the area of Indian Writing in English with an emphasis on partition literature, romanticism and comparative literature.

Someshwar Sati is presently an Associate Professor at the Department of English, Kirori Mal College, University of Delhi. He has done his MPhil and PhD from CES, JNU, on the Indian English Novel. His research areas include Postcolonial Theory, The Indian English Novel: Midnight's Children and After, Disability Studies and Theory, Disability in Translation, Translation Studies, The Victorian English Novel and the 20th-century English Novel. He has also been awarded the CDN Prize for the best paper presented at the IACLALS 2016 conference organized by IACLALS and the Department of English, Kakatiya University, Warangal.

Rukmini Sen is an Associate Professor at School of Liberal Studies, Ambedkar University Delhi. She teaches courses in law and society, relationships and affinities, women's movements, gender and society. She has been actively associated with various women's rights and disability rights organizations in Kolkata and Delhi. She is professionally attached to the Indian Association for Women's Studies, Indian Sociological Society and Law and Social Science Research Network. She is currently part of a UGC UKERI research project Teaching Feminisms, Transforming Lives that Ambedkar University Delhi and University of Edinburgh, UK, are collaboratively pursuing. One of her most recent publications is 'Women with Disabilities: Cartographic Encounters with Legal Interstices', *Indian Anthropologist* (2016, 46 [2]: 75–91).

Suchaita Tenneti is currently pursuing an MPhil in sociology from the JNU, New Delhi. She is specializing in disability studies with a focus on educational issues pertaining to disability and queer disability studies.

Shubhangi Vaidya is a sociologist by training and teaches at the School of Inter-Disciplinary and Trans-Disciplinary Studies at the Indira Gandhi National Open University, Delhi. She has published in the areas of disability and gender studies and is the author (with Anu Aneja) of *Embodying Motherhood: Perspectives from Contemporary India* (SAGE Yoda Press, 2016) and *Autism and the Family in Urban India* (2016).

Index

activists, 7
advocacy activities, 5
All India Confederation of the Blind (AICB), 6
anecdotes of joy, 198

Blind and the Welfare Society for the Disabled, 6
Boats Club, 6
building daily rhythms
   experiences with professionals, 210–211

care and companionship
   legal understanding, 402
      abortion & utilitarian view, 416–418
      construction of family, 406–408
      interdependence, 408–409
      right to equal opportunity, 419–421
      rights based legislation, 403–406
      social support systems, 418–419
caring and caregiving
   community, 147–152
   family and gender, 147–152
Centring Corporeal Difference, 285–288
Child Development professionals, 203
Child Study Centre, 203
children of deaf adults (CODA), 62
chronic sorrow, 197
community-based rehabilitation (CBR), 23
compulsory ableness, 42

conceptualizing culture, 245
consistency and continuity, 205
Convention on the Rights of Persons with Disabilities (CRPD), 385
corporeality and culture
   corporeal difference, 270–271
   normative notions, 263–265
   reconceptualizing treatment, 266–270
   standardized normative treatment, 265–266
Critical Intersectionality, 355–356
cross-disability
   demands, 24–25
   movement, 23
cultural statement, 102

Deaf Pride and Autistic Neurodiversity, 246, 246
Demonstration on GoI Methi Chowk, 1989, 8
Dialogic Imagination
   Four Essays, 221
Disability Nationalism in Crip Times, 120
disability rights movement in India
   charity to self-advocacy, 22
   cross-disability movement, 23–31
   methodology, 23
   tactics and tools, 31–33
   origin, contesting views, 12–16
Disability Studies (DS), 86–89
   agencies and services, 81

CRPD, 386–387
   law making, 394–397
   MHA, 393–394
   NTA, 390–393
   people and organizations in lawmaking, 397–399
   PWDA, 388–390
   RCI Act, 387–388
   epistemological re-visioning, 89–92
   estrangement, 76–77
   folklore, construction, 298
   formalising estrangement, 94–96
   governmental policies, 84
   interdisciplinary nature, 350–352
   inversion, 92–94
   lawmaking, 383
   non-governmental agencies, 83
   phenomenological research, failure, 79–80
   possibility in India, 92
   resistance', 77–79
   spirit, 75
disability
   cross-cultural perspective, 248–254
   cultural construct, 246–248
   culture
      new mobilisations and movements, 254–259
   employment, 360–362
   human diversity, 413–414
   social construct, 414–416
disability–sexuality epistemological framework, 119
Disabled Persons' Organisations (DPOs), 85
   private sector, 85–86
   service providers, 85
Disabled Rights Group (DRG), 21
disablism, 39
dyadic relation encountered, 202

enactment of disability rights 1995, 4–5

femininity
   abilism, 102
   contextualizing experience, 103–105
   desired body, 112–115
   labouring body, 109–112
   normalcy and beauty, 105–109
Feminist Disability Studies, 102

general elections, 9

hunger strike, 8

inclusion and disadvantage
   stories, 208
inclusive education in India, 332–335
   nature, 331–332
   realizing inclusion, 338–341
   school, 341–346
   sources of knowledge, 335–338
Indian disability scholars, 64
Indian political theorising-, 63

Jataka Katha, 295
journey
   birth and afterwards, 183–187
   life post school, 192–195
   school life and beyond, 187–192
justice theories, 60–62

Kesari, Sita Ram, 11

Linda Ware, 349
   limitations of teacher agency, 356–357
   teacher awareness, disability structural matrix, 353–355
localised epistemologies, 325
   northern mo(ve)ments, 120–122
   overlapping movements, 119
localized epistemologies
   sexuality/disability, 118
loyal and hardworking employees, 365–366

Mandal Commission Report, 10
Mehta's, Ved
  continent of India, 227
  blind autobiographer and essayist, 227
  blind child, 233
  Continents of Exile, 237
  cosmopolitan ideas, 235
  Disability Studies (DS), 228
  idiosyncratic experiences, 240
  karmic life cycle, idea, 237
  ledge and twin cosmologies, 228–233
  Virya, 239
  visible cosmos, 234
metaphor role, 297
Ministry of Personnel and Grievances, 11
Ministry of Social Welfare, 6, 11
mobilizing factors, 24
Monsoon Session
  legislation, 7
  parliament, 7

National Centre for Promotion of Employment for Disabled People (NCPEDP), 22
nature of work, 363–365

Panchatantra, 295
parental diffidence
  self-regulation, 206–207
political theory
  disability critiques
    Rawlsian Theory of Justice, 67–73
  disability critiques strengthens binaries, 64
  disabled subject, 58–59
  dynamic interaction, 65
post-colonial Indian English fiction, 278
  growing global, 289–291
  impairment, 282–284
  localizing the universal, 291–293
  prosthetic allegory, 280–282
  power of language, 298–299
  prevalence of proverbial, 299
  print expertise, culture, 209
PWD Act, 23

qualitative study
  child
    expression, 322–323
  child
    labels as giving to outsiders, 319–322
    member of the family, 317–319
    skill like rolling, 323–324
  families and disability epistemologies, 314–316
  method, 316–317

Rawlsian Theory of Justice, 67–73
reasonable accommodation, 368–369
reinforcement of stereotype, 300–304
representing disability, 362–363

Sacks, Oliver W.
  Awakenings, 222
  Disablility Studies (DS), 218
  essay from Sara Newman, 220
  imaginative element, 222
  life writing, 216
  medico-humanistic concerns, 224
  modern qualities, 215
  recounting of life stories, 217
  The Nation's, 224
social identity
  stories, 208
social initiative
  involving and engaging, 207
South Asian epistemologies, 122
  anomalous embodiments, categorical generation, 123–126
  care and power, 159–160
  care ethics as public, 160

caregiving, 156–157
colonial eugenics and discursive
    nationalisms, 126–131
critique of care
    disability, 158–159
disability, 152–154. 1
disposing and producing bodies,
    138–141
ethics of care, 158
Indian scenario, 154–156
metropolitan moves and local
    expressions, 138
society, 152–154
state, 152–154
stronghold of ableism, 366–367
Studies in Ableism (SiA)
    refocus and paradigm shift
        divisions, 44–49
    refocus and paradigm shift
        normativity, 49–52
    phenomenological studies,
        52–54
    project, 41–44
Tong, Feminist Rosemary, 38
supercrips, 369–370

teacher education programmes in
    India, 198
Temporarily Able Bodies (TAB), 196
The Blind Men and The Elephant,
    297
The Disabled Demand Legislation,
    1989, 6
*The Production of Disability and
    Abledness*, 42
theoretical conceptualization, 199

unifying disability and diversity
    voice, 422–429

Winter Session of Parliament, 11
women's and disability rights move-
    ments in India, 167, 168–171
    accommodations and normalcy,
        174–175
    cross disability work, 178–180
    inclusion and intersectionality,
        172–174
    voices and leadership, 175–178